COMPLEMENTARY AND ALTERNATIVE CARDIOVASCULAR MEDICINE

CONTEMPORARY CARDIOLOGY

CHRISTOPHER P. CANNON, MD
SERIES EDITOR

COMPLEMENTARY AND ALTERNATIVE CARDIOVASCULAR MEDICINE

Edited by

RICHARD A. STEIN, MD

Associate Chairman of Medicine
Beth Israel Medical Center;
Chief of Medicine
The Singer Division of Beth Israel Medical Center
New York, NY

and

MEHMET C. OZ, MD

Cardiovascular Institute
Columbia Presbyterian Medical Center
New York, NY

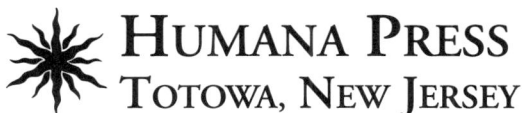

HUMANA PRESS
TOTOWA, NEW JERSEY

© 2004 Humana Press Inc.
999 Riverview Drive, Suite 208
Totowa, New Jersey 07512

www.humanapress.com

For additional copies, pricing for bulk purchases, and/or information about other Humana titles, contact Humana at the above address or at any of the following numbers: Tel.: 973-256-1699; Fax: 973-256-8341, E-mail: humana@humanapr.com; or visit our website: www.humanapress.com

Production Editor: Jessica Jannicelli.
Cover design by Patricia F. Cleary.

This publication is printed on acid-free paper. ∞
ANSI Z39.48-1984 (American National Standards Institute) Permanence of Paper for Printed Library Materials.

e-ISBN: 1-59259-728-9
Printed in the United States of America. 10 9 8 7 6 5 4 3 2 1
Library of Congress Cataloging-in-Publication Data
Complementary and alternative cardiovascular medicine / edited by
Richard A. Stein, Mehmet C. Oz.
        p. ; cm. -- (Contemporary cardiology)
    Includes bibliographical references and index.
    ISBN 1-58829-186-3 (alk. paper)
    1. Cardiovascular system--Diseases--Alternative treatment.
    [DNLM: 1. Cardiovascular Diseases--therapy. 2. Complementary
Therapies--methods. WG 166 C737 2004] I. Stein, Richard A., M.D.
II. Oz, Mehmet, 1960- III. Series: Contemporary cardiology (Totowa,
N.J. : Unnumbered)
    RC684.A48C65 2004
    616.1'06--dc22
                                2003027924

PREFACE

As health care providers, we spend our lives searching for treatments that reduce suffering and lengthen the lives of our patients. Sometimes we find solutions in surprising places. Although we all have hopes for advancements in technology, the future of medicine is also about challenging preconceptions as we change our healing biases. In many ways, this is the natural evolution of "global medicine." We have global communications and global banking; however, until recently medicine has remained remarkably provincial. Traditionally, healers arose from their local culture with the same biases as their patients. As a result, only recently have Western physicians become aware of the mysteries and opportunities of Eastern approaches. Yet, in the context of our honest commitment to evidence-based medical care, our reaction is to view these options with skepticism, because the important "gold standard" of proof, the large randomized clinical trial, is not accessible to us.

Nevertheless, patients are experimenting already with many unconventional treatments. The increasing use of complementary and alternative medical (CAM) therapies by patients to prevent or treat cardiovascular disease and the ineffective communication between patient and physicians in this regard are documented by repeated population surveys in the United States. The finding that less than one half of the more than 50% of our patients who use CAM therapies share this information with their doctor is the basis for an increasing concern. How can we prevent or even monitor potential adverse events and poor clinical outcomes resulting from drug–supplement interactions or failure by the patient to comply with traditional medical care? Even more provocatively, how will we learn about the benefits of CAM approaches if we are unaware of their use? We, as health care providers, are challenged to acquire the knowledge base to be effective communicators and counselors to our patients. *Complementary and Alternative Medicine in Cardiovascular Disease* addresses these challenges for cardiovascular medicine.

The charge given to each expert author was to address, where relevant, history, theoretical basis, philosophy, practical application and the specific therapies, pharmaceuticals, diets and supplements of the selected CAM therapy or practice. In addition, each author was directed to review and critique, as appropriate, the relevant clinical evidence. The guiding principal was to provide information regarding CAM that the physician or other health care provider "should know" in caring for and counseling patients with, or at risk of, cardiovascular diseases.

The topics covered in *Complementary and Alternative Medicine in Cardiovascular Disease* range from the more commonly encountered use of herbs, vitamins and other supplements, dietary and supplemental fats and oils, meditation, prayer, and acupuncture to less familiar areas such as homeopathy, massage, chelation therapy, aromatherapy, and energy therapies. We also asked committed practitioners to describe their fields to allow readers to acquire the "flavor" of their patient's CAM experience.

Our goal was to provide a resource that would form the basis of an ever-increasing personal knowledge base in CAM and cardiovascular disease for the physician, nurse, and other health care provider. The quality of the chapters contributed by the authors has permitted us to produce a remarkable text that we are confident will be of continued value to the reader.

Richard A. Stein, MD
Mehmet C. Oz, MD

CONTENTS

CONTRIBUTORS

DENNIS V. C. AWANG, PhD, FCIC • *MediPlant Consulting, Inc., White Rock, BC, Canada*

SOEREN BALLEGAARD, MD • *The Ballegaard Acupuncture Center, Hellerup, Denmark*

JANE BUCKLE, PhD, RN • *R. J. Buckle Associates, LLC*

PATRICIA CADOLINO, LMT, CIMI • *Massage Therapy Services, Stony Brook University Hospital, Stony Brook, NY*

SUZANNE W. CRATER, RN, ANP-C • *Duke Clinical Research Institute, Duke University Medical Center, Durham, NC*

TERRY D. ETHERTON, PhD • *Dairy and Animal Science Department, The Pennsylvania State University, University Park, PA*

VALERIE K. FISHELL, MS • *Department of Nutritional Science, The Pennsylvania State University, University Park, PA*

STEVEN C. HALBERT, MD • *Director of Protocol Development, Jefferson Center for Integrative Medicine; and Department of Medicine, Thomas Jefferson University, Philadelphia, PA*

KARI D. HECKER, PhD, RD • *Department of Nutritional Science, The Pennsylvania State University, University Park, PA*

WAHIDA KARMALLY, PhD, RD, CDE • *The Irving Center for Clinical Research, Columbia University, New York, NY*

PENNY M. KRIS-ETHERTON, PhD, RD • *Department of Nutritional Science, The Pennsylvania State University, University Park, PA*

FREDI KRONENBERG, PhD • *Richard and Hinda Rosenthal Center for Complementary and Alternative Medicine, Department of Rehabilitation Medicine, College of Physicians & Surgeons, Columbia University, New York, NY*

MITCHELL W. KRUCOFF, MD, FACC • *Division of Cardiology, Duke Clinical Research Institute, Duke University Medical Center, Durham, NC*

TIERAONA LOW DOG, MD • *Executive Advisory Board, NIH National Center for Complementary and Alternative Medicine; Department of Medicine, Program in Integrative Medicine, University of Arizona, Tucson, AZ*

ROBERT S. MCCALEB • *Herb Research Foundation, Boulder, CO*

WOODSON C. MERRELL, MD • *Department of Medicine, College of Physicians & Surgeons, Columbia University, New York, NY*

ERIN L. OLIVO, PhD • *Department of Psychiatry, College of Physicians & Surgeons, Columbia University, New York, NY*

MEHMET C. OZ, MD • *Associate Professor of Surgery, Cardiovascular Institute, Columbia Presbyterian Medical Center, New York, NY*

GLEN REIN, PhD • *Quantum Biology Research Lab, Huntington, NY*

AMY ROTHENBERG, ND, DHANP • *The New England School of Homeopathy, Amherst, MA*

ARSHAD M. SAFI, MD • *Division of Cardiology, The Brooklyn Hospital Center, Brooklyn, NY*

CYNTHIA A. SAMALA, RD • *Department of Patient Services, Veterans Affairs New York Harbor Health Care System, Brooklyn, NY*

RICHARD A. STEIN, MD • *Associate Chairman of Medicine, Beth Israel Medical Center; Chief of Medicine, The Singer Division of Beth Israel Medical Center, New York, NY*

MARIA SYLDONA, PhD • *Transpersonal MindBody Healing Center, Northport, NY*

JACQUELINE C. WOOTTON, MEd • *Richard and Hinda Rosenthal Center for Complementary and Alternative Medicine, Department of Rehabilitation Medicine, College of Physicians & Surgeons, Columbia University, New York, NY*

JONATHAN E. E. YAGER, MD • *Division of Cardiology, Duke Clinical Research Institute, Duke University Medical Center, Durham, NC*

VALUE-ADDED eBook/PDA

This book is accompanied by a value-added CD-ROM that contains an eBook version of the volume you have just purchased. This eBook can be viewed on your computer, and you can synchronize it to your PDA for viewing on your handheld device. The eBook enables you to view this volume on only one computer and PDA. Once the eBook is installed on your computer, you cannot download, install, or e-mail it to another computer; it resides solely with the computer to which it is installed. The license provided is for only one computer. The eBook can only be read using Adobe® Reader® 6.0 software, which is available free from Adobe Systems Incorporated at www.Adobe.com. You may also view the eBook on your PDA using the Adobe® PDA Reader® software that is also available free from Adobe.com.

You must follow a simple procedure when you install the eBook/PDA that will require you to connect to the Humana Press website in order to receive your license. Please read and follow the instructions below:

1. Download and install Adobe® Reader® 6.0 software
   You can obtain a free copy of the Adobe® Reader® 6.0 software at www.adobe.com
   Note: If you already have the Adobe® Reader® 6.0 software installed, you do not need to reinstall it.
2. Launch Adobe® Reader® 6.0 software
3. Install eBook: Insert your eBook CD into your CD-ROM drive
   PC: Click on the "Start" button, then click on "Run"
   At the prompt, type "d:\ebookinstall.pdf" and click "OK"
   Note: If your CD-ROM drive letter is something other than d: change the above command accordingly.
   MAC: Double click on the "eBook CD" that you will see mounted on your desktop. Double click "ebookinstall.pdf"
4. Adobe® Reader® 6.0 software will open and you will receive the message "This document is protected by Adobe DRM" Click "OK"
   Note: If you have not already activated the Adobe® Reader® 6.0 software, you will be prompted to do so. Simply follow the directions to activate and continue installation.

Your web browser will open and you will be taken to the Humana Press eBook registration page. Follow the instructions on that page to complete installation. You will need the serial number located on the sticker sealing the envelope containing the CD-ROM.

If you require assistance during the installation, or you would like more information regarding your eBook and PDA installation, please refer to the eBookManual.pdf located on your CD. If you need further assistance, contact Humana Press eBook Support by e-mail at ebooksupport@humanapr.com or by phone at 973-256-1699.

*Adobe and Reader are either registered trademarks or trademarks of Adobe Systems Incorporated in the United States and/or other countries.

1 Complementary and Alternative Medicine in the Prevention and Treatment of Cardiovascular Disease

An Introduction

Richard A. Stein, MD,
and Mehmet C. Oz, MD

CONTENTS

The knowledge base required to diagnose and treat cardiovascular disease (CVD) is large and rapidly expanding, although the amount of time available to physicians and other health care providers to acquire this information is finite and shrinking. As clinicians, we are required to triage new information with respect to its importance and value to our clinical mission and to the time and effort required to learn and incorporate it into our practices. Thus, three important questions to address at the beginning of this book are: (1) "Why do I need to know about complimentary and alternative medicine (CAM)?" (2) "What do I need to know

From: *Contemporary Cardiology*
Complementary and Alternative Cardiovascular Medicine
Edited by: R. A. Stein and M. C. Oz © Humana Press Inc., Totowa, NJ

about CAM and CVD?" and (3) How do I assess multiple reports and studies on CAM and CVD for best evidence to provide effective and sensitive patient counseling?

WHY THE NEED FOR A KNOWLEDGE BASE REGARDING CAM?

A significant and growing percentage of our patients use some form of CAM, making it a critically important aspect of the health care environment. The surveys performed by Eisenberg and colleagues from Harvard in 1990 *(1)* and again in 1997 *(2)* provided surprising data concerning CAM. The investigators used telephone interviews to survey English-speaking households in the United States. They defined CAM as medical interventions not taught widely at US medical schools or generally available at US hospitals. They found that the percentage of the US population estimated to be currently using at least one CAM therapy, either independently or through practitioners, was 34% in 1990 and 42% in 1997 (a 25% increase). If we extrapolate this data trend to today, we are at or beyond the point where most of our patients are currently using some form of CAM. Equally important is the finding that most (72% of the people using CAM in the 1997 Eisenberg survey) did not share this information with their physicians.

Wootton and Sparber *(3)* reviewed six national surveys performed from 1990 to 2000 and found that the Eisenberg data were supported by the findings of a large market survey sponsored by Landmark Health Care Inc. *(4)* and in a survey by Astin *(5)* of a randomly drawn subsample of the National Family Opinion survey performed in 1994. Other studies performed during this same time period have reported smaller percentages of the populations using CAM. The differing percentages likely relate, in part, to the structure of the surveys and the questions. In one such large random survey, CAM was defined as unconventional therapies and the questions were restricted to the use of practitioner-directed therapies as opposed to self-care *(6)*.

The sociodemographic characteristics of patients who are most likely to use CAM note a small preponderance of women vs men and greater use in middle-aged, higher educated, and higher income populations. However, these findings may reflect sampling issues, because smaller studies that have focused on underserved populations note a similar high percentage of CAM use as reported in higher socioeconomic groups.

Liu and colleagues surveyed 376 consecutive patients admitted for cardiovascular surgery to Columbia University–New York Presbyterian Hospital *(7)*. They obtained a 70% response rate and noted that 77% of the patients reported using CAM therapies, which was reduced to 44% if vitamins and prayer were excluded. Their findings that only 17% of patients using CAM therapies discussed this with their physician and that neither age, gender, race or education level predicted usage are consistent with prior studies of the general population. Equally importantly, most patients responded that they did not wish to reveal their CAM use even when directly prompted. It is clearly not possible for a clincan, using socioeconomic information, to predict the likelihood of their patients using CAM for cardiovascular disease. Given the prevalence of its usage, cardiovascular physicians face this challenge on a daily basis.

Additionally, health care providers need to know about CAM, because patient use in the context of physician-directed conventional therapy may represent a source of conflict between a patient requesting CAM therapies and a clinician advising against or rejecting such treatments. An obvious source of conflict is patient risk of harm from CAM treatment related adverse events or supplement—drug interactions with conventional therapy. In addition, the failing, by the physician, to provide informed counsel could result in the patient forgoing a safe CAM form that would be beneficial. Such benefits may be related directly to the use of the CAM therapy or may be a result of the integration of safe CAM therapies with conventional treatments, permitting a better fit of the overall treatment plan to a patient's belief system and affording the patient a proactive role and sense of control in his or her health care.

Once clinicians are convinced of the importance of CAM, they are faced with the question: "What do I need to know?" Unfortunately, physicians often cannot adhere to evidence-based medicine for many CAM therapies since the gold standard of evidence-based care—the large, randomly assigned, blinded, placebo-controlled study (clinical trials)—does not exist. Therefore, the health care provider must use best available evidence to determine safety and efficacy and must practice with the knowledge that such "best" evidence may be refuted by future studies. A recent example of this occurence is sentiments concerning conventional medical treatment using hormone replacement therapy (HRT) for women who are postmenopausal *(8)*. Large case cohort studies suggested clinical efficacy, but subsequent clinical trials demonstrated lack of efficacy and, in some instances, increased cardiovascular and noncardiovascular events and mortality.

Unfortunately, some CAM therapies, despite widespread use and, occasionally, substantial historical recognition and supportive anecdotal reports, will not be the subject of large well-designed clinical trails in the United States in the near future. As discussed in the text, the cost of such trials is prohibitive to a for-profit source that cannot have patent protection for the product or therapy. The National Institutes of Health (NIH) and foundations with a focus on CAM are initiating such studies, but these studies are occurring at a limited pace.

WHAT THE PHYSICIAN MUST KNOW REGARDING CAM AND CVD

Effective physician counseling of patients regarding the CAM use for the prevention and treatment of CVD requires, at a minimum, that physicians be familiar with the available evidence regarding the more common alternative therapies and be able to classify them, with respect to their safety and efficacy. In their recent review of ethical considerations of CAM therapies in conventional medical settings, Adams and colleagues *(9)* note that a physician must be able to classify that a CAM therapy has evidence that (1) supports safety and efficacy, (2) supports safety but is inconclusive concerning efficacy, (3) supports efficacy but is inconclusive concerning safety, or (4) indicates serious risk or inefficacy.

Weiger and colleagues *(10)* recently proposed criteria for using existing data to provide evidence-based advice on CAM therapies to patients with cancer. These criteria and guidelines are not disease specific and can, in part, be used as a template for developing a guideline format that is appropriate for counseling patients who are on CAM for CVD. Thus, CAM therapies would be classified by, the described evidence criteria, into four physician-response categories:

1. Recommend—The best evidence supports both efficacy and safety. This classification requires more than three adequate quality random clinical trials of 50 or more subjects, with 75% of trials supporting efficacy and evidence supporting efficacy coming from more then one clinical research team.
2. Accept; May Consider Recommending—The best evidence supports both efficacy and safety. This requires more than one randomized clinical trial to evaluate efficacy, with more than 50% of trials supporting efficacy and evidence fails to meet criteria for the Recommend classification.
3. Accept—The best evidence on efficacy is inclusive, but evidence supports safety. The evidence on efficacy is inconclusive or is inadequate to support efficacy. The data fail to meet criteria for Recommend classification but does not meet criteria for Discourage/Reject classification.
4. Discourage/Reject—The best evidence indicates either inefficacy or serious risk. The criteria for this classification include more than two adequate clinical trials of 50 or more subjects in which 67% of trials suggest that the therapy is effective or there is evidence or a reasonable theoretical potential that this treatment is not safe.

The criteria for classification of a CAM therapy as safe are the absence of documented significant adverse events associated with the CAM therapy and the absence of an obvious theoretical model for significant adverse events. In our judgment, these criteria are not suitable for some cardiovascular CAM therapies, because in a CVD prevention and treatment program, such therapies are likely to be used for an extended time period (sometimes decades) and be used with prescribed medications that change over time. The recent unexpected adverse events associated with HRT indicate that large studies lasting 3 yr or longer are often necessary to document safety. Because such studies are not presently available for most CAM therapies described in this book (e.g., herbal, vitamin, and nutraceutical supplements), physicians should consider advising patients that in the absence of strong data supporting safety, we are basing our recommendations on the studies to date that have not demonstrated significant adverse events. However, the lack of large studies of appropriate duration leaves the issue of safety uncertain.

A TEMPLATE FOR ASSESSING INFORMATION ON CAM

A thorough evaluation of the rapidly expanding medical literature regarding CAM and CVD requires an assessment of the quality of the source and the publication (print or Web), the type of study (research design), the significance and limitations of the findings (statistics and possible sources of bias), and relevance of the findings to patient. Groups of investigators with quality research experience or an academic background are often sources of high-quality studies. Respected peer-reviewed journals represent the greatest likelihood that a critical, unbiased evaluation of the study, the data, and the presentation has preceded publication. Studies performed by individuals with something to gain from the outcome (i.e., manufacturers of the product being studied) require careful scrutiny by a peer-reviewed journal or the reader before integrating such findings in best evidence-based analysis. Abstracts, even those that are presented at highly respected national meetings, have only been superficially critiqued concerning study methods, and a clinician's assessment of the findings presented should await peer-reviewed publication. This is particularly difficult in the current information environment where the findings of positive studies are often presented to the public (patients) via television, radio, or print media within days, even hours, of presentation. The patient may not easily accept the appropriate wait-and-see attitude.

The research study design (often referred to as the type of study) plays a major role in determining the importance of the findings to evidence-based medical decision making. The least valuable contributors to evidence-based decision making are descriptive studies (published as case reports or clinical series); however, they may be critically important in the recognition of a medical illness or a treatment option. For example, one of the earliest important papers that helped in the recognition of the human immunodeficiency virus (HIV) was a case series of a cluster of Kaposi sarcoma cases in men who were homosexual *(11)*.

Explanatory study designs seek to examine the cause of a disease or the efficacy of a treatment by using comparison. Studies that are observational—where the investigators observe nature to reach conclusions—include case-control studies, cohort or follow-up studies, and cross-sectional studies.

In a case-control study, one begins with a group of subjects (cases) who have the disease in question and identifies a group that is similar in all regards except for the disease (controls). Investigation determines if a proposed factor is significantly more or less prevalent in the history of the cases or the controls. For example, to determine if antioxidant vitamins are cardioprotective, a case cohort study would identify men with myocardial infarction in a studied cohort and a control group and survey them regarding previous and present use of antioxidant vitamins. A significantly higher use of such vitamins in controls compared to cases would support the hypothesis that antioxidant vitamins protect patients from myocardial infarction.

The cohort or follow-up study involves the evaluation of a group of subjects without the disease and incorporate a long follow-up period so that sufficient cases of the disease to develop. The objective is usually to determine if the presence or absence of a given factor measured at the initial evaluation was predictive of the likelihood of developing the disease. The Framingham Heart Study is of this design. Here a large part of the population of Framingham, Massachusetts, served as the cohort. This study is responsible, in large part, for our understanding of both the traditional and newer coronary heart disease risk factors.

In a cross-sectional study, a study population is divided into those with a disease (or outcome) and those without a disease. The population is evaluated regarding risk factors or the use of preventive strategies for the disease. Results are determined by a correlation of the risk factor/preventive strategy with the presence or absence of the disease.

These three observational study designs can identify correlations and strongly suggest an effect of the factor being measured on the studied outcome. They are generally, except in the case of large, long-term cohort studies, less expensive and shorter than clinical trials. However, they are subject to variables such as selection bias, subject bias, and observer bias. An example of such bias would be an antioxidant-heart disease case-control study where subjects who were identified as using antioxidant vitamins also consumed known (and unknown) cardioprotective dietary substances to a greater extent than the control group. Selecting a control group that was matched for smoking, serum cholesterol, and blood pressure would miss these and other important variables.

Another important bias occurs when factors that are not appropriately considered in the interpretation of the findings could distort the outcome of observational research design studies. This is the basis for the reliance on large, randomized, controlled, and blinded clinical trials of appropriate duration. This is the gold standard of research design. The random assignment to the experimental or control group should eliminate selection bias, and the blinding of the patient and the team that is collecting the data about which patients are receiving the product or treatment vs placebo should eliminate patient and observer bias. The size and duration of the trial should allow for the determination of a statistically significant difference in outcome (based on reasonable clinical projections) in the experimental vs the control group. Such studies are essential to arrive at an evidenced-based decision regarding the safety and efficacy of any treatment options, including CAM.

Large clinical trails of sufficient duration to prove or disprove efficacy and determine the type and frequency of adverse events are expensive, both financially and in investigator effort. However, there is no substitute for the findings of such a study, and, as clinicians, although we counsel in the present based on best available evidence, we must lobby strongly for the funding of appropriate clinical trials of CAM therapies in the near future.

A scoring system for published CAM articles is essential for assessing the relative values of such studies to the clinician. The US Agency for Heath Care Policy Research (AHCPR) has produced valuable evidence-based clinical guidelines for cardiovascular care during the last decade. For each such guideline, the expert committee has presented the criteria to score published studies regarding their value. These guidelines are useful to the clinician who must assimilate data from studies on CAM and CVD to determine his or her own counseling guidelines.

The editor's recommendations to the authors of this text are based on the Strength-of-Evidence Ratings section in the US Department of Health and Human Services *AHCPR Clinical Practice Guideline number 17: Cardiac Rehabilitation (12)*. We consider this a practical scoring system for clinicians and suggest that when combined with the criteria proposed by Weiger and colleagues (with an awareness of the issue of safety as it applies to CAM treatment of CVDs), it will provide the clinician with a rational, evidenced-based, and patient need-responsive system. The scoring system was incorporated into our instructions to the chapter authors of this book.

> *The approach suggested in this text on CAM and CVD is to collect the relevant published studies and reviews (from computer searches of MEDLINE and appropriate alternative medicine databases, websites, reference texts, and other sources) and to grade them according to AHCPR criteria used for the Cardiac Rehabilitation Guidelines as follows:*
>
> > *A. Well-designed and well-conducted clinical trials of sufficient size and duration.*
> >
> > *B. Observation studies and small clinical trials.*
> >
> > *C. Expert opinions and panel consenses.*
>
> *If class A studies exist (e.g., vitamin E and coronary heart disease [CHD] event rate and mortality), then these should be noted and briefly described with a clear outcome statement. If only type B studies exist, then these should be noted and size, follow-up period, and possible confounding factors also noted. In the absence of class A and B studies, expert opinion and consensus data (e.g., German Commission E Monographs) should be noted.*
>
> *If there are class A and B studies of the treatment approach that are important but do not address cardiovascular medicine (e.g., clinical trials of homeopathic remedies for allergic rhinitis), these should, especially in the absence of studies addressing CVD, be noted, because they will be of interest and possible value to the clinician who will be counseling patients. Also for consensus statements, the type of panel or individuals, and the basis of the recommendations (personal experience and collected experiences or review of literature and studies) should be noted.*
>
> *The goals of the clinical evidence section or aspect of your chapter are to provide the reader with the clinical evidence (if it exists) and the collected wisdom of practioners and societies. Negative studies and recommendations should be noted, as well as positive ones. If the data do not provide a basis for arriving at a conclusion regarding efficacy (and safety), then this should be stated.*

CONCLUSION

The use of alternative therapies for the prevention and treatment of CVD is increasing. As a result, physicians will need to obtain the knowledge and skills to counsel patients regarding these therapies. In our final analyses, we must provide specific and nonjudgmental honest and evidence-based counsel so that our patients will continue to discuss and, hopefully, increasingly discuss these therapies with us.

REFERENCES

1. Eisenberg DM, Kestrel RCA, Foster C, Norlick FE, Calkins DR, Delbanco TL. Unconventional medicine in the United States: prevalence, costs, and patterns of use. N Engl J Med 1993;328:246–252.
2. Eisenberg DM, Davis RB, Ettner SL, et al. Trends in alternative medicine use in the United States, 1990–1997: Results of a follow-up national survey. JAMA 1998;280:1569–1575.
3. Wootton JC, Sparber A. Surveys of complementary and alternative medicine: Part. general trends and demographic groups. J Altern Complement Med 2001;7:195–208.
4. Landmark Health Care. The Landmark Report on Public Perceptions of Alternative Care. Landmark Healthcare Inc., Sacramento, CA, 1998.
5. Astin JA. Why patients use alternative medicine: results of a national survey. JAMA 1998;279:1548–1553.
6. Paramore LC. Use of alternative therapies: estimates from the 1994 Robert Wood Johnson Foundation National Access to Care Survey. J Pain Symptom Manage 1997;13:83–89.
7. Liu EH, Turner LM, Lin SX, et al. Use of alternative medicine by patients undergoing cardiac surgery. J Thorac Cardiovasc Surg 2000;120:335–341.
8. Blakely JA. The heart and estrogen/progestin replacement study revisited: hormone replacement therapy produced net harm, consistent with the observational data. Arch Intern Med 2000;160:2897–2900.
9. Adams KE, Cohen MH, Eisenberg D, Johnsen AR. Ethical considerations of complementary and alternative medical therapies in convention medical settings. Ann Intern Med 2002;137:660–664.
10. Weiger WA, Smith M, Boon H, Richardson MA, Kaptchuk TJ, Eisenberg DM. Advising patients who seek complementary and alternative medical therapies for cancer. Ann Intern Med 2002;137:889–903.
11. Hymes KB, Greene JB, Marcus A. Kaposi's sarcoma in homosexual men—a report of eight cases. Lancet 1981;2:598–602.
12. *Clinical Practice Guideline Number 17: Cardiac Rehabilitation.* US Department of Health and Human Services, Public Health Service, Agency for Health Care Policy and Research, National Heart, Lung and Blood Institute. AHCPR Publication No. 96-0672. October 1995.

2 History, Regulation, Integrity, and Purity of Herbs and Supplements

Robert S. McCaleb
and Fredi Kronenberg, PhD

CONTENTS

HISTORY OF HERBS IN MEDICINE AND PHARMACY

Herbs were our first source of medicine, and their use predates written history by several thousand years. No one knows when humans first used plants for medicine, but pollens of at least six medicinal plants were found in a Neanderthal burial site estimated to be at least 60,000 yr old *(1)*.

From: *Contemporary Cardiology*
Complementary and Alternative Cardiovascular Medicine
Edited by: R. A. Stein and M. C. Oz © Humana Press Inc., Totowa, NJ

11

The early history of medicine parallels the history of herbal medicine: the first books written about medicine were also the first books written about herbs, including Chinese texts from 5000 yr ago, such as the famous herbal of the Yellow Emperor and the Egyptian text *Ebers papyrus*, written 3500 yr ago. In Western medicine, the father of modern medicine, Theophrastus, is also the father of modern botany. Theophrastus published the first book describing plants in detail in 320 BC, which was also the first Western book about their medicinal uses.

Herbal medicine has been at the heart of medicine in every culture in the world and at every time throughout history. Today, according to the World Health Organization (WHO), more than 80% of the world's population relies on traditional medicines, mostly plant based, as their main source of health care *(2)*. This figure includes not only the large populations of China and India and all of the less developed countries of the world but also many modern nations. Even in the United States, approx 25% of our prescription medicines are still extracted from plants or are synthetic copies of plant chemicals *(3)*, and at least 57% of our top prescription medicines are derived in some way from plants, including *semisynthetics*, in which plant chemicals are used as building blocks for synthetic drugs *(4)*. A semisynthetic drug made from a plant chemical doesn't necessarily resemble anything naturally found in the plant, but it could not be made without the plant chemical as a starting point.

Making drugs in the laboratory is a newer practice than most people realize. The first synthetic chemical was produced in the mid-19th century, and the widespread use of synthetic drugs began during the last 70 yr. In the United States, natural remedies were replaced by powerful synthetic or highly purified "wonder drugs." However, in our haste to embrace "scientific" medicine, we quickly forgot the contributions nature made and still makes to medicine. Most synthetic drugs are duplicates or modifications of the same plant chemicals that make herbs work. For example, the world's oldest known cultivated medicinal plant is the Chinese herb *ma huang*, or *Ephedra*, which is grown for more than 5000 yr in China for treating respiratory disease, including asthma. Ephedra is the source of ephedrine, which is still used today to treat asthma, and pseudoephedrine, which is used as a nasal decongestant. These compounds can be made synthetically in a laboratory but are no more effective than extracts of the plant.

The focus of research in the 20th century shifted from the study of whole plants toward single "active principles" and synthetic chemicals. Plant drug research in the United States came to a virtual standstill as doctors and scientists turned increasingly to laboratory-made medicines.

Because pharmacists and doctors no longer needed to know about the plants themselves, courses on plant medicines disappeared from medical and pharmacy schools. Public funding for medical research focused primarily on cancer and later on AIDS, leaving little support for research on innovations in natural medicines. Drug companies focused their research efforts on developing synthetic drugs they could own through patent protection (*see* Government Regulation of Herbal Products section).

The nexus of medicinal plant research shifted to places where they were still considered an important part of health care, such as Europe and Asia. In the United States and Western Europe, researchers concentrated on isolated plant constituents rather than whole herbs or crude extracts. For example, until recently, there was hardly any research on the health effects of green tea, but there were thousands of studies on caffeine. Although numerous studies exist for ephedrine and pseudoephedrine, there are few on the plant ephedra or its extracts.

Medicinal herb research in Europe accelerated rapidly from the 1960s to the present. The best herb research was performed in Europe, primarily because modern medicine in Europe continued the use of complex or "crude" plant drugs and their extracts. With favorable treatment from European governments, phytomedicine flourished and European companies developed sophisticated herb extracts, sponsored research, and built the European phytomedicine empire that is changing medicine worldwide. American doctors, scientists, and regulators decried the lack of sound evidence for medicinal herbs, whereas European scientists conducted the studies that made phytomedicine a dominant form of therapy there.

CURRENT WORLDWIDE USE OF HERBS

Herbal medicines are government approved and sold with medicinal claims throughout Europe and most of Asia, as well as in Australia, Mexico, and Canada. In other countries, limited health claims based on traditional uses are allowed. In an informal review by the United States. Commission on Dietary Supplement Labels, 11 of the 14 countries reviewed had an abbreviated method for allowing informative medicinal label claims on herbal products.

Technologically advanced nations' attempts to control and regulate herbal medicines in the same way as synthetic drugs, sometimes improving the reliability of these time-honored treatments but occasionally creating unforeseen problems.

The most widely used system of herbal medicine in the world is probably traditional Chinese medicine (TCM), used not only in China but also throughout Asia and, as a form of alternative medicine, in the United States and Europe. TCM is probably used to some extent by more than one-third of the world's population. However, the best accepted forms of herbal therapy today are those that are supported by modern clinical research, usually involving semipurified, standardized extracts of single herbs or simple combinations of fewer than six herbs, in contrast to the complex mixtures characteristic of TCM remedies. The highest quality research is on single-herb extracts, such as ginkgo, St. John's wort, and saw palmetto.

GOVERNMENT REGULATION OF HERBAL PRODUCTS

Although many believe that herbal medicine was displaced by safer or more effective medicines, the truth is that synthetics overtook natural medicines in the pharmacy because of economics and regulation, not science and medicine. In the early 20th century, the US Congress, alarmed by questionable "patent medicines," established the Food and Drug Administration (FDA) and required foods and drugs to be proven safe before they could be sold. As more sophisticated and expensive research methods were devised, it became increasingly expensive to establish the safety of drugs. In 1962, Congress passed the additional requirement that drugs be proven effective, further increasing the cost of drug approval. Drug industry statistics set the cost at an average of $350 million to prove that a drug is safe and effective, and it can take 5–12 yr or more to gain approval. Drug companies can recover research and approval costs through the sale of the drug but only if the company has the exclusive right to sell it. However, herbal medicines are rarely patentable, denying companies the exclusive right to sell them. Patent law prevents people from claiming that they invented substances or technologies that were already known. Common substances such as ice or ginseng, have been known for too long to be patentable. If a company choses to spend $350 million to prove that ginseng is safe and effective, anyone could sell it as a safe and effective drug. The effect of regulation and economics on plant-based pharmaceuticals has been chilling. Since 1962, not a single new complex plant drug has been approved in the United States. Because herbs could not be sold as medicines, they were regulated as foods or occasionally as food chemicals (additives). Today, herbs, as well as vitamins and minerals, are regulated as dietary supplements in the United States.

The Introduction of DSHEA

The relationship between the FDA and the American herb industry has been highly adversarial for the past 30 yr. In 1994, the US Congress unanimously passed a bill called the Dietary Supplement Health and Education Act (DSHEA), which defined dietary supplements as special nutritionals and forbade the FDA from treating them as food chemicals or as drugs unless manufacturers made drug claims for their products. DSHEA allows dietary supplements to bear health-benefit claims called "statements of nutritional support," commonly referred to as *structure/ function claims*, because they may describe the effect of the supplement on the structure or function of the body. These statements must be truthful and not misleading and must be supported by scientific evidence. Labels must carry a disclaimer that the product is not intended for treating, curing, or preventing disease. With the passage of DSHEA, the United States changed virtually overnight from one of the most hostile regulatory environments in the world for herbs to one of the most permissive. DSHEA allows fairly informative labeling of products without previous government approval, yet it requires a scientific basis and truth in labeling, which the FDA is empowered to enforce. However, there have been some abuses of the new law because of both opportunists making exaggerated claims and inadequate FDA scrutiny.

DSHEA is clearly a compromise solution to the regulation of herbs for health care. Better models allowing more frank and informative labeling of herbal products will surely arise. There is still no regulatory framework for traditional forms of herbal medicine that are not based on scientific research, for example TCM and Ayurvedic medicine. The German regulatory system also lacks an appropriate mechanism for those remedies, whereas the systems used in France, the United Kingdom, and Canada may work somewhat better. These systems focus on informing the public about traditional uses rather than expecting strong scientific backing of all remedies.

The European regulatory model has provided greater research incentives for herbs than the FDA model provides, which crippled American medicinal plant research. European regulations made European drug companies the leaders in natural product medicine. The changes in US supplement regulation have finally opened the doors to better research funding for natural products and more informative labels and labeling for products.

TYPES OF HERBAL PRODUCTS

Herbal products span a range of different forms, from jars of dried leaves, flowers, and roots to glossy, full-color boxes of blister-packed, coated tablets that look much like conventional drugs. The most popular forms of herbal products in the United States are capsules and tablets. Most of these products contain standardized herb extract.

Other ancient types of herbal products are also still available. Many health-food stores continue to carry hundreds of herbs in the original bulk form, that is, dried herbs usually displayed in glass jars and sold by the ounce. Herbal teas, also called infusions, can be found in nearly every restaurant and hotel in the world. Herbal products also include liquid extracts or tinctures, cough syrups, and lozenges.

ABOUT EXTRACTS

The leading products on the market today are standardized extracts, meaning that every dose of the extract contains the same level of important compounds. Doctors and pharmacists favor standardized extracts, because they add a level of consistency that appeals to professionals, and, in many cases they are among the best researched products. However, they are somewhat controversial, too, because they are highly processed, and, in many cases, we do not fully understand which constituents in an herb contribute to its activity.

Plants contain a complex mixture of thousands of substances, including water and fiber, chlorophyll, starches, fats, and proteins, plus unique phytochemicals that give each plant its particular physiological effects. Manufacturers make extracts by grinding the herb and using a solvent, such as alcohol, to dissolve beneficial compounds from the herb. Some herbs do not need to be extracted, but for several reasons, some are best used in extract form.

- Concentration: Some herbs are so mild that it is unrealistic to use them without concentration. Bilberry is a good example. The dark-blue pigments in bilberry fruit are responsible for its antioxidant benefits, but to get enough of these compounds into a few capsules, it is necessary to concentrate them by 100 times. To get an effective dose of simple dried bilberry fruit in a capsule, we would need to take up to 100 capsules a day. Instead, we take a concentrate. This concentrate is called a 100-to-1 concentrate and is usually written 100:1.
- Selection: When a concentrate is made, something is omitted from the extract. The largest part of what is excluded is the insoluble fiber. Extraction procedures can be designed to select for extraction of particular beneficial compounds or elimination of undesirable or toxic compounds.

Standardized Extracts

To standardize an extract, the manufacturer tests for key compounds in the plant and adjusts the strength of the extract to ensure that the level of these compounds remains consistent. For instance, if a company processes a batch of ginseng that is lower in the active ginseng compounds (the ginsenosides), the company can either further concentrate the extract or use more ginseng.

One problem with standardizing extracts is that we often do not know which chemicals in an herb contribute to its health benefits. Only a few of the hundreds of herbs on the market are standardized to known active principles. Examples include kava, senna, ginseng, ephedra, cola, and maté. Other extracts are standardized to "marker" compounds, which may not be critical to the plant's effectiveness. Markers are chosen based on some evidence that if the extract contains enough of the marker compound, it will be effective. St. John's wort is a good example. Its standardized extracts have well-researched antidepressant effects, despite that the marker compound to which extracts are standardized, hypericin, is not the "active principle" in this antidepressant herb *(5)*. However, clinical trials prove that an extract (made in a certain way) that has enough hypericin is effective against depression *(6)*. Whichever chemical or chemicals are responsible for this effect are extracted along with the hypericin, so the hypericin serves as a good marker.

One of the risks of standardizing extracts to a single chemical compound is the possibility of an unscrupulous manufacturer boosting the level of the marker compound with a cheap, synthetic chemical. This is called "spiking" and is believed to be uncommon for most herbs, partly because cheap synthetic sources of most marker compounds are not available. There is sound evidence of spiking in ephedra products (inexpensive ephedrine is available), but this is a dangerous practice for manufacturers because it is both unethical and illegal.

A larger problem is that in independent tests, some products have failed to contain the levels of marker compounds that are stated on the label. In some cases, no marker compounds were found in these tests, indicating that the product may not have included any of the labeled herb. In either case, this could result from either poor quality control or intentional fraud.

Hydroalcoholic Extracts (Tinctures)

The simplest extracts on the market are hydroalcoholic extracts, sometimes called tinctures, which are sold in dropper bottles. These are usually labeled with a ratio that tells you how much of the herb is present in a given quantity of an extract. The ratio is a measure of the weight of herb (the first number) used to make a certain amount of extract (the second number). If 1 kg of herb is extracted to produce 1 kg of extract, the extract is a "one-to-one," or 1/1, extract. An extract labeled 1/1 is roughly equivalent to an equal weight of the herb. One dropperful usually contains approx 1 mL of extract, which weighs approx 1 g, so 1 dropperful of a 1/1 extract is approximately equal to 1 g of the herb. In a 1/5 extract, 1 g of herb is present in 5 g (5 mL) of extract. It takes 5 dropperfuls of a 1/5 extract to equal 1 g of the herb, and 1 dropperful of a 2/1 extract is equal to 2 g of herb.

To extract an herb with high levels of nonpolar compounds which are not water soluble, manufacturers use more alcohol, up to 80%. Approximately 25% alcohol is necessary to prevent an extract from spoiling, but the alcohol content in extracts will vary from 25% to 80% alcohol, depending on the requirements of the herb being extracted. The flavor components and pungent principles in ginger are all soluble in alcohol, so ginger extracts may contain 80% alcohol. In other cases, such as green tea extract, the beneficial components are soluble in water, and only enough alcohol is used to preserve the extract. Some extract makers use other solvents, including acetone and hexane, and, in these cases, it is important for the manufacturer to test for solvent residues.

GUIDELINES FOR CHOOSING PRODUCTS

Choosing herbal products is one of the major challenges to using these supplements. Dozens of brands are available, and each claims to be the best. Frequent stories in the media proclaim that the herb industry is "unregulated" and warn that products may not contain the ingredients they claim. Actually, the FDA does have the power to regulate, but to date, its enforcement of the regulations has been weak. The resulting confusion leaves the pharmacist, the physician, and the general public wondering how to select the highest quality product. The herb industry, like other businesses, includes companies committed to quality with high ethical standards and also opportunists with only profit in mind.

The Importance of Quality, Testing,
and Good Manufacturing Practices

Three things are essential to any product used for health purposes, whether it is a drug, a vitamin, or an herbal product: safety, effectiveness, and quality.

Good manufacturing practices (GMPs) refer to the steps a company takes to ensure quality in manufacturing its products. GMPs include guidelines for proper sanitation, good record keeping, laboratory testing, and the use of appropriate raw materials and processing equipment. When GMPs are followed, the risk of a critical failure in quality, safety, or effectiveness is reduced.

Laboratory testing is an important part of the manufacture of herbal products, especially for the more sophisticated extracts. An overwhelming failure of GMPs and laboratory testing occurred only a few years ago, when at least seven companies sold products that were labeled as containing mild, harmless plantain leaves (*Plantago major*), but they actually contained the powerful heart drug *Digitalis lanata*. Proper testing should have uncovered the problem long before it reached the retail shelf. The type of testing needed to ensure quality depends on the specific product.

- Identity: The first essential quality parameter in making an herbal product is plant identity. This can be verified in whole herbs by botanical features (leaf shape, types of flowers, fruits, etc.), by microscopic inspection and by chemical profiling or "fingerprinting." However, the more processed the product, the fewer ways there are to test it. A powdered herb can be tested microscopically or chemically, but an extract can only be examined chemically.
- Purity: Assuming it is the right plant, the batch may contain some weed leaves, small amounts of a completely different herb, or perhaps the wrong part of the herb being purchased, such as hawthorn leaves mixed in with hawthorn berries. Purity also means freedom from contaminants, which may include pesticides, heavy metals, dirt, disease-causing bacteria, mold, or animal or insect contamination, to name a few.
- Potency: Even if it is the right plant and free from any serious contaminants, is it strong enough to be effective? For the few herbs whose most active constituents are known, manufacturers can test for those compounds, but for the many herbs whose active principles are not known, we can only test for markers or assess potency in some other way.

Reputation and Trust

There are many manufacturers who make high-quality herbal products. Unfortunately, some product marketers sell inferior products, by either accident or intentional fraud. It is difficult to generalize about issues of reputation and trust, because there are ethical and unethical herb companies of all sizes.

Large companies that are household names have the most to lose from lapses in quality. However, small companies can also make good products; many use the same ingredient suppliers as their better established competitors, and some large companies have faltered on quality. Since 1996, several newspapers and magazines have published exposés on herbal products based on laboratory testing of products sampled from retail store shelves. These included *The Boston Globe*, *Los Angeles Times*, *Consumer Reports*, and *HerbalGram*, among others. An Internet publisher, ConsumerLab.com, has also tested retail samples of herbal products. There have been some problems with methodology in these programs, because journalists who were unfamiliar with the complexities of natural products selected inexperienced laboratories for testing.

In some cases, the laboratories used different testing methods than those used by the product manufacturers. Nonetheless, each publication reported a significant number of products that failed to meet label claim. This highlighted problems of consistency and probably ethics in the industry and considerably damaged public confidence in herbal products. To date, the herb industry has been unable to implement effective self-regulation, and the FDA has simply failed to act against products that fail to meet label claim, although it is its responsibility to do so. FDA spokesmen claim that the problem is the industry is "unregulated," but in a hearing before a congressional subcommittee, FDA Commissioner Jane Henney, MD, affirmed that the FDA has adequate authority and bears responsibility for regulating supplements, including herbal products.

INTERPRETING SUPPLEMENT LABELS
Claims

In the United States, supplement marketers can make "statements of nutritional support," often called "structure/function claims," because they describe the way an herb affects the structure or function of the body. Wellness claims about maintaining healthy body functions are acceptable, if there is evidence to support such claims, and drug claims that the product is intended to treat or mitigate disease are not allowed. For example, consider possible label claims for garlic. A garlic product might claim "helps maintain healthy cholesterol levels" or "helps maintain heart health," but, if the label claimed that the herb "helps prevent heart disease," the product would be considered a mislabled drug. Here are some more examples:

- Saw palmetto is effective against prostate enlargement. Illegal drug claim: "Relieves symptoms of prostate enlargement." Legal statement of nutritional support: "Helps maintain prostate health."
- Echinacea stimulates the immune system and reduces the frequency and duration of colds. Illegal drug claim: "For colds and flu." Legal statement: "Boosts natural resistance."

Other countries employ similar compromises. In England, products may be labeled "a traditional herbal remedy for (insert condition: sleep, menstrual disorders, etc.)." In France, herbs may be labeled "traditionally used for (condition)."

People are capable of understanding the difference between "take two aspirins for headache" and "a traditional herbal remedy for headache." The American situation is more complex, but people can understand that herbal dietary supplements are not the same as conventional medicines, although they may have similar uses in health care.

United States supplement law requires that statements be truthful and not misleading and that they be supported by scientific evidence. The exact wording of claims and the amount of evidence required are not detailed. In some cases, health-benefit claims may be exaggerated or carry implications that are not supported by sound evidence. In the United States, dietary supplements that make structure/function claims must carry the following disclaimer:

> *This statement has not been evaluated by the Food and Drug Administration. This product is not intended to diagnose, treat, cure or prevent any disease.*

The FDA's purpose in requiring the statement is to alert the buyer that the FDA has not reviewed or approved the claim and that the product should not be considered an approved drug.

INGREDIENTS

United States supplement laws now require full disclosure of ingredients, including binders, fillers, and other inert ingredients, that are used to make tablets and other herbal products. Some companies explain what each compound is for; others do not. The key ingredients in a supplement—the herbs or nutrients included—are listed in a special place on the package, which is called the "Supplement Facts" panel. This panel lists the required information about the ingredients, including what part of the plant is used, the genus and species, and the content of key ingredients. For reasons of confidentiality, companies are allowed to use mixtures in which the exact quantity of each ingredient is not disclosed. Such a product might be labeled "a blend of..."

Potency claims are sometimes difficult to interpret. Careful reading is necessary to determine the strength of the product. For example, one product may contain a concentrated and standardized extract of an herb, whereas another might contain just powdered whole herb, which, although it seems to provide more of the herb, actually delivers less of the relevant constituents.

With hundreds of herbal products available, it is not easy to choose the best herbal products. The key is to be armed with a basic understanding of the types of products and differences between them, to ask lots of focused and probing questions, and to determine to buy based on top quality, not low price. Avoid companies that make extravagant claims and those who use tricky wording to describe the strength or potency of the product. The best attitude with which to approach the herbal marketplace is open-minded skepticism.

INTERNET RESOURCES

Consumer Lab
http://consumerlab.com

FDA Center for Food Safety & Applied Nutrition
http://www.cfsan.fda.gov

NIH National Center for Complementary and Alternative Medicine
http://nccam.nih.gov

NIH Office of Dietary Supplements
http://dietary-supplements.info.nih.gov

The Richard and Hinda Rosenthal Center for Complementary and
Alternative Medicine, Columbia University
http://cpmcnet.columbia.edu/dept/rosenthal

The American Herbal Pharmacopoeia
http://www.herbal-ahp.org
U.S. Pharmacopeia
http://www.usp.org

OTHER RESOURCES

American Botanical Council
PO Box 201660
Austin, TX 78720-1660
(512) 331-886 (800)-373-7105
http://www.herbalgram.org

Herb Research Foundation
1007 Pearl Street, Suite 200
Boulder, CO 80302
(303) 449-2265 (Office)
(800) 748-2617 (VoiceMail)
(303) 449-7849 (Fax)
http://www.herbs.org

PERIODICALS

Alternative Therapies in Women's Health
American Health Consultants
3525 Piedmont Rd., NE
Bldg. 6, Suite 400
Atlanta, GA 30305
800-688-2421

HerbalGram
PO Box 144345
Austin, TX 78714-4345
(512) 926-4900

Journal of Alternative & Complementary Medicine
Mary Ann Liebert, Inc. Publishers
2 Madison Ave
Larchmont, NY 10538
(914) 834-3100
(800) MLIEBERT
info@liebertpub.com
http://www.liebertpub.com

Journal of Ethnopharmacology
Elsevier Science
PO Box 945
New York, NY 10159-0945
(212) 633-3730

Journal of Natural Products
PO Box 3337
Columbus, OH 43210
(614) 447-3776
(800) 333-9511

Medical Herbalism
PO Box 20512
Boulder, CO 80308
(303) 541-9552

Phytomedicine
Stockton Press
Houndmills, Basingstoke
Hants RG 21 6XS
United Kingdom
(800) 747-3187

Center for Medical Consumers
HEALTHFACTS
130 MacDougal Street
New York, NY 10012-5230
http://www.medicalconsumers.org
medconsumers@earthlink.net

COURSES FOR HEALTH CARE PROVIDERS

Botanical Medicine in Modern Clinical Practice
Offered annually at Columbia University, College of Physicians &
Surgeons
New York, NY; http://rosenthal.hs.columbia.edu/
(212) 342-0101

GENERAL HERBAL MEDICINE REFERENCES

McGuffin M, Hobbs C, Upton R, Goldberg A (eds.). Boca Raton, FL, Botanical Safety Handbook. CRC Press, 1997.

Blumenthal M, Busse WR, Goldberg A, et al. (eds.). The Complete German Commission E Monographs: Therapeutic Guide to Herbal Medicines. American Botanical Council, Austin TX, 1998.

Commission E monographs (published by the German government's Commission E, an expert committee of physicians, pharmacologists, toxicologists and other authorities, charged with writing monographs on commonly used herbal medicines) have been translated by and are available from the American Botanical Council

Blumenthal M, Goldberg A, Brinckmann J (eds.). Herbal Medicine: Expanded Commission E Monographs. Integrative Medicine Communications, Newton, MA, 2000.

Brinker F. Herb and Drug Contraindications and Interactions, Eclectic Institute, Sandy, OR, 1997.

De Smet PAGM. (ed.). Adverse Effects of Herbal Drugs (Vols. 1-3), Springer-Verlag, Berlin, 1992, 1993, 1995.

Duke JA. The Green Pharmacy. Rodale/St. Martin's Press, 1997.

Foster S, Tyler VE. The Honest Herbal. Haworth Herbal Press, Inc., New York, 1999.

Graedon J, Graedon T. The People's Pharmacy Guide to Home and Herbal Remedies. St. Martin's Press, New York, 1999.

Hocking GM. A Dictionary of Natural Products. Plexus Publishing, Medford, NJ, 1997.

McCaleb RS, Leigh E, Morien K. The Encyclopedia of Popular Herbs. Prima Health, Roseville, CA, 2000.

Miller LG, Murray WJ (eds.). Herbal Medicinals: A Clinician's Guide. Pharmaceutical Products Press, New York, 1998.

Murray M, Werbach M. Botanical Influences on Illness. Third Line Press, Tarzana, CA, 1994.

PDR for Herbal Medicines. Gruenwald J, Brendler T, Jaenicke C (eds.). Medical Economics Co., Montvale, NJ, 2001.

Pierce A. The American Pharmaceutical Association Practical Guide to Natural Medicine. William Morrow, New York, 1999.

Robbers J, Tyler V. Tyler's herbs of choice: The therapeutic use of phytomedicinals. The Haworth Herbal Press, Binghamton, NY, 1998.

Schulz V, Hansel R, Tyler V. Rational phytotherapy: A physicians's guide to herbal medicine. Springer-Verlag, Berlin, 1998.

The Prescriber's Letter. Natural Medicines Comprehensive Database. From the editors of the Prescriber's Letter. Therapeutic Research Faculty, Stockton, CA.

US Pharmacopeia. USP Monographs. http://www.usp.gov; 800-822-8772.

WHO monographs on Selected Medicinal Plants, Vol. 1. WHO, Geneva, 1999.

REFERENCES

1. Soleck RS, Shanidar IV. A Neanderthal flower burial in Northern Iraq. Science 1975;190:880.
2. Farnsworth NR, Akerele O, Bingel AS, et al. Medicinal plants in therapy. Bull World Health Org 1985;63:965–981.
3. Farnsworth NR. The role of medicinal plants in drug development. In: Krogsgaard-Larsen P, Christensen SB, Kofod H, eds. Natural Products and Drug Development. Munksgaard, Copenhagen,1984, pp. 17–30.
4. Grifo F, Newman D, Fairfield AS, et al. The origins of prescription drugs. In: Grifo F, Rosenthal J, eds. Biodiversity and Human Health. Island Press, Washington, DC, 1997, pp. 131–163.
5. Lenoir S, Degenring FH, Saller R. A double-blind randomised trial to investigate three different concentrations of a standardised fresh plant extract obtained from the shoot tips of Hypericum perforatum L. Phytomedicine 1999;6:141–146.
6. Linde K, Ramirez G, Mulrow CD, et al. St. John's wort for depression—an overview and meta-analysis of randomized clinical trials. Br Med J 1996;313:253–258.

3 Botanical Medicine and Cardiovascular Disease

Tieraona Low Dog, MD

CONTENTS

The role of plant medicine in the treatment of cardiovascular disorders has been a long and distinguished one. Our first effective treatments for hypertension and congestive heart failure (CHF) were derived from plants. Plant sterols effectively reduce cholesterol and are now added to food products as part of a heart-healthy dietary approach. Flavonoids, which are responsible for the colors of flowers, fruit, and, occasionally, plant leaves are believed to reduce the risk of coronary artery disease (CAD) by inhibiting platelet aggregation, reducing injury from ischemia

From: *Contemporary Cardiology*
Complementary and Alternative Cardiovascular Medicine
Edited by: R. A. Stein and M. C. Oz © Humana Press Inc., Totowa, NJ

and reperfusion, reducing plasma cholesterol levels, and/or inhibiting low-density lipoprotien (LDL) oxidation (1,2). The monounsaturated fat in olive oil and multiple constituents in garlic are beneficial for the cardiovascular system when consumed as part of a healthy diet. Other botanicals, such as hawthorn, guggul, red yeast rice, and globe artichoke, show promise for several cardiovascular conditions.

Although the data are intriguing, outcome studies that demonstrate the extent to which these botanicals reduce morbidity and mortality in those with cardiovascular disease (CVD) have yet to be conducted; thus, the formal recommendation of many of these plants is premature as primary treatment for most cardiovascular conditions. Practitioners are cautioned to be diligent in their care and follow-up of patients who choose to use herbal therapies in place of prescription drug therapy. In addition, the quality of botanical medicines available in the United States can be anywhere from excellent to awful. Adulteration, contamination, and substitution of herbs are not uncommon, making it imperative to choose supplements that have proven themselves in clinical trials (usually produced in Europe) or from companies that have gone through a quality certification program, such as the US Pharmacopeia (USP) or the National Sanitation Foundation (NSF), and bear the quality seal on their label.

ARTICHOKE (CYNARA SCOLYMUS)
Category 3 for Dyslipidemia

Globe artichoke leaf has been used as a treatment for dyspepsia since ancient times. More recently, researchers have found that the leaf extract has lipid-lowering activity. In vitro research indicates that the mechanism of action is an indirect inhibition of 3-hydroxy-3-methylglutaryl coenzyme A (HMG-CoA) reductase (3). Although there are likely multiple active constituents, luteolin exerted the highest inhibitory potency and effectively blocked the stimulation of cholesterol biosynthesis by insulin. Artichoke extracts also enhance biliary cholesterol excretion (4), which may also contribute to its lipid-lowering effects.

An older study of 17 outpatients with familial type IIa or IIb hyperlipoproteinemia was conducted to determine the efficacy of an isolated constitutent from artichoke, cynarin, for lowering lipids in this population. The patients were treated with either 250 mg/d or 750 mg/d of cynarin for 3 mo. There were no significant changes noted in serum cholesterol and triglyceride levels (5). Of course, this study used an isolated constituent from artichoke, which, at least according to recent in vitro data, is not the main lipid-lowering agent.

A recent randomized, placebo-controlled multicenter trial examined the efficacy and tolerability of 450 mg per tablet artichoke dry extract (drug/extract ratio 25–35/1, aqueous extract, CY450) vs placebo for the treatment of hyperlipidemia. The study enrolled 143 adult patients with initial total cholesterol of greater than 280 mg/dL and randomized them to receive either 1,800 mg artichoke dry extract per day or placebo for 6 wk. Changes of total cholesterol and LDL cholesterol from baseline to the end of treatment showed a statistically significant superiority ($p = 0.0001$) of artichoke dry extract over placebo. The decrease of total cholesterol in the CY450 group was 18.5%, compared to 8.6% in the placebo group. The LDL cholesterol decrease in the CY450 group was 22.9% and 6.3% for placebo. LDL/high-density lipoprotein (HDL) ratio showed a decrease of 20.2% in the CY450 group and 7.2% in the placebo group. No adverse events were noted in the study *(6)*.

The adverse effect profile for artichoke in the literature is good. The only contraindication at this time is for use in those who have a bile duct obstruction because of the choleretic activity of the extract. Given the short duration of the English trial and the lack of confirmatory studies, the true effectiveness of globe artichoke leaf for the treatment of hyperlipidemia is currently not known.

BISHOP'S WEED (AMMI VISNAGA)
Class 3 for Mild Angina

The fruit of this plant has been used since ancient times for its medicinal properties. Papyrus writings from Egypt describe the use of *Ammi visnaga* to treat asthma, painful kidney stones, and angina. In more modern times, there has been a growing body of research on the furanochromones and coumarin derivatives and their effects on the cardiovascular, respiratory, and gastrointestinal (GI) systems.

Visnagin, a constituent of bishop's weed, has demonstrated vasodilating activity in vitro and in animal studies *(7)*, likely by inhibiting phosphodiesterase *(8)*. Intravenous administration of visnagin resulted in dose-related decreases in blood pressure, with no significant changes in heart rate *(9)*.

Khellin accounts for much of the antispasmodic effects of *Ammi visnaga*, relaxing vascular smooth muscle through a nonspecific inhibition of calcium flux *(10)*. This is in contrast to visnadin, which preferentially inhibits contractile responses mediated by Ca^{2+} entry through L-type Ca^{2+} channels *(11)*, resulting in peripheral and coronary vasodilation. Both *Ammi visnaga* and the isolated constituent visnadin are still used in Europe to treat angina pectoris *(12)*. The German Commission E approved the use of *Ammi visnaga* to treat mild anginal symptoms. Standardized preparations of this herb may prove useful for mild angina, especially in those patients who cannot tolerate nitroglycerin.

Khellin exerts lipid-lowering effects in animal studies *(13)*. A study of khellin in 20 nonobese men with normal lipid levels found a significant increase in HDL cholesterol levels, although total cholesterol and triglyceride concentrations were unchanged. Unfortunately, nausea and vomiting caused four volunteers to withdraw, and elevation of liver enzymes caused an additional two participants to withdraw *(14)*. These side effects are not generally noted with standardized preparations of the whole fruit.

Generally, recommended standardized extracts provide an equivalent of 20 mg khellin/d. Prolonged use or overdose of the herb may lead to nausea, vertigo, constipation, anorexia, headache, pruritus, and sleeplessness *(15)*. Elevated liver enzymes and vomiting have been noted when the isolated constituents were administered alone.

CARDIAC GLYCOSIDES
Class I for Congestive Heart Failure

The role of botanical medicine in the treatment of congestive heart failure (CHF) is a long and interesting one. Plants containing cardiac glycosides have been used for centuries for the treatment of "dropsy," the old term for CHF. The primary plants used for this purpose include foxglove, squill, strophanthus, and lily of the valley. The ancient Egyptians used squill as a cardiac medicine, whereas the Romans employed the herb as a diuretic, heart tonic, emetic, and rat poison. Foxglove was mentioned in 1250 in the writings of Welsh physicians.

William Withering (1741–1799) first learned the value of foxglove (*Digitalis purpurea*) from an old woman in Shropshire, England, "who had sometimes made cures after the more regular practitioners had failed. . . . This medicine was composed of 20 or more different herbs; but it was not very difficult to perceive that the active herb could be no other than the foxglove." Withering, an observant physician, not only accurately described the efficacy of foxglove but also its toxicity, more than 200 yr ago. When given in large and quickly repeated doses, foxglove causes sickness, vomiting, purging giddiness, confused vision, objects appearing green or yellow, increased secretion of urine, slow pulses (as low as 35 beats in a minute), cold sweats, convulsions, syncope, and death."

Digitalis glycosides exert a positive inotropic effect via two mechanisms: direct inhibition of membrane-bound Na^+, K^+-activated adenosine triphosphatase (Na^+, K^+-ATPase), which leads to an increase in the intracellular concentration of Ca^{2+}, and an associated increase in a slow inward Ca^{2+} current during the action potential (AP).

Digitalis also lowers the heart rate (negative chronotrope), impedes stimulus conduction (negative dromotrope), and promotes myocardial excitability (positive bathmotrope) *(16)*. Although the suitability of digitalis for CHF has been questioned with more recent advances in pharmacological interventions, a recent Cochrane review found that the literature indicates that digitalis has a useful role in the treatment of patients with CHF who are in normal sinus rhythm *(17)*.

Even though many physicians are familiar with digitalis, most are not aware that other countries have used and continue to use several cardiac glycoside-rich plants to treat mild CHF. The inner scales of the bulb from white squill (*Urginea maritima*), a common plant of coastal Mediterranean regions that, depending on its origin, as well as time and manner of harvest and drying, contains 0.15–2.0% cardioactive glycosides. The primary glycosides are scillaren A and proscillaridin. The product is typically standardized to 0.2% proscillariden, with a standard dose being 0.1–0.5 g/d *(18)*. The German Commission E monograph (revised 1989) approved the use of squill for milder cases of heart insufficiency and also for diminished kidney capacity. The monograph lists nausea, vomiting, stomach disorders, diarrhea, and irregular pulse as side effects *(19)*.

Lily of the valley (*Convallaria majalis*) remains popular among herbalists throughout the world as a treatment for minor CHF. The aerial parts of the plant are gathered and dried during flowering. The herb contains more than 30 different cardioactive glycosides, namely convallatoxin and convallatoxol. Lily of the valley has primarily the same activity as digitalis (positive inotrope, negative chronotrope, negative dromotrope, and positive bathmotrope). The German Commission E monograph (revised 1990) approved the use of the herb for mild cardiac insufficiency, heart insufficiency resulting from old age, and chronic cor pulmonale. The dose listed in the monograph is 0.6 g/d standardized lily-of-the-valley herb *(19)*.

Note: Cardiac glycosides have a low therapeutic index and care must be taken when prescribing. Given the variability of glycoside levels in the herbs, only standardized products are recommended. It should go without saying that any cardiac glycoside-containing botanical be administered only by qualified health care professionals who are well versed in the management of patients with cardiac illnesses.

DANDELION (*TARAXACUM OFFICINALE*)
Class 3 as a Diuretic for Hypertension

Folk healers throughout most of the world regard dandelion leaf and root as effective diuretics. Herbalists often add dandelion leaf to hypertension formulas to reduce intravascular volume. However, other than some older animal data *(20)*, there is basically no research available for review that can allow one to determine the diuretic strength of the herb. Although not completely understood, the purported diuretic activity is believed to be associated with the sesquiterpene lactones found in the plant, along with high potassium levels. Because the leaf contains approx 4% potassium, the potassium depletion often associated with diuretics is generally not a problem with this botanical. The German Commission E recognizes the root and leaf for the stimulation of diuresis *(19)*.

The dose is generally 3 g/d. Dandelion has a low risk of toxicity when used appropriately. Even though dandelion leaf is a rich source of potassium, practitioners should monitor patients who take the herb for prolonged periods for possible hypokalemia.

GARLIC *(ALLIUM SATIVUM)*
Class 2 for Dyslipidemia, Class 3 for Hypertension

Garlic is the best known of the lipid-lowering herbs among the lay public. The lipid-lowering effects of garlic have been demonstrated in both animal studies and human clinical trials. Several meta-analyses have been performed during the years, demonstrating a reduction in total cholesterol of 5–12% *(21–24)*. The lipid-lowering effects of garlic are believed to result from inhibition of HMG-CoA reductase *(25)* and increased catabolism of fatty acid containing lipids, particularly triglycerides *(26)*.

Although the evidence does support a small but statistically significant decrease in lipid levels at 3-mo follow-up, pooled analyses of placebo-controlled trials failed to demonstrate significant reductions of total cholesterol at 6 mo. Contradictory results are likely the result of methodological shortcomings and the use of different garlic formulations and different time scales used in the studies *(27)*. A recent report by the Agency for Healthcare Research and Quality (AHRQ) concluded "it is not clear if statistically significant positive short-term effects—but negative longer term effects—are due to: systematic differences in studies that have longer or shorter follow-up durations; fewer longer term studies; or time-dependent effects of garlic" *(28)*.

Most garlic supplements are standardized to allicin potential and are enteric coated to prevent gastric acid inactivation of the allicin-producing enzyme, alliinase. A recent evaluation of garlic powder tablets used in clinical trials (1989–1997) found that the there was great variation in the amount of allicin released when subjected to the USP acid disintegration test (724A). Older batches were more resistant to acid disintegration and released three times more allicin (44% vs 15% of their potential, $p < 0.001$) than newer lots. Conflicting trial results may be the result of lower amounts of bioavailable allicin in some products. A recent evaluation of garlic products found that 23 out of 24 brands tested released only 15% of their stated allicin potential when subjected to the USP testing method. To ensure greater bioavailability, some researchers argue that garlic powder supplements should no longer be standardized to allicin potential but on dissolution allicin release (29,30). Until test products can be assured of containing and making bioavailable the key active constituents in garlic, conducting and evaluating clinical trials will be extremely difficult.

The benefits of long-term garlic consumption might best be viewed as a tonic effect on the cardiovascular system. Garlic has been shown to have mild antihypertensive (31), antiarrhythmic (32), antithrombotic, and antiatherogenic activites. The latter properties result from platelet aggregation inhibition, cholesterol biosynthesis inhibition and enhancing fibrinolysis (33,34). Garlic oil, aged garlic, fresh garlic, and garlic powder inhibit platelet aggregation via interference with the cyclooxygenase mediated thromboxane synthesis pathway (35). Raw garlic inhibited cyclooxygenase activity noncompetitively and irreversibly (36). After 26 wk of garlic consumption, there was roughly an 80% reduction in serum thromboxane in healthy male volunteers eating 3 g fresh garlic daily (36). Cooked garlic has a lower inhibitory effect on platelet aggregation than raw garlic (37).

The antiatherogenic activity of garlic has been demonstrated in a clinical study conducted in Europe. A randomized, double-blind, placebo-controlled trial was conducted with 152 men and women who were diagnosed with advanced plaque accumulation and one other cardiac risk factors (high cholesterol and hypertension). Patients were randomized to take 900 mg garlic (Kwai®) or placebo for 48 mo. Ultrasound was used to measure plaque in carotid and femoral arteries at 0, 16, 36, and 48 mo. At 48 mo: a 2.6% reduction in plaque volume was noted in the garlic group, compared to a 15.6% increase in the placebo group (38).

In addition to widespread belief in the lipid-lowering effects of garlic, many lay people also consider garlic a useful treatment for high blood pressure (39). Research demonstrates that animals that were fed garlic, along with a high-cholesterol diet, had reduced blood pressure and lower elevations in cholesterol than control animals (40). However, many of the animal studies that show the antihypertensive activity of garlic are difficult to interpret, as the garlic was often administered intravenously.

In one pilot study in humans, the antihypertensive activity of garlic was noted to occur within 5 h of administration of a single dose of 2400-mg dried garlic, with the effect lasting roughly 14 h (41). A meta-analysis of the efficacy of garlic and blood pressure found a mean difference in the absolute change (from baseline to final measurement) of systolic blood pressure that was greater in the subjects who were treated with garlic than those treated with placebo. The effect on diastolic blood pressure was not as significant *(21)*. In a prospective, 4-yr clinical trial of adults with atherosclerosis, standardized garlic powder supplementation (900 mg/d) lowered blood pressure by 7% ($p < 0.05$) *(32)*. However, the AHRQ concluded in its report that there is no evidence that garlic has a beneficial effect on blood pressure *(28)*.

Reported adverse events associated with garlic include cases of postoperative bleeding during augmentation mammaplasty *(42)* and transurethral resection of the prostate *(43)* in patients taking garlic before surgery. There is also a report of spontaneous spinal epidural hematoma *(44)*. None of the patients was taking warfarin, and a direct interaction with warfarin has not been found *(45)*. However it is well known that antiplatelet agents can increase the risk of major bleeding when combined with warfarin. Practitioners should be watchful of patients who are stable on warfarin and who add large amounts of raw garlic or garlic tablets to their diet.

In conclusion, garlic has mild, yet beneficial, effects on the cardiovascular system and should be considered part of a heart healthy diet. Patients who enjoy eating garlic should be encouraged to continue to do so. The lipid-lowering effects are mild and may not be sustained, thus garlic should be not be considered a primary therapy for patients with moderate to severe dyslipidemia. Data are lacking to recommend garlic as a primary therapy for hypertension.

GINKGO (*GINKGO BILOBA*)
Class 2 for Peripheral Vascular Disease

Standardized extracts of ginkgo are often recommended to treat intermittent claudication. In vitro studies have demonstrated that ginkgo extract stimulates the release of nitric oxide (NO), which induces vasodilation by activating guanylate cyclase in the vascular smooth muscle. Increased release of prostacyclin (PGI2) has also been demonstrated with administration of ginkgo extracts.

Fifteen controlled trials have been conducted on ginkgo to treat intermittent claudication—only two were considered of good quality in a 1992 meta-analysis. It was noted that all the trials, including the two best, showed positive results in increased pain-free walking distance when compared to placebo *(46)*. A recent double-blind, placebo-controlled multicenter trial of 111 patients with intermittent claudication found that after 3 mo of taking a ginkgo extract (EGb 761), patients experienced nearly a 50% increase in pain-free walking distance, compared to roughly 25% in the placebo group. However, adherence to taking the active or placebo was good only seven patients (three in active and four in placebo group) adhered to the walking exercise program *(47)*.

The dose typically used for the treatment of peripheral artery disease is 120–160 mg/d of an extract standardized to 24% ginkgolides and 6% terpenes. The German Commission E lists occasional GI upset, headache, and allergic skin reactions as side effects of ginkgo and contraindicates the herb in patients with a hypersensitivity to ginkgo preparations. The leaf has a relatively low risk of toxicity when used appropriately. The LD50 is 7.7 g/kg of standardized ginkgo extract when given orally to mice. No evidence of chronic toxicity was noted when doses up to 500 mg/kg/d were given to mice for a 27-wk period (48).

Concerns have been raised regarding the potential risk of bleeding in patients who are taking gingko alone or in combination aspirin or warfarin. Spontaneous ocular hymphema was noted in a patient who was taking ginkgo and aspirin (49), intracerebral hemorrhage when ginkgo was taken with warfarin for 2 mo (50), bilateral subdural hematoma in a 33-yr-old woman who had been taking 120 mg/d of ginkgo for 2 yr (51), and subarachnoid hemorrhage in a 61-yr-old man with mildly prolonged bleeding time who had been taking 120–160 mg/d ginkgo for 6 mo (52). An additive effect on platelet inhibition was noted in normal and thrombosis-induced rats when given a combination of ticlopidine (50 mg/kg/d) and EGb 761 (40 mg/kg/d of a proprietary standardized extract of ginkgo that contains 24% ginkgoflavones and 6% terpenes). Bleeding time was prolonged by 150% (53), but this study used a ginkgo dose much higher than the recommended therapeutic dose. Although the true risk of interaction with warfarin or antiplatelet agents is not known (45), patients should be monitored if taking these medications. However, given the tens of millions of doses of ginkgo that have been consumed in Europe and the United States, risk of hemorrhage is relatively small.

Walking is considered one of the best self-help treatments for peripheral artery disease, but many people suffer extreme pain after walking even for short periods. While we await more conclusive evidence on the efficacy of ginkgo for this condition, practitioners may wish to do a trial of this herb for 8 wk (if not contraindicated) in conjunction with a walking program to see if ginkgo increases the distance the participants are able to walk free of pain or discomfort.

GUGGUL (*COMMIPHORA MUKUL*)
Class 3 for Dyslipidemia

The guggul tree grows in dry areas of India, Pakistan, and Afghanistan, where it has been used by indigenous medical practitioners to treat obesity, rheumatic conditions, and other ailments. Since the 1960's, research has focused on its lipid-lowering activity, and today, it is commonly used as a lipid-lowering agent in India. Although it is known that guggul prevents LDL oxidation *(54)*, more recent research indicates that the guggulsterones (4,17,20-pregnadiene-3, 16-dione) found in guggul are highly efficacious antagonists of the farnesoid X receptor (FXR), a nuclear hormone receptor that is activated by bile acids. The FXR controls cholesterol by regulating the level of bile acids in the body. Blocking the action of FXR helps the body to rid itself of more cholesterol. Guggulsterone treatment decreased hepatic cholesterol in mice fed a high-cholesterol diet but was not effective in mice without the FXR *(55)*.

Older studies have demonstrated a reduction in total serum cholesterol, LDL cholesterol, very low-density lipoprotein (VLDL) and triglycerides, with an increase in HDL cholesterol *(56,57)*. One trial found guggul to be as effective as clofibrate in reducing cholesterol levels *(58)*, whereas another study of 61 patients with hypercholesterolemia found 50 mg guggulsterones bid to be superior to placebo in reducing lipids during a 24-wk period. Guggul decreased total cholesterol levels by 11.7%, LDL cholesterol by 12.5% and triglycerides by 12.0%, with no change noted in HDL cholesterol *(59)*.

Given the in vitro, animal, and human data, this herb warrants further study, because it may prove to be a beneficial, well-tolerated, and cost-effective treatment for dysplipidemia. However, to date, the studies suffer from significant methodological flaws, making any definitive conclusion about lipid-lowering effects premature.

The purified, standardized extract of the plant is better tolerated than the crude herb, which has been reported to cause numerous side effects, including abdominal pain, diarrhea, and skin rash. Most extracts are standardized to 5% guggulsterone content, and the therapeutic dose is 500 mg taken three times per day to provide 25 mg guggulsterone tid.

Side effects reported in clinical trials were minor and included diarrhea, mild nausea, headache, and restlessness *(59)*. Guggul is contraindicated during pregnancy because of purported uterine-stimulating properties *(60)*. Guggul has been reported to reduce the effectiveness of propranolol and diltiazem *(61)*.

HAWTHORN (*CRATAEGUS OXYACANTHA*, *C. LAEVIGATA*, AND *C. MONOGYNA*)
Class 2 for New York Heart Association; Class 1 and 2 Congestive Heart Failure; Class 3 for Hypertension, and Class 3 for Dyslipidemia

Hawthorn is a fruit-bearing shrub that has been used in European and Asian medicine to treat several complaints, including digestive disorders, dyspnea, urinary complaints, and CVD. People throughout the world have consumed the fruit as a food and to make wine and jams.

Today, most research focuses on the cardiovascular effects of hawthorn fruit, leaves, and flowers.

Hawthorn is rich in flavonoids, oligomeric procyanidins, and triterpenes; substances all known to exert beneficial effects on the cardiovascular system. Hawthorn is a positive inotrope, although controversy surrounds the mechanism. It was previously believed to result from cyclic adenosine monophosphate (cAMP) phosphodiesterase; however, the L-type calcium current is not affected, as previously believed *(62)*. More recent research indicates that the positive inotropic action of hawthorn is cAMP-independent and similar to the activity of cardiac glycosides *(63)*. Crataegus extract blocks repolarizing potassium currents in ventricular myocytes, similar to the action of class III antiarrhythmic drugs, and might be the basis for hawthorn's antiarrhythmic effect *(61)*. The flavonoids and proanthocyanidins in hawthorn possess angiotensin-converting enzyme inhibiting (ACEI) activity *(64)*.

Standardized extracts of hawthorn (providing a daily dose of 9 mg or more of oligomeric procyanidins) are beneficial for mild cases of CHF (New York Heart Association [NYHA] stages I and II) in 14 clinical trials, and 1 trial assessed its benefit in patients with NYHA stage III. Sixteen weeks of treatment with a hawthorn extract (WS 1442; 1800 mg/d), in addition to diuretic drug therapy, improved exercise tolerance in a randomized, placebo-controlled, three-arm study (placebo and 900 mg and 1800 mg hawthorn extract) of 209 patients with NYHA class III heart failure *(65)*.

A randomized, double-blind, placebo-controlled study ($n = 60$) found a reduction in myocardial ischemia and improvement in angina pectoris with increased physical performance in patients who had been diagnosed with stable angina when given 180 mg/d of standardized hawthorn extract *(66)*. Another study found hawthorn equivalent in effectiveness to 37.5 mg/d captopril in 132 patients with NYHA class II cardiac insufficiency *(67)*. A standardized hawthorn extract (WS 1442) was superior to placebo in a double-blinded, placebo-controlled study of 136 patients with NYHA stage II cardiac insufficiency. The primary target parameter was the change in the difference of the pressure, heart rate product (systolic blood pressure × heart rate/100) (PHRP 50 W load vs rest) measured at the beginning and end of treatment. A clear improvement in the performance of the heart was shown in the group receiving the test substance, whereas the condition of the placebo group progressively worsened. The therapeutic difference between the groups was statistically significant *(68)*.

Improvement in exercise tolerance, quality of life, and dyspnea-fatigue index was greater in the patients receiving a fresh Crataegus fruit extract compared to placebo in a 3-mo randomized, double-blind, placebo-controlled trial of 88 patients with NYHA stage II CHF *(69)*.

The German Commission E recognized hawthorn for the treatment of mild CHF. However, at this time, hawthorn should be seen primarily as an adjunctive therapy for all but the mildest cases of CHF, because a clear reduction in morbidity and mortality has been seen with the use of angiotensin-converting enzyme (ACE) inhibitors, which should remain, if appropriate, a first-line treatment for CHF.

Hawthorn's flowers, leaves, and berries often find their way into antihypertensive formulas. It has been postulated that the mild hypotensive activity of hawthorn may result from inhibition of ACE *(70)*. Ex vivo studies indicate that the flavonoids induce endothelium-dependent NO-mediated relaxation *(71)*.

However, reductions in systolic and diastolic blood pressures in humans are small with the use of hawthorn *(67,72)*. Therefore, hawthorn should not relied on as a sole therapy for hypertension treatment. Herbalists typically combine hawthorn with a diuretic agent (i.e., dandelion leaf), a nervine (i.e., valerian), and peripheral vasodilators (i.e., ginger). Because this type of individualized combination therapy has not been subjected to randomized trials, its efficacy is unknown.

Hawthorn reduces cholesterol in rabbits that were fed a high-cholesterol diet *(73,74)*. The study by Zhang et al. *(73)* found that hawthorn fruit does not affect the activities of HMG-CoA reductase or cholesterol 7-alpha-hydroxylase (CH) but does suppress the activity of intestinal acyl CoA:cholesterol acyltransferase (ACAT) ($p < 0.05$). The authors conclude that the lipid-lowering effects of hawthorn may, in part, result from the inhibition of cholesterol absorption mediated by downregulation of intestinal ACAT activity.

Although hawthorn is often found in dietary supplements that are designed to reduce cholesterol, there are no human clinical trials available to determine if the fruit, leaves, or flowers lower lipids humans, and, if they do, to what extent and at what dose.

The dose typically given for hawthorn leaf with flower is 2.0–3.5 g/d as an infusion or decoction or equivalent dose in tincture. Standardized extracts are also available and generally provide 30–168.7 mg procyanidins, calculated as epicatechin, or 3.5–19.8 mg flavonoids, calculated as hyperoside taken in two or three individual doses *(19)*. The majority of studies have been conducted on two distinct preparations of hawthorn. Special extract WS 1442 (Dr. Willmar Schwabe Pharmaceuticals) contains 80 mg hawthorn leaf with a 5/1 (w/w) dry flower extract standardized to 18.75% oligomeric procyanidins (15 mg) per capsule.

Extract LI132 (Lichtwer Pharma GmbH) contains 95 mg hawthorn leaf, 55 mg hawthorn fruit, and 45 mg hawthorn flower, plus 30 mg dry cold macerate 5:1 (w/w) of hawthorn leaf with flower per tablet.

Hawthorn has a low risk of toxicity when used appropriately. No organ toxicity was noted at 100 times the human dose of a hawthorn extract standardized to 18.76% oligomeric procyanidins (75). Hawthorn is considered to be quite safe when used appropriately; however, practitioners should be aware that hawthorn preparations may potentiate the activity of cardiac glycoside medications, such as digitalis (60).

HORSE CHESTNUT (*AESCULUS HIPPOCASTANUM*)
Class 2 for Chronic Venous Insufficiency

Horse chestnut tree seeds and bark have been used as traditional medicines in Europe for at least the past four centuries. The seed was primarily used for the treatment of varicose veins, hemorrhoids, phlebitis, neuralgia, and rheumatic complaints. The seeds contain several active constituents, including flavonoids and a combination of approx 30 unique pentacyclic triterpene diester glycoside saponins, collectively referred to as escin.

Horse chestnut seed extracts (HCSE) likely work through numerous mechanisms. In vitro research indicates that the extract inhibits the activity of elastase and hyaluronidase, which are enzymes involved in degrading the proteoglycan matrix, which comprises part of the capillary endothelium (76). Animal data suggest that HCSE shifts the balance away from degradation and toward proteoglycan synthesis, thus reducing vascular permeability and leakage (77).

A recent systematic review was published that examined 16 randomized controlled trials using HCSE for the treatment of chronic venous insufficiency (CVI). Eight of the studies were considered to be of good quality. Side effects noted in clinical trials included pruritus, nausea, and gastric complaints. Although the authors note that none of the studies was flawless, they do conclude that their critical literature review suggests that HCSE is an effective therapy for CVI (77).

HCSE are widely used in Europe, with a low incidence of adverse effects. Esculin exerts antithrombin activity and may lead to an increased bleeding time (78). Although the clinical significance of this interaction is not known when patients use therapeutic doses of the extract, practitioners should be mindful of patients who are taking anticoagulant medications. Standardized HCSE contains 16–20% triterpene glycosides, calculated as escin. The usual recommended daily dose is 100–150 mg of escin equivalent, or approx 500–750 mg HCSE containing 20% escin.

PLANT STEROLS
Class 1 for Cholesterol Reduction

Even though cholesterol is the sterol of mammalian cells, phytosterols are the sterols produced by plants. Although plant sterols are similar to the structure of cholesterol, they differ by possessing a methyl or ethyl group in their side chains, making them poorly absorbed. Plant-derived sterols have been shown to decrease total cholesterol levels for more than 50 yr. Their success as pharmaceutical agents were never fully realized because the introduction of more powerful drugs, but plant sterols have now become part of a public health strategy for maintaining healthy lipid levels by adding them to foods, such as margarine and salad dressing.

Because their structural similarity with cholesterol, phytosterols impair intestinal absorption of cholesterol, resulting in a 10–15% reduction in LDL cholesterol, with daily intakes of 2–3 g *(79)*. The ability of plant sterols to displace cholesterol from micelles in the small intestine is part of the mechanism that inhibits cholesterol absorption *(80)*. Esterification of these sterols increases their solubility in fat and their efficacy in lowering LDL cholesterol *(81)*, and most products on the market today are esterified to unsaturated fatty acids (sterol esters) or saturated fat (stanol esters). Studies have shown that both products work equally well in reducing LDL cholesterol *(82)*, but neither offers any reduction in triglycerides or increase in HDL cholesterol.

Patients who are taking cholesterol-lowering medications may experience additional benefit when consuming phytosterol-rich margarines or spreads. A recent study of 167 patients who were stable on statin medications for at least 3 mo found a further reduction of total cholesterol by 12% at 8 wk, compared with a reduction in the placebo group of 5% ($p < 0.0001$) and a reduction of LDL cholesterol of 17%, compared with a 7% reduction in the placebo group ($p < 0.0001$) *(83)*.

The use of phytosterol-rich margarines and spreads does not adversely affect the taste of food, and extensive toxicological studies have failed to reveal any significant harmful side effects with the use of these functional foods *(79)*. There are reports in the literature of decreased serum levels of β-carotene, α-tocopherol, and/or lycopene as a result of eating foods that contain stanol and sterol esters. Additional supplementation of these nutrients may be necessary. The American Heart Association and the National Cholesterol Education Program Expert Panel recommend plant sterols as adjunct therapy for the reduction of LDL.

RAUWOLFIA (*RAUWOLFIA SERPENTINA*)
Reserpine: Class 1 for Hypertension

The root of *Rauwolfia serpentina* has been used in India for centuries to treat anxiety, insanity, and venomous bites. The antihypertensive activity of the root was noted as early as 1918. The isolated alkaloid, reserpine, revolutionized the management of hypertension in Western medicine in the 1950s. Reserpine depletes adrenergic neurons of norepinephrine, resulting in decreased sympathetic tone and vasodilation. These effects occur in the central nervous system (CNS), peripheral nervous system, and adrenal glands. Rauwolfia's depletion of selected neurotransmitters in the CNS likely explain its traditional use in the treatment of certain psychiatric illnesses.

The antihypertensive effects of reserpine may take up to 2 wk to be observed. Smaller doses of reserpine should be used if a diuretic is concomitantly prescribed. In comparative studies, low doses of reserpine (0.25 mg/d) given concurrently with thiazide were as effective as sustained-release nifedipine (20 mg/d) in a study of black African patients who were with diagnosed hypertension (84). Other studies comparing low-dose reserpine (0.1 mg/d) plus a diuretic show that this combination is as effective as calcium channel blockers (85). A study in Germany found that low-dose reserpine (0.1 mg/d) given concurrently with clopamide (5 mg/d) was significantly more effective in reducing blood pressure than enalapril (5 mg/d). After 3 wk of treatment, mean systolic and diastolic blood pressure reduction from baseline (24 h after last medication intake) in the reserpine/diuretic group was –19.6/–17.0 mmHg and –6.1/–9.5 mmHg for the enalapril group (between-group comparison: $p < 0.01$ for both parameters). The normalization rates for diastolic blood pressure (<90 mmHg) were 64.1% for the reserpine/diuretic and 28.6% for enalapril ($p < 0.01$). Adverse events that were considered possibly or definitely drug related by the investigator were noted in 11 patients (17.2%) in the reserpine/diuretic group and 9 patients (14.3%) in the enalapril group. Two patients in the enalapril group discontinued the study prematurely because of coughing and skin eruptions (86).

Although low-dose reserpine plus a diuretic is fairly well tolerated in many patients, central side effects of sedation, nasal stuffiness, and severe depression have limited its continued use for the treatment of hypertension in the United States. However, other countries have continued to consider reserpine as a second-line treatment for hypertension when there is no evidence of end-organ damage (87). The use of low-dose reserpine when diuretics are not sufficient to control blood pressure in several countries, is likely, in part, based on its low cost. Yet the side-effect profile of this alkaloid makes the use of reserpine in older patients less than desirable. Rauwolfia is still used by some naturopathic practitioners in nonstandardized preparations. Given the variability of alkaloid levels in the root, this practice should not be encouraged.

RED YEAST RICE (*MONASCUS PURPUREUS*)

Class 3 for Dyslipidemia

The product sold as red yeast rice is prepared from cooked, nonglutinous white rice fermented by the yeast *Monascus purpureus*, which is then sterilized, dried, ground and encapsulated. Red yeast rice is a dietary staple in many Asian countries, with typical dietary consumption ranging from 14 to 55 g/d *(88)*. In addition to its medicinal properities, red yeast rice has been used to make rice wine and as a food preservative for maintaining the color and taste of fish and meat *(89)*.

The primary active ingredient in red yeast rice is believed to be monacolin K (also known as mevinolin and lovastatin). Monacolin K inhibits the enzyme that initiates cholesterol biosynthesis, HMG-CoA reductase. It is highly unlikely that the small amount of monacolin K present in red yeast rice fully accounts for the beneficial effects on lipids seen in clinical trials, because it is presently only 0.2%. Red yeast rice also contains other potential lipid-lowering agents, such as 10 other monacolin analogs, omega-3 fatty acids, isoflavones, and plant sterols (ß-sitosterol, campesterol, stigmasterol, and sapogenin) *(90)*.

A randomized double-blind, placebo-controlled study of 83 men and women found that those taking 2.4 g/d red yeast rice significantly lowered their cholesterol from 250 mg/dL to 208 mg/dL (17%) after 8 wk, compared to controls *(88)*. LDL cholesterol levels dropped from 173 to 134 (22%), triglycerides dropped from 133 to 118 (12%), and HDL cholesterol levels remained the same. Dietary intake was monitored, and there were no significant differences between the two groups in total calories, total fat, saturated fat, monounsaturated fat, polyunsaturated fat, or fiber. No changes in liver function tests or other serious adverse events were reported.

A pilot trial of red yeast rice was conducted with 14 individuals with dyslipidemia related to human immunodeficiency virus (HIV). Patients were randomly assigned to receive either 1200 mg/d of red yeast rice or placebo for 8 wk in a double-blind fashion. At the conclusion of the trial, there was a statistically significant reduction in total cholesterol ($p = 0.01$) and LDL cholesterol ($p = 0.01$) in the group receiving red yeast rice compared to placebo. No changes were noted in HDL cholesterol or triglycerides, and no adverse effects were reported *(91)*.

A recent study of commercial red yeast rice products found that there is tremendous variation in quality among products. Findings from clinical trials demonstrating significant and clinically relevant cholesterol reduction using a defined Chinese red yeast rice preparation (Cholestin) cannot be generalized to other commercially available preparations that do not contain the same levels and profile of monacolins. Citrinin, a toxic fermentation byproduct, was found at measurable concentrations in seven of the nine preparations *(92)*.

It should be noted that the proprietary red yeast rice product used in the clinical trial by Heber et al., Cholestin, is no longer available as a dietary supplement in the United States. The FDA claimed that the manufacturer was selling lovastatin, a patented lipid-lowering drug. After several years of battling in court, the dietary supplement company lost the fight and Cholestin was removed from sale; however, other red yeast rice products can still occasionally be found on the shelves of health food stores. Patients continue to order the product from Canada and other countries via the Internet. This may have as much to do with price as preference for a "natural" product. The current cost for cholesterol-lowering drugs is approx $120–300/mo, with an average cost of $187/mo. The red yeast rice product used in the clinical trial cost approx $25–35/mo.

TEA (*CAMELLIA SINENSIS*)
Class 3 for Dyslipidemia and Cardiac Protection

Tea is second only to water as the most common beverage in the world. Green tea from *Camellia sinensis* lowers plasma cholesterol in animal models with hypercholesterolemia *(93)*. Prospective studies have suggested that the polyphenolic flavonoids in tea may exert a protective effect against cardiovascular disease (CVD). A potential mechanism put forth for such an effect has been inhibition of lipid peroxidation by polyphenolic antioxidants. However, a recent study challenges this hypothesis, because the polyphenolic compounds from tea failed to inhibit in vivo lipid peroxidation *(94)*. Other researchers have suggested that tea increases the expression of the hepatic LDL cholesterol receptor, a cell surface protein involved in the control of plasma cholesterol *(95)*, and increases the fecal excretion of bile acids and cholesterol *(96)*. The purported beneficial effects might also be explained by the ability of green tea catechins and gallate esters to reduce intestinal cholesterol absorption and inhibit platelet aggregation *(97)*.

A meta-analysis of tea consumption in relation to stroke, myocardial infarction, and all coronary heart disease (CHD) was conducted based on 10 cohort studies and 7 case control studies *(98)*. The authors concluded that the incidence rate of myocardial infarction is estimated to decrease by 11% with an increase in tea consumption of 3 c/d (fixed-effects relative risk estimate = 0.89, 95% confidence interval: 0.79, 1.01) (1 c = 237 mL). However, evidence of bias toward preferential publication of smaller studies that suggest protective effects urges caution in interpreting this result." The study-specific effect estimates for stroke and CHD were too heterogeneous to allow for summarization.

The authors clearly point out the limitations of their findings. When evaluating studies, they found that many failed to precisely identify the type of tea being used or consumed—studies referring to the test item simply as tea. This represents a significant problem with evaluating the evidence, because tea actually represents a heterogeneous group of beverages, which can include fermented black tea, half fermented oolongs, unfermented green tea, and sweetened or unsweetened ice tea and other distinct herbal teas. Also lacking in most studies was a description of how the tea was prepared, including steeping time and whether milk was added *(98)*.

REFERENCES

1. Aviram M, Fuhrman B. Polyphenolic flavonoids inhibit macrophage-mediated oxidation of LDL and attenuate atherogenesis. Atherosclerosis 1998;137:S45–S50.
2. Xia J, Allenbrand B, Sun GY. Dietary supplementation of grape polyphenols and chronic ethanol administration on LDL oxidation and platelet function in rats. Life Sci 1998;63:383–390.
3. Gebhardt R. Inhibition of cholesterol biosynthesis in primary cultured rat hepatocytes by artichoke *(Cynara scolymus L.)* extracts. J Pharmacol Exp Ther 1998;286:1122–1128.
4. Kirchhoff R, Beckers CH, Kirchhoff GM, Trinczek-Gärtner H, Petrowitz O, Reimann H-J. Increase in choleresis by means of artichoke extract. Results of a randomised placebo-controlled double-blind study. Phytomedicine 1994;1:107–115.
5. Heckers H, Dittmar K, Schmahl FW, Huth K. Inefficiency of cynarin as therapeutic regimen in familial type II hyperlipoproteinaemia. Atherosclerosis 1977;26:249–253.
6. Englisch W, Beckers C, Unkauf M, Ruepp M, Zinserling V. Efficacy of Artichoke dry extract in patients with hyperlipoproteinemia. Arzneimittelforschung 2000;50:260–265.
7. Duarte J, Perez-Vizcaino F, Torres AI, Zarzuelo A, Jimenez J, Tamargo J. Vasodilator effects of visnagin in isolated rat vascular smooth muscle. Eur J Pharmacol 1995;286:115–122.
8. Duarte J, Lugnier C, Torres AI, Perez-Vizcaino F, Zarzuelo A, Tamargo J. Effects of visnagin on cyclic nucleotide phosphodiesterases and their role in its inhibitory effects on vascular smooth muscle contraction. Gen Pharmacol 1999;32:71–74.
9. Duarte J, Torres AI, Zarzuelo A. Cardiovascular effects of visnagin on rats. Planta Med 2000;66:35–39.
10. Ubeda A, Villar A. Relaxant actions of khellin on vascular smooth muscle. J Pharm Pharmacol 1989;41:236–241.
11. Duarte J, Vallejo I, Perez-Vizcaino F, Jimenez R, Zarzuelo A, Tamargo J. Effects of visnadine on rat isolated vascular smooth muscles. Planta Med 1997;63:233–263.
12. Rauwald HW, Brehm O, Odenthal KP. The involvement of Ca^{2+} channel blocking mode of action in the pharmacology of Ammi visnaga fruits. Planta Med 1994;60:101–105.
13. el Naser H, Abdel Ghaffar E, Mahmoud SS. Hypocholesterolemic effect of khellin and methoxsalen in male albino rats. Arzneimittelforschung 1992;42:140–142.

14. Harvengt C, Desager JP. HDL-cholesterol increase in normolipaemic subjects on khellin: a pilot study. Int J Clin Pharmacol Res 1983;3:363–366.
15. Wichtl M. Herbal Drugs and Phytopharmaceuticals. Bisset NG, ed. CRC, Boca Raton, FL, 1994, pp. 67–69.
16. Belz GG, Breithaupt-Grogler K, Osowski U. Treatment of congestive heart failure-current status of digitoxin. Eur J Clin Invest 2001;31(suppl 2):10–17.
17. Hood WB, Dans A, Guyatt GH, Jaeschke R, McMurray JV. Digitalis for treatment of congestive heart failure in patients in sinus rhythm (Cochrane Review). Cochrane Database Syst Rev 2001;3:CD002901.
18. Schulz V, Hansel R, Tyler VE. Rational Phytotherapy: A Physicians's Guide to Herbal Medicine. Springer-Verlag, Berlin, 1998, pp. 100–101.
19. Blumenthal M, Busse W, Goldberg A, et al., eds. The Complete German Commission EMonographs: Therapeutic Guide to Herbal Medicines. Integrative Medicine, Boston, 1998.
20. Racz-Kotilla E, Racz G, Solomon A. The action of Taraxacum officinale extracts on the body weight and diuresis of laboratory animals. Planta Med 1974;26:212–217.
21. Silagy CA, Neil HA. A meta-analysis of the effect of garlic on blood pressure. J Hypertens 1994;12:463–468.
22. Warshafsky S, Kamer RS, Sivak SL. Effect of garlic on total serum cholesterol. A meta-analysis. Ann Intern Med 1993;119:599–605.
23. Stevinson C, Pittler MH, Ernst E. Garlic for treating hypercholesterolemia. Ann Intern Med 2000;133:420–429.
24. Ackermann RT, Mulrow CD, Ramirez G, et al. Garlic shows promise for improving some cardiovascular risk factors. Arch Intern Med 2001;161:813–824.
25. Gebhardt R. Multiple inhibitory effects of garlic extracts on cholesterol biosynthesis in hepatocytes. Lipids 1993;28:613–619.
26. Lawson LD. Garlic: A review of its medicinal effects and indicated active compounds. In: Lawson LK, Bauer R, eds. Phytomedicines of Europe: Chemistry and Biological Activity. American Chemical Society, Washington DC, 1998, pp. 176–209.
27. Rahman K. Historical perspective on garlic and cardiovascular disease. J Nutr 2001;131:977S–979S.
28. Agency for Healthcare Research and Quality. Garlic: Effects on Cardiovascular Risks and Disease, Protective Effects Against Cancer, and Clinical Adverse Effects. Summary, Evidence Report/Technology Assessment: Number 20. Rockville, Md: Agency for Healthcare Research and Quality; October 2000: AHRQ Publication No. 01-E022. Available at: http://www. ahrq. gov/clinic /garlicsum.htm. Accessed August 24, 2001.
29. Lawson LD, Wang ZJ, Papadimitriou D. Allicin release under simulated gastrointestinal conditions from garlic powder tablets employed in clinical trials on serum cholesterol. Planta Med 2001;67:13–18.
30. Lawson LD, Wang ZJ. Low allicin release from garlic supplements: a major problem due to the sensitivities of alliinase activity. J Agric Food Chem 2001;49:2592–2599.
31. Silagy CA, Neil HA. Garlic as a lipid lowering agent—a meta-analysis. J R Coll Physicians Lond 1994;28:39–45.
32. Siegel G, Walter A, Engel S, Walper A, Michel F. Pleiotropic effects of garlic. Wien Med Wochenschr 1999;149:217–224.
33. Legnani C, Frascaro M, Guazzaloca G, et al. Effects of a dried garlic preparation on fibrinolysis and platelet aggregation in healthy subjects. Arzneimittelforschung 1993;43:119–122.

34. Gadkari JV, Josh VDJ. Effect of ingestion of raw garlic on serum cholesterol level, clotting time and fibrinolytic activity in normal subjects. J Postgrad Med 1991;37:128–131.

35. Lawson LD, Ransom DK, Hughes BG. Inhibition of whole blood platelet-aggregation by compounds in garlic clove extracts and commercial garlic products. Thromb Res 1992;65:141–156.

36. Ali M, Thomson M. Consumption of a garlic clove a day could be beneficial in preventing thrombosis. Prostaglandins Leukot Essent Fatty Acids 1995;53:211–212.

37. Ali M, Bordia T, Mustafa T. Effect of raw versus boiled aqueous extract of garlic and onion on platelet aggregation. Prostaglandins Leukot Essent Fatty Acids 1999;60:43–47.

38. Koscielny J, Klussendorf D, Latza R, et al. The antiatherosclerotic effect of Allium sativum. Atherosclerosis 1999;144:237–249

39. Wilson RP, Freeman A, Kazda MJ, et al. Lay beliefs about high blood pressure in a low- to middle-income urban African-American community: an opportunity for improving hypertension control. Am J Med 2002;112:26–30

40. Ali M, Al-Qattan KK, Al-Enezi F, Khanafer RM, Mustafa T. Effect of allicin from garlic powder on serum lipids and blood pressure in rats fed with a high cholesterol diet. Prostaglandins Leukot Essent Fatty Acids 2000;62:253–259

41. McMahon FG, Vargas R. Can garlic lower blood pressure? A pilot study. Pharmacotherapy 1993;13:406–407

42. Burnham BE. Garlic as a possible risk for postoperative bleeding. Plast Reconstruc Surg 1995;95:213.

43. German K, Kumar U, Blackford HN. Garlic and the risk of TURP bleeding. Br J Urol 1995;76:518.

44. Rose KD, Croissant PD, Parliament CF, Levin MB. Spontaneous spinal epidural hematoma with associated platelet dysfunction from excessive garlic consumption: a case report. Neurosurgery 1990;26:880–882.

45. Vaes LP, Chyka PA. Interactions of warfarin with garlic, ginger, ginkgo, or ginseng: nature of the evidence. Ann Pharmacother 2000;34:1478–1482.

46. Kleijnen J., Knipschild P. *Ginko biloba*. Lancet 1992;340:1136–1139

47. Peters H, Kieser M, Holscher U. Demonstration of the efficacy of Ginkgo biloba special extract Egb761 on intermittent claudication—a placebo-controlled, double-blind multicenter trial. VASA 1998;27:106–110.

48. DeFreudis FV. *Ginko biloba Extract (Egb761)*: Pharmacological Activities and Clinical Applications. Elsevier, Amsterdam, 1991, pp. 133–134

49. Rosenblatt M, Mindel J. Spontaneous hyphema associated with ingestion of *Ginko biloba* extract. N Engl J Med 1997;336:1108.

50. Matthews MK. Association of *Ginko biloba* with intracerebral hemorrhage. Neurology 1998;50:1933.

51. Rowin J, Lewis SL. Spontaneous bilateral subdural hematomas associated with chronic *Ginkgo biloba* ingestion. Neurology 1996;46:1775–1765.

52. Vale S. Subarachnoid haemorrhage associated with Ginko biloba. Lancet 1998;352:36.

53. Kim YS, Pyo MK, Park KM, et al. Antiplatelet and antithrombotic effects of a combination of ticlodipine and Ginkgo biloba ext (Egb761). Thromb Res 1998;91:33–38.

54. Singh K, Chandler R, Kapoor NK. Guggulsterone, a potent hypolipidaemic, prevents oxidation of low density lipoprotein. Phytother Res 1997;11:291–294.

55. Urizar NL, Liverman AB, Dodds DT, et al. A natural product that lowers cholesterol as an antagonist ligand for the FXR. Science 2002;296:1703–1706.
56. Nityanand S, Kapoor NK. Hypocholesterolemic effect of *Commiphora mukul* resin (Guggal). Indian J Exp Biol 1971;9:367–377.
57. Nityanand S, Srivastava JS, Asthana OP. Clinical trials with gugulipid—a new hypolipidemic agent. J Assoc Phys India 1989;37:323–338.
58. Malhotra SC, Ahuja MMS, Sundarum KR. Long-term clinical studies on the hypolipidemic effect of *Commiphora mukul* (guggul) and clofibrate. Ind J Med 1977;65:390–395.
59. Singh RB, Niaz MA, Ghosh S. Hypolipidemic and antioxidant effects of *Commiphora mukul* as an adjunct to dietary therapy in patients with hypercholesterolemia. Cardiovasc Drug Ther 1994;8:659–664.
60. McGuffin M, Hobbs C, Upton R, Goldberg A. American Herbal Products Association's Botanical Safety Handbook. CRC, Boca Raton, FL, 1997.
61. Dalvi SS, Nayak VK, Pohujani SM, Desai NK, Kshirsagar NA, Gupta KC. Effect of gugulipid on bioavailability of diltiazem and propanolol. J Assoc Phys Ind 1994;42:454–455.
62. Muller A, Linke W, Klaus W. Crataegus extract blocks potassium currents in guniea pig ventricular cardiac myocytes. Planta Med 1999;65:335–339.
63. Schwinger RH, Pietsch M, Frank K, et al. Crataegus special extract WS 1442 increases force of contraction in human myocardium cAMP-independently. J Cardiovasc Pharmacol 2000;35:700–707.
64. Lacaille-Dubois, Franck U, Wagner H. Search for potential angiotensin converting enzyme (ACE)-inhibitors from plants. Life Sci 2000;67:121–131.
65. Tauchert M. Efficacy and safety of crataegus extract WS 1442 in comparison with placebo in patients with chronic stable New York Heart Association class-III heart failure. Am Heart J 2002;143:910–915.
66. Hanack T, Bruckel MH. The treatment of mild stable forms of angina pectoris using Crataegutt Novo: a double-blind study using placebo as control. Therapiewoche 1983;33:4331–4333.
67. Tauchert M, Ploch M, Hubner WD. Efficacy of hawthorn extract LI 132 in comparison with captopril: multicentre double-blind study on 132 patients with cardiac insufficiency of NYHA Grade II. Munch Med Wschr 1994;136:27–33.
68. Weikl A, Assmus KD, Neukum-Schmidt A, et al. Crataegus Special Extract WS 1442. Assessment of objective effectiveness in patients with heart failure (NYHA II). Fortschr Med 1996;1142:291–296.
69. Rietbrock N, Hamel M, Hempel B, Mitrovic V, Schmidt T, Wolf GK. Actions of standardized extracts of Crataegus berries on exercise tolerance and quality of life in patients with congestive heart failure. Arzneimittelforschung 2001;51:793–798.
70. Stitcher O, Meier B. Hawthorn (Crataegus): Biological activity and new strategies for quality control. In: Lawson LK, Bauer R, eds. Phytomedicines of Europe: Chemistry and Biological Activity. American Chemical Society, Washington, DC, 1998, pp. 241–262.
71. Kim SH, Kang KW, Kim KW, Kim ND. Procyanidins in crataegus extract evoke endothelium-dependent vasorelaxation in rat aorta. Herz 1999;24:465–474.
72. Leuchtgens H. Crataegus special extract WS 1442 in cardiac insufficiency NYHA II. Fortschr Med 1993;111:20–21.
73. Zhang Z, Ho WK, Huang Y, James AE, Lam LW, Chen ZY. Hawthorn fruit is hypolipidemic in rabbits fed a high cholesterol diet. J Nutr 2002;132:5–10.

74. Rajendran S, Deepalakshmi PD, Parasakthy K, Devaraj H, Devaraj SN. Effect of tincture of Crataegus on the LDL-receptor activity of hepatic plasma membrane of rats fed an antherogenic diet. Atherosclerosis 1996;123:235–241.
75. Mills S, Bone K. Principles and Practice of Phytotherapy. Churchill Livingstone, London, 2000, pp. 439–447.
76. Facino RM, Carini M, Stefani R, Aldini G, Saibene L. Anti-elastase and antihyaluronidase activities of saponins and sapogenins from *Hedra helix*, *Aesculus hippocastanum*, and *Ruscus aculeatus*: factors contributing to their efficacy in the treatment of venous insufficiency. Arch Pharm 1995;328:720–724.

4 Herb and Dietary Supplement Interactions With Cardiovascular Drugs

Dennis V. C. Awang, PhD, FCIC

CONTENTS

INTRODUCTION

In the wake of a remarkable increase in popularity of herbal products and their attendant commercial success in the 1990s has come a wave of publicity over the potential for detrimental effects of mixing herbs with conventional drugs. Several alarmist articles in both the popular press and medical journals ignore that herbs are generally less toxic than pharmaceuticals and that currently there have been no deaths reported from untoward herb–drug interactions. The majority of published herb–drug interactions are based on case reports or extrapolation from in vitro observations, and few are based on clinical studies, making it extremely difficult to evaluate their soundness. Nonetheless, some prominent herbs, such as garlic, ginkgo, and St. John's wort, can have a significant influence on coadministered medication. Herbal medicines may mimic,

From: *Contemporary Cardiology*
Complementary and Alternative Cardiovascular Medicine
Edited by: R. A. Stein and M. C. Oz © Humana Press Inc., Totowa, NJ

decrease, or increase the action of prescribed drugs, which is especially important for drugs with narrow therapeutic windows, such as numerous cardiovascular drugs, and in sensitive patient populations, such as the elderly, chronically ill, and those with compromised immune systems.

The dramatically increased popularity of herbal products in North America in the 1990s (1) has led to increased scrutiny of commercial products for quality and conformity to label claims, as reflected in numerous analytical surveys sponsored by media and consumer organizations. Also, recently a plethora of articles in scientific, mainly medical, publications have appeared addressing the question of herb–drug interactions (2–4); two books on the topic were published in 1998 from the same publishing company (5,6). Particular attention has been directed to the potential for adverse consequences in the treatment of chronic conditions (7), effected by preoperative herbal use (8), especially regarding homeostasis (9). Several recent publications have focused on the potential for adverse effects of herbal medicinals on cardiovascular drugs (10–12).

Assessment of the potential for adverse consequences, resulting from either the intrinsic pharmacological effect of botanicals or their influence on the activity of prescription medications, has been criticized on mainly two counts. First, many of the reports of herb-induced interactions are unreliable, because they are based on poorly documented case reports (2) or theoretical extrapolations from in vitro activity (7); a review of the published clinical evidence on interactions between herbal and conventional drugs evaluated 108 cases of suspected interactions and classified 68.5% as unable to be evaluated, 13% as well-documented, and 18.5% as possible interactions (13).

Concern over the potential adverse effects of dietary supplements, and also of some food items, is exacerbated by a conviction in some regions of the country that the dearth of adverse-event reports may reflect a combination of underreporting and the pervasive belief of herbal enthusiasts in the general benignity of natural products (2), with a consequent lack of causality attribution. Furthermore, it has been expressed that the likelihood of herb–drug interactions could be higher with herbs than with prescription drugs, which usually contain single chemical entities, whereas herbs contain an array of constituents with varied pharmacological activity (13). It has been highlighted that the potential importance of herb–drug interactions warrants an increased research effort because of the paucity of reliable information in this area (14). Herbs, as well as nutritional items, may influence treatment of patients with cardiac problems by directly affecting either the cardiovascular system, the absorption, and/or metabolism of cardiovascular drugs.

Several herbs have exhibited varied potential for improving cardio-vascular conditions *(11)*, particularly hawthorn, garlic, ginkgo, and horse chestnut. Hawthorn (*Crataegus* spp.) leaves, flowers, and berries are the most widely used cardiotonic preparations in Europe; the plant is used primarily for angina, cardiac dysrhythmias and mild hypertension *(5)*. Garlic (*Allium sativum*), which is claimed to impart several health ben-efits *(15–18)* is most promising for its antithrombotic effect *(19)*. Ginkgo (*Ginkgo biloba*) has been used for treating arterial occlusive disease *(20)* and judged particularly effective for intermittent claudication *(21)*. Horse chestnut (*Aesculus hippocastanum*) is effective in treating chronic venous insufficiency (CVI) *(22)*. In addition, the nonherbal endogenous antioxi-dant, coenzyme Q10 (CoQ10 or ubiquinone), is beneficial in treating heart failure, angina, and essential hypertension *(23)*; in 1974 the Japanese gov-ernment approved its use to treat congestive heart failure (CHF).

Numerous medicinal herbs, including garlic and ginkgo, as well as CoQ10, have been implicated as having potential for adverse drug-inter-action effects. These last three substances have been cited for their pos-sible interference with the blood-clotting process, which is relevant for patients who are at risk for bleeding or taking anticoagulants. This is an important consideration, particularly when drugs with narrow therapeu-tic windows are involved, such as the anticoagulant warfarin (Coumadin) and the cardiac glycoside, digoxin.

ANTICOAGULANT–ANTIPLATELET INTERACTIONS

The potential for interaction of coumarin anticoagulants with a host of medicinal herbs has been advanced. Many of the proposed cautions relate to herbs for which some type of in vitro activity has been observed, which may have an influence on the blood-clotting process: one or more of the vascular, platelet, and coagulation phases. The anticoagulant potentials of feverfew (*Tanacetum parthenium*), ginger (*Zingiber officinale*), and especially Asian ginseng (*Panax ginseng*), which is often advanced in the company of ginkgo, are highly questionable and likely inconsequential in the clinical context. Although feverfew extracts and its sesquiterpene lactone constituents, notably parthenolide, inhibit plate-let aggregation by inhibiting serotonin release, among other actions *(24)*, no reports can be found in the literature of bleeding episodes or alter-ations in bleeding time that are associated with feverfew consumption. A similar situation obtains for ginger, which also inhibits platelet aggre-gation in vitro, because it is a potent inhibitor of arachidonic acid, epi-nephrine, adenosine diphosphate, and collagen *(25)*. Although there is no evidence for an interaction of either feverfew or ginger with coumarin anticoagulants, there has been one case report that associates Asian ginseng use with a decreased anticoagulation effect of warfarin *(26)*. A subsequent in vivo study with rats revealed no pharmacodynamic or pharmacokinetic interactions of single-dose or steady-state ginseng on warfarin *(27)*. A clear resolution of this ginseng case report is difficult, particularly because there has been widespread acceptance of ginseng as an antiplatelet medicinal, based on the observation that its constituent ginsenoside Rg2 inhibits platelet aggregation, whereas ginsenoside Ro inhibits conversion of fibrinogen to fibrin *(28)*. However, although the identity of this ginseng preparation is not in question, the patient was taking several other medications, which could have complicated the interaction arena. A lowered international normalized ratio (INR) was restored to normal level 2 wk after cessation of the patient's thrice-daily ingestion of capsules of the proprietary extract of *P. ginseng (26)*; one case report *(29)* has associated use of ginger (marmalade with 15% raw ginger) with inhibited platelet aggregation, which was restored to normalcy 1 wk after discontinuing ginger, with no symptoms noted. Until further clarification of this situation, those taking warfarin or related coumarin anticoagulants should refrain from consuming ginseng or have their clotting time regularly monitored.

There is also no evidence for an interaction of either garlic or ginkgo with warfarin; however, both herbals interfere with platelet function. Garlic, which inhibits platelet aggregation and fibrinolytic activity in both patients with coronary illnesses *(30)* and healthy subjects *(31)*, has been associated with postoperative bleeding *(32,33)* and spontaneous spinal epidural hematoma *(34)*. Ginkgo, whose constituent ginkgolides are potent antagonists of platelet activating factor (PAF), has also been associated with spontaneous and increased bleeding, even in the absence of anticoagulant drugs *(2)*. The effects of garlic and ginkgo, like those of coumarin-containing plant preparations, such as dong quai *(danggui, tang kuei) (Angelica sinensis* syn *A. polymorpha)*, have been regarded as not true herb–drug interactions but simply additive anticoagulant effects *(13)*. A 46-yr-old black American woman with atrial fibrillation who was stabilized on warfarin registered a greater than twofold elevation in prothrombin time (PT) and INR after taking dong quai concurrently for 4 wk. The patient's coagulation values returned to normal 1 mo after discontinuing the herb *(35)*. However, in a study with rabbits, dong quai, an herb especially popular in China to treat gynecological disorders, did not affect warafin's kinetics because no decrease in plasma concentration of the drug was observed *(36)*. Although dong quai extract alone did not alter baseline PT, mean PT values were decreased significantly from 24 to 48 h postdose after the herbal treatment, returning to control levels after 72 h. In the absence of any observed effect on protein binding or warfarin metabolism, the mechanism of this pharmacodynamic interaction and toxicity on coadminstration of dong quai and warfarin remains cryptic.

Another Chinese herb, danshen (*Salvia miltiorrhiza*), also interferes with platelet function, constituting an apparent true herb–drug interaction. A case of profound anticoagulation was reported that involved an interaction between warfarin and danshen, in a patient who had undergone mitral valve replacement *(37)*. The patient on discharge was being medicated with digoxin, captopril, furosemide, and warfarin; a stabilized INR approx 3.0 was elevated to 8.4 after 6 wk, along with an activated partial thromboplastin time of more than 120 s, when the patient reported to the emergency department complaining of chest pain and increasing dyspnea. After approx 2 wk of withdrawal from danshen and warfarin, the latter was gradually reintroduced and INR was stabilized.

St. John's Wort

St. John's wort (*Hypericum perforatum*), the popular herbal remedy for the treatment of mild to moderate depression, is now widely regarded as profoundly affecting the clearance and consequent bioavailability of several drugs. Chronic administration (8–14 d) of St. John's wort induces the cytochrome P450 (CYP 450) enzyme system, as well as the adenosine triphosphate (ATP)-dependent P-glycoprotein (Pgp) pump. CYP 3A4, the most abundant hepatic enzyme, oxidizes more than half of all medications that are subject to oxidative metabolism *(38)*.

Both CYP2C9 and Pgp are involved in warfarin's metabolism. Seven cases of reduced anticoagulant effect of warfarin have been reported in patients using St. John's wort *(39)*. Although no patients developed thromboembolic complications, the INR decrease was regarded as clinically significant; INR returned to target values after discontining St. John's wort. However, no case report of hemorrhage associated with use of the herb has been published.

Cyclosporine, the drug that is commonly administered to mitigate transplant rejection, is a substrate of both CYP3A4 and Pgp and highly susceptible to St. John's wort, which causes significant reduction in plasma levels of the drug. Two cases of acute heart transplant rejection have been reported in men in their 60s who were being maintained on cyclosporine 3 wk after initiation of daily dosing with a standardized St. John's wort preparation (300 mg, tid) *(40)*. The St. John's wort interaction with cyclosporine has such pronounced potential that coadministration of the two agents should be scrupulously avoided *(38)*.

Two interesting recent publications described the safety and efficacy of a proprietary St. John's wort preparation, Ze 117, that effectively treats depression *(39)*, but has low hyperforin content, which is the phloroglucinol derivative formerly regarded as the chief active antidepressant constituent of St. John's wort. Clinical pharmacokinetic studies have shown that Ze 117 does not interact appreciably with either CYP3A4 or Pgp *(40)*, whereas hyperforin induces hepatic CYP3A4 via the pregnane X receptor *(41)*. This raises the prospect of developing an efficacious hyperforin-free St. John's wort preparation; such products would not increase the clearance of those therapeutically important drugs seriously affected by the usual hyperforin-charged St. John's wort preparations.

Coenzyme Q10

Reports of CoQ10 interacting with warfarin, producing a decreased response to the anticoagulant, have been discredited in a recent randomized, double-blind, placebo-controlled crossover trial *(42)*. The effects of CoQ10 and ginkgo on warfarin dosage were assessed; no statistically significant influence on the response to warfarin was detected for either substance. The authors of the study suggest that the interaction observed in the case reports resulted from either health problems of the subjects involved or impurities in the products used.

FOOD PLANTS/NUTRIENTS

Many food plants can also interact with warfarin. For example, its anticoagulant effect can be diminished by vitamin K in greens *(43)* and broccoli *(44)*, as well as by large amounts of avocado *(45)*. One case report documents a significantly decreased INR in a 44-yr-old man who consumed 1.13–3.75 L of green tea *(Camellia sinensis)* daily for approx 1 wk, while being maintained on warfarin *(46)*.

The juice of Seville (sour) orange *(Citrus aurantium)*, which is popular as a promoter of weight loss and used to knock out intestinal CYP 450 3A4 isoenzyme in bioavailability studies, can cause cardiac disturbances in individuals with severe hypertension and tachyarrythmias. The sympathomimetic amines *m*-synephrine (phenylephrine) and octapine have been indicted as the agents responsible for adverse effects, but further studies are needed to confirm such speculation *(47)*. The hemodynamics of normotensive subjects were not significantly affected.

Red wine decreases the bioavailability of cyclosporine by as much as 50%, both area under the concentration-vs-time curve (AUC) and peak concentration being significantly reduced *(48)*.

Grapefruit Juice

Grapefruit acts on the drug transporter Pgp and, as well, is a potent inhibitor of cytochrome P450 enzymes *(49)*, producing greatly increased AUC of a considerable number of medications, notably the calcium channel blockers amlodipine, felodipine, nifedipine, nimodipine, nosoldipine, nitredipine *(50)*, and verapamil *(51)*, used for hypertension, angina, and certain arrythmias. Grapefruit also increases blood concentrations of cyclosporine *(52)* and the antiarrythmic quinidine *(53)*. The mechanism of action of grapefruit is claimed to chiefly involve selective downregulation of CYP3A4 in the small intestine *(54)*. The active agents are naringenin *(55)*; the aglycone of naringin, the major bioflavonoid and bitter principle in grapefruit juice; and two furanocoumarins, 6',7'-dihydroxybergamottin (DHB) *(56)* and an uncharacterized other (FC726) *(57)*; DHB exerts multiple effects, whereas FC726 works specifically on CYP3A4.

LAXATIVE HERBS AND DRUGS

Bulk-forming laxative herbs, such as the hydrocolloidal fiber-containing guar (*Cyamopsis tetragonolobus*) gum, psyllium (*Plantago* spp.), konjac (*Amorphophallus rivieri*), and others, taken in sufficient quantity can delay gastric emptying and reduce the rate of absorption of carbohydrates and drugs, including digoxin *(61)*.

Laxative herbs that contain stimulant anthranoids, including senna species (*Cassia senna*, *C. acutifolia*, and *C. angustifolia*), Chinese rhubarb (*Rheum officinale*), cascara sagrada (*Rhamnus purshiana*), frangula or alder buckthorn (*Rhamnus frangula*), yellow dock (*Rumex crispus*), and drug aloe, the leaf exudates of *Aloe vera*, can decrease the absorption of intestinally absorbed drugs resulting from an increased rate of intestinal transit *(62)*.

CONCLUSION

Patients who are on anticoagulants should avoid consuming ginkgo, ginseng, dong quai, and danshen products. Those who consume other herbs, particularly those for which there is any indication of potential for affecting platelet function, should have their bleeding times monitored *(2)*. Anyone who is taking critical chronic medication should not use St. John's wort, because the herb reduces the bioavailability of many drugs. The effect of herbal laxatives in decreasing absorption of drugs should also be considered.

Finally, because North America has no effective regulatory program to provide assurance of either the identity or the quality of herbal products, pregnant or lactating women would be well advised to refrain from their use.

REFERENCES

1. Eisenberg D, David RB, Ettner SL, et al. Trends in alternative medicine use in the United States, 1990–1997. JAMA 1998;280:1569–1575.
2. Fugh-Berman A. Herb-drug interactions. Lancet 2000;355:134–138.
3. Ernst E. Possible interactions between synthetic and herbal medicinal products. Part 1: a systematic review of the indirect evidence. Perfusion 2000;13:4–15.
4. Izzo AA, Ernst E. Interactions between herbal medicines and prescribed drugs. Drugs 2001;61:2163–2175.
5. Brinker F. Herb Contraindications and Drug Interactions. Eclectic Medical Publications, Sandy, OR, 1998.
6. Meletis CD, Jacobs T. Interactions Between Drugs and Natural Medicines. Eclectic Medical Publications, Sandy, OR, 1998.
7. Awang DVC, Fugh-Berman A. Herb-drug interactions in chronic conditions. Alt Ther Women's Health 2002;4:57–60.
8. Ang-Lee MK, Moss J, Yuan C-S. Herbal medicines and perioperative care. JAMA 2001;286:208–216.
9. Shaw HS, Kroll DJ. The convergence of herb pharmacodynamics and herb-drug interactions on hemostasis. Alt Ther 2001;7:46–47.
10. Aggarwal A, Ades PA. Interactions of herbal remedies with prescription cardiovascular medications. Coronary Artery Dis 2001;12:581–584.
11. Valli G, Giardina E-GV. Benefits, adverse effects and drug interactions of herbal therapies with cardiovascular effects. J Amer Coll Cardiol 2002;39:1083–1095.
12. Awang DVC, Fugh-Berman A. (2002) Herbal interactions with cardiovascular drugs. J Cardiovasc Nurs 2002;16:64–70.
13. Fugh-Berman A, Ernst E. Herb-drug interactions: review and assessment of report reliability. J Clin Pharmacol 2001;52:587–595.
14. Ernst E. Herb-drug interactions: potentially important but woefully under-researched. Eur J Clin Pharmacol 2000;56:523–524.
15. Orekhov AN, Grünwald J. Effects of garlic on atherosclerosis. Nutrition 1997;13:656–663.
16. Prasad K, Mantha SV, Kalra J, Lee P. Prevention of hypercholestorelomic atherosclerosis by garlic, an antioxidant. J Cardiovasc Pharmacol Ther 1997;2:309–320.
17. Jepson RG, Kleijnen J, Leng GC. Garlic for peripheral arterial occlusive disease. Cochrane Database Syst Rev 2000;4:CD 000095.
18. Koscielny J, Klubendorf D, Latza R, et al. The anti-atherosclerotic effect of *Allium sativum*. Atherosclerosis 1999;144:237–249.
19. Brace LD. Cardiovascular benefits of garlic (*Allium sativum* L). J Cardiovasc Nurs 2002;16:33–49.
20. Kleijnen J, Knipschild P. Ginkgo biloba. Lancet 1992;340:1136–1139.
21. Pittler MH, Ernst E. Ginkgo biloba extract for the treatment of intermittent claudication: a meta-analysis of randomized trials. Amer J Med 2000;108:276–281.
22. Pittler MH, Ernst E. Horse-chestnut seed extract for chronic venous insufficiency. A criteria-based systematic review. Arch Dermatol 1998;134:1356–1360.

23. Sarter B. Coenzyme Q10 and cardiovascular disease: a review. J Cardiovasc Nurs 2002;16:9–20.

24. Groenewegen WA, Heptinstall SA. (1990) Comparison of effects of an extract of feverfew and parthenolide, a component of feverfew, on human platelet activity in vitro. J Pharm Pharmacol 1990;42:553–557.

25. Lumb AB. Effect of dried ginger on human platelet function. Thromb Haemost 1994;71:110–111.

26. Janetzky K, Morreale AP. Probable interaction between warfarin and ginseng. Am J Health Syst Pharm 1997;54:692–693.

27. Zhu M, Chan KW, Ng LS, Chang Q, Chang S, Li, RC. Possible influences of ginseng on the pharmacokinetics and pharmacodynamics of warfarin in rats. J Pharm Pharmcol 1999;51:175–180.

28. Jung KY, Kim DS, Oh SR, et al. Platelet activating factor antagonistic activity of ginsenosides. Biol Pharm Bull 1998;21:79–80.

29. Dorso CR, Levin RI, Eldor A, Jaffe EA, Weksler BB. Chinese food and platelets (letter). N Engl J Med 1980;303:756–757.

30. Bordia A, Verma SK, Srivastava KC. (1998) Effect of garlic (*Allium sativum*) on blood lipids, blood sugar, fibrinogen and fibrinolytic activity in patients with coronary artery disease. Prostaglandins Leukot Essent Fatty Acids 1998;58:257–263.

31. Legnani C, Frascaro M, Guazzaloca G, Ludovici S, Cesarano G, Coccheri S. Effects of a dried garlic preparation on fibrinolysis and platelet aggregation in healthy subjects. Arzneimittelforschung 1993;43:119–122.

32. German K, Kumar U, Blackford HN. Garlic and the risk of TURP bleeding. Br J Urol 1995;76:518.

33. Burnham BE. (1995) Garlic as a possible risk for postoperative bleeding. Plast Reconstr Surg 1995;95:213.

34. Rose KD, Croissant PD, Parliament CF, Levin M.B. (1990) Spontaneous spinal epidural hematoma with associated platelet dysfunction from excessive garlic consumption: a case report. Neurosurgery 1990;26:880–882.

35. Page RL, Lawrence JD. Potentiation of warfarin by dong quai. Pharmacotherapy 1999;19:870–876.

36. Lo ACT, Chan K, Yeung JHF, Woo KS. Danggui (*Angelica sinensis*) affects the pharmacodynamics but not the pharmacokinetics of warfarin in rabbits. Eur J Drug Metab Pharmacokin 1995;20:55–60.

37. Izzat MB, Yim APC, Hazem El-Zufar M. A taste of Chinese medicine! Ann Thorac Surg 1998;66:941–942.

38. Cott J. (2000) Drug interactions with St. John's wort. Alt Ther Women's Health 2000;4:60–64.

39. Kaufeler R, Meier B, Brattström A. Efficacy and tolerability of Ze 117 St. John's wort extract in comparison with placebo, imipramine and flouxotine for the treatment of mild to moderate depression according to ICD-10. An overview. Pharmacopsychiatry 2001;34(suppl 1):S49–S50.

40. Brattström A. St. John's wort extract Ze 117: efficacy and safety. Deutsche Apotheker Zeitung, in press.

41. Moore LB, Goodwin B, Jones SA, et al. (2000) St. John's wort induces hepatic drug metabolism through activation of the pregnane X receptor. Proc Natl Acad Sci USA 2000;97:7500–7502.

42. Engelsen J, Nielsen JD, Winther K. (2002) Effect of coenzyme Q10 and Ginkgo biloba on warfarin dosage in stable, long-term warfarin treated outpatients. A

randomised, double blind, placebo-crossover trial. Thromb Haemost 2002;87:1075–1076.

43. Walker FB. Myocardial infarction after diet-induced warfarin resistance. Arch Intern Med 1984;144:2089–2090.

44. Kempin SJ. (1983) Warfarin resistance caused by broccoli. N Engl J Med 1983;308:1229–1230.

45. Wells PS, Holbrook AM, Crowther NR, Hirsch J. Interactions of warfarin with drugs and food. Ann Intern Med 1994;121:676–683.

46. Taylor J, Wilt V. Probable antagonism of warfarin by green tea. Ann Pharmacother 1999;33:426–428.

47. Penzak SR, Jann MW, Cold JA, Hon YY, Desai HD, Gurley BJ. Seville (sour) orange juice: synephrine content and cardiovascular effects in normotensive adults. J Clin Pharmacol 2001;41:1059–1063.

48. Tsunoda SM, Harris RZ, Christians U, et al. Red wine decreases cyclosporine bioavailability. Clin Pharmacol Ther 2001;70:462–467.

49. Bailey DG, Malcolm J, Arnold O, Spence JD. Grapefruit juice-drug interactions. Br J Clin Pharmacol 1998;46:101–110.

50. McInnes K. (1998) Drug interactions with grapefruit juice. Can Pharm J 1998;131:30–32.

51. Bailey DG, Arnold JMO, Spence JD. Grapefruit juice and drugs: how significant is the interaction? Clin Pharmacokinet 1994;26:91–98.

52. Yee GC, Stanley DL, Pessa LJ, et al. Effect of grapefruit juice on cyclosporin concentration. Lancet 1995;345:955–956.

53. Min DI, Ku YM, Geraets DR, et al. Effect of grapefruit juice on the pharmacokinetics and pharmacodynamcis of quinidine in healthy volunteers. J Clin Pharmacol 1996;36:469–476.

54. Lown KS, Bailey DG, Fontana RJ, et al. Grapefruit juice increases felodipine oral availability in humans by decreasing intestinal CYP3A protein expression. J Clin Invest 1997;99:2545–2553.

55. Fuhr U, Kummert AL. The fate of naringin in humans: a key to grapefruit juice-drug interactions? Clin Pharmacol Ther 1995;58:365–373.

56. Evans AM. Influence of dietary components on the gastrointestinal metabolism and transport of drugs. Ther Drug Monitor 2000;22:131–136.

57. Wilkins D. University of Michigan Medical Center press release. November 19, 1997.

58. Brinker F. Interactions of pharmaceutical and botanical medicines. J Naturopath Med 1997;7:14–20.

59. McRae S. Elevated serum digoxin levels in a patient taking digoxin and Siberian ginseng. Can Med Assoc J 1996;155:293–295.

60. Awang DVC. Siberian ginseng toxicity may be case of mistaken identity. Can Med Assoc J 1996;155:1237.

61. Brown DD, Juhl R, Warner SL. Decreased bioavailability of digoxin due to hypocholesterolemic interventions. Circulation 1978;58:164–172.

62. Westendorf J. Anthranoid derivatives—general discussion. In: DeSmet PAGM, Keller K, Hänsel R, Chandler R., eds. Adverse Effects of Herbal Drugs (vol 2). Springer, Berlin, 1993, pp. 105–118.

5 Vitamin Therapy for Cardiovascular Disease

Wahida Karmally, PhD, RD, CDE

Contents

INTRODUCTION
ANTIOXIDANT NUTRIENTS
VITAMINS AND ENDOTHELIAL FUNCTION
REFERENCES

INTRODUCTION

Recently, much public and scientific interest has been directed toward the role of vitamins and other nutrients in health promotion and disease prevention. It is estimated that 40% of the US population takes vitamin supplements *(1)* in varying doses to prevent or treat diseases, such as cardiovascular disease (CVD) and cancer. Vitamins have significant health effects beyond preventing deficiency diseases, namely their antioxidant functions. In this chapter, the role of vitamin therapy for CVD is reviewed; the evidence affecting cardiovascular health is also discussed. The vitamins included in the discussion are vitamins E, C, B_6, B_{12}, folic acid, niacin, and beta-carotene.

ANTIOXIDANT NUTRIENTS

The Institute of Medicine defines a dietary antioxidant as a "substance in foods that significantly decreases the adverse effects of reactive species, such as reactive oxygen and nitrogen species, on normal physiological function in humans" *(2)*. There is much evidence to support that

From: *Contemporary Cardiology*
Complementary and Alternative Cardiovascular Medicine
Edited by: R. A. Stein and M. C. Oz © Humana Press Inc., Totowa, NJ

high levels reactive oxygen and nitrogen species can be damaging to cells and contribute to disease. Among the chronic diseases in which oxidative stress plays a significant role is CVD. It has been proposed that oxidation of low-density lipoproteins (LDLs) may be a key step in the development of atherosclerosis (3–5). Oxidized LDL cholesterol is believed to have different properties than LDL that is not oxidized. Oxidized LDL accumulates in the cells that line the blood vessels. These lead to fatty streaks and later to atherosclerotic lesions. The concept that oxidatively modified LDL is proatherogenic and exists in vivo is supported by a growing body of data. In animal models, antioxidant supplementation inhibits atherosclerosis progression (6). The nutrients studied in these experiments were ascorbic acid, α-tocopherol and β-carotene.

Vitamin C

The prospective studies that relate ascorbic acid (Vitamin C) to CVD are not consistent. A significant inverse relationship was found between plasma vitamin C and coronary artery disease (CAD) in epidemiological studies (7). Ascorbate concentrations were also lower in the aortas of people with atherosclerosis, diabetes, and CAD and in smokers and nonsmokers when compared with unaffected controls. It has been hypothesized that low ascorbate concentrations in the arterial wall may predispose LDL to oxidation, which could promote atherogenesis. In the NHANES Study, which included 11,349 US men and women, there was an inverse association between cardiovascular mortality and ascorbic acid intake of at least 50 mg/d through diet or supplement (8). A large, more than 4-yr prospective study of 19,496 men and women in Norfolk, United Kingdom, showed that plasma ascorbic acid was inversely related to mortality from all causes and from CVD and ischemic heart disease in men and women (9). Studies such as these have several confounders: elevation of plasma ascorbic acid might indicate that foods that contribute vitamin C may also contribute nutrients, such as potassium, folate, calcium, magnesium, and isoflavones, that might confer cardiovascular benefits. Studies conducted on large cohorts (10,11) did not show association between vitamin C intake and mortality.

Observational studies suggest that vitamin C plays a role in the etiology of CVD, but there are no completed interventional trials of this vitamin alone. The Recommended Dietary Allowance (RDA) for vitamin C is 75 mg/d for women and 90 mg/d for men. The recommendation for smokers is an additional 35 mg/d because of increased oxidative stress and other metabolic differences. The Upper Limit (UL) for vitamin C is 2000 mg/d (12).

There is no established evidence for the use of vitamin C supplementation in CVD prevention.

Vitamin E

Alpha-tocopherol is the predominant lipophilic antioxidant in plasma membranes and tissue and is the most abundant antioxidant in LDL. On average, there are six molecules of α-tocopherol per LDL particle; they can function as antioxidants by trapping free radicals. In prospective studies *(11,13)*, α-tocopherol supplementation reduced the risk of coronary events in both men and women. In the female Nurses' Health Study, with a cohort of 87,000 women, there was an inverse association between CAD events and vitamin E intake *(13)*. Reduced risk was seen with a vitamin E consumption of at least 100 IU/d. In a randomized, placebo-controlled study in men, the LDL oxidation kinetics in a group supplemented with 800 IU was similar to the group that received combined supplementation with 1.0 g ascorbate, 30 mg beta-carotene, and 800 IU α-tocopherol. There was a 40% decrease in the oxidation rate after 3 mo of supplementation. Plasma vitamin E levels are significantly lower in patients (both men and women) with active variant angina than in patients without coronary spasm *(14)*. In a cohort of 34,486 postmenopausal women *(10)*, dietary vitamin E was protective in women in the highest quintile of dietary vitamin E intake. Randomized clinical trials investigating the effect of antioxidant intake on CAD have shown mixed results. In the alpha-tocopherol, beta carotene (ATBC) Cancer Prevention Study *(15,16)*, there was no benefit with respect to CAD for α-tocopherol or β-carotene. This trial was conducted in more than 29,000 Finnish male smokers. However, the dose of α-tocopherol (50 mg/d) was below the protective range suggested by the Nurses' Health Study.

In the Cambridge Heart Antioxidant Study (CHAOS), in which 2002 British men and women with angiographically proved CAD were included, there was a 77% reduction in nonfatal myocardial infarction in subjects who were taking vitamin E, compared with those on placebo *(17)*, but there was an increase in cardiovascular and overall mortality.

Among the large trials, the Heart Outcomes Prevention Evaluation (HOPE) study (with 2545 women and 6996 men ≥ 55 yr) was designed to test the hypotheses that two preventive intervention strategies, namely angiotensin-converting enzyme (ACE) inhibition or vitamin E (400 IU), would improve morbidity and mortality in patients at high risk of cardiovascular events, compared with placebo for 4–6 yr. There were no significant differences between vitamin E and placebo in myocardial infarction, stroke, or death from CVD *(18)*. In a substudy of the HOPE trial, Study to Evaluate Carotid Ultrasound changes in patients treated with Ramipril and 400 IU vitamin E (SECURE), which lasted more than 4.5 yr, ramipril had a beneficial effect and vitaminE had a neutral effect on atherosclerosis progression *(19)*.

The GISSI-Prevenzione trial randomly assigned 11,324 patients who survived recent (≤3 mo) myocardial infarction (MI) to supplements of ω-3 fatty acids (1.0 g/d), vitamin E (300 mg), both, or placebo on top of optimal pharmacological treatment and lifestyle advice *(20)*. This was a multicenter trial conducted in Italy for 3 to 5 yr. Supplements of ω-3 fatty acids significantly decreased mortality and sudden death. Vitamin E had no significant effects on cardiovascular deaths and /or nonfatal MI.

The Heart Protection Study (HPS) recently published *(21)* the findings of a large trial with 20,536 UK adults (aged 40–80 yr) with coronary disease, other occlusive arterial disease, or diabetes. The subjects were randomly allocated to receive antioxidant vitamin supplementation (600 mg vitamin E, 200 mg vitamin C, and 20 mg β-carotene daily) or matching placebo in a 5-yr treatment period. Primary outcomes were major coronary events (for overall analysis) and fatal or nonfatal vascular events (for subcategory analyses), with subsidiary assessment of cancer and other major morbidity. Although these vitamins increased blood vitamin concentrations substantially, they did not show significant differences in all-cause mortality or deaths resulting from vascular and nonvascular causes. There were significant differences in nonfatal MI or coronary death, nonfatal or fatal stroke, or coronary or noncoronary revascularization. For the first occurrence of any of these "major vascular events," there were no differences. Among these high-risk subjects, antioxidant vitamins were safe.

The HPS provided unequivocal evidence about the net effects of several years of such treatment on total mortality among high-risk patients. A "2 × 2 factorial" design was used to allow all patients to contribute fully to the assessment of the separate effects of the cholesterol-lowering drug and the vitamin supplement, as well as provide information about their combined effects.

However, it can be argued that assessing the effect of antioxidants, such as vitamin E, for a 4- to 6-yr period may not be long enough *(22)*. The findings for vitamin E in the Primary Prevention Project (PPP) could be regarded as a false-negative result, because of the inadequate power of a study that was stopped prematurely with the evidence of aspirin's benefit *(23)*. The study was conducted in 4495 people with at least one major recognized risk factor for CVD. This was a randomized controlled open 2×2 factorial trial to investigate the effects of 100 mg aspirin and 300 mg vitamin E in the CVD events.

The RDA for vitamin E for men and women is 15 mg/d and the UL is 1000 mg/d *(12)*.

CONCLUSION STATEMENT

Vitamin E intake has been associated with decreased risk for cardiovascular death and nonfatal MI in cohort and cross-sectional studies and in trials with relatively healthy subjects consuming ≥ 100 IU vitamin E/d for at least 2 yr. However, there was no significant effect of vitamin E supplementation (400 and 600 IU/d) during 4–6 yr in high-risk patients.

Grade II: The conclusion is supported by fair evidence.

β-*Carotene*

β-carotene inhibits oxidation of LDL and Lp(a) *(24)*. Smokers have lower LDL β-carotene levels relative to nonsmokers. However, the Physicians' Health Study did not demonstrate benefit from 50 mg β-carotene supplementation on alternate days when compared to placebo *(25)*. The ATBC trial showed that β-carotene supplementation with 20 mg/d increased total mortality and lung cancer significantly and showed a nonsignificant increase in mortality from CVD after 6.5 yr of supplementation.

The Beta-Carotene and Retinol Efficacy Trial (CARET) was stopped 21 mo early because the β-carotene group had 285 more lung cancer cases and 17% more deaths than the control group *(26)*. Cardiovascular mortality was also increased in the β-carotene group.

CONCLUSION STATEMENT

Randomized studies assessing supplementation with β-carotene have shown no benefit; in smokers, the risk of developing lung cancer and overall mortality increased.

Folate and Vitamins B_6 and B_{12}

Elevated levels of homocysteine (Hcy) in the bloodstream have been associated with an increased risk of CVD *(27)*. Clinical studies have linked moderate hyperhomocysteinemia to peripheral vascular, cerebrovascular, and coronary heart disease (CHD). These metabolic defects can be related to genetic reasons or nutritional deficiency of vitamin B_6 or B_{12} or folate that are cofactors to the enzymes in Hcy metabolism *(28)*.

A prospective study of male physicians indicated that plasma Hcy concentrations of 17 μmol/L or 12% more than the UL of normal were associated with a threefold to fourfold increase in the risk of acute myocardial infarction *(29)*. A high plasma Hcy concentration and low levels of folate and vitamin B_6, through their role in Hcy metabolism, were also associated with an increased risk of extracranial carotid artery stenosis.

Hcy's effect is independent of the established risk factors, such as hyperlipidemia and hypertension. Elevated Hcy level may reflect inadequate availability of folate and vitamins B_6 and B_{12}. The female Nurses' Health Study *(30)* demonstrated a significant inverse relationship between dietary intakes of folate and vitamin B_6 and mortality and morbidity from CVD. The Kuopio Ischemic Heart Disease Risk Factor Study, which was conducted for 10 yr in Finnish men, showed a significant inverse association between quantitatively assessed moderate to high folate intakes with 4-d food records and incidence of acute coronary events in men *(31)*. The mean daily dietary intake of folate in this population was only 259 μg/d. The proportion of subjects who suffered an acute coronary event during the follow-up was 12% in persons in the lowest folate intake quintile and 8.1% in persons in the highest folate intake quintile. There was an increased intake of vitamins B_6 and B_{12} from the lowest quintile to the highest quintile of folate intake. Supplementation with these vitamins, particularly folic acid, may normalize plasma Hcy levels.

Dietary supplementation with folic acid is a safe and an effective treatment for lowering Hcy levels and possibly a prevention of CVD, based on epidemiological studies. In the United States, as mandated by its government, grain products are fortified with folic acid (140 μg/100 g) since 1998 to prevent neural tube birth defects *(32)*. The potential positive impact of this program was studied in 747 subjects from the original Framingham cohort *(33)*. It was estimated that the percentages of those with elevated Hcy levels could drop from 26% to 21%. It has also been shown that current levels of fortification do raise folate levels in 75 women and men with CAD *(34)*. The effect of folic acid fortification in Framingham Offspring cohort showed a significant decrease in the prevalence of hyperhomocysteinemia from 18.7% to 9.8% *(35)*.

Ongoing studies with folate supplementation in the United States, United Kingdom, Norway, and Australia in patients with CAD may provide information on Hcy as a risk factor for cardiovascular heart disease and the role of folate in secondary prevention.

Folate may have protective effects that are independent of Hcy lowering because of enhanced vascular NO activity *(36,37)* and could prevent endothelial dysfunction associated with a fat load or an oral administration of methionine. Other studies did not show enhancement of endothelial function *(38)*. A direct protective effect of folate on LDL cholesterol oxidation has also been demonstrated *(39)*.

A prospective, double-blind, randomized trial with a combination of 1 mg of folic acid, 400 µg vitamin B_{12}, and 10 mg of pyridoxine or placebo administered to 205 patients for 6 mo after successful coronary angioplasty demonstrated that vitamins significantly reduced Hcy levels and decreased the rate of restenosis and the need for revascularization of the target region (40). The extension of this study (41) provided data to show that Hcy-lowering therapy with folic acid, vitamin B_{12}, and pyridoxine was effective in controlling excessive restenosis mechanisms 1 yr after successful coronary angioplasty. The benefit obtained obtained at 6 mo was maintained at 1 yr, despite cessation of the vitamin therapy at 6 mo. The authors recommend this combination of vitamins as an adjunctive therapy for patients who are undergoing coronary angioplasty.

In a study investigating the association of serum Hcy levels, as well as folate and vitamin B_{12} levels, to the rate of in-stent restenosis after 6 mo did not show a relationship (42).

CONCLUSION STATEMENT

Some cohort studies show an inverse relationship between folate status (dietary folate, serum folate) and serum total homocysteine and risk for CHD. No RCT have been completed to determine the outcome of folate supplementation on incidence of MI, stroke or death from CVD.

Grade II The conclusion is supported by fair evidence.

VITAMINS AND ENDOTHELIAL FUNCTION

The vascular endothelium is the primary site of dysfunction in many diseases, particularly CVD. Research suggests that vitamins E and C and folic acid have beneficial effects on vascular endothelial function in patients who are at high risk of CVD, as well as in healthy people (43). These studies used 300 IU, 600 IU, or 1000 IU of vitamin E or 500 mg, 1 g, or 2 g of vitamin C. The studies showed a decrease in monocyte adhesion or an improvement in flow-mediated dilation (FMD) of the brachial artery. A randomized, crossover study of 25 men and 25 postmenopausal women showed that degradation of endothelial function after the acute high-fat meal ingestion was mitigated by a concomitant ingestion of 800 IU of vitamin E (44).

Most studies support a role for vitamins C and E in the improvement of endothelial function in healthy subjects (45), as well as patients with diabetes (46) or lipid abnormalities (47). Similar effects of chronic consumption of vitamins E or C on endothelial function have not been demonstrated. Therefore, the clinical significance of these acute effects is not clear.

The acute effects of 3 g of vitamin C infusion *(48)* was studied in 11 subjects with idiopathic dilated cardiomyopathy. The authors demonstrated that endothelium dysfunction can be acutely reversed. Vitamin C is a water-soluble antioxidant and is an efficient scavenger of oxygen free radicals, suggesting an increased availability of NO.

The administration of vitamin C suppresses endothelial cell apoptosis (programmed cell death), suggesting the functional benefit of vitamin C supplementation on endothelial function *(49)*. Patients were randomized to receive vitamin C (2.5 g) or placebo, according to a sequential administration protocol combining iv bolus with oral application of the treatment (2 g vitamin C) and placebo for 3 d to patients with CHF.

Vitamins have been studied in combinations, particularly vitamins C and E. In a double-blind prospective study *(50)*, 40 patients (0–2 yr after cardiac transplantation) were randomly assigned vitamin C 500 mg plus 400 IU vitamin E twice daily ($n = 19$) or placebo ($n = 21$) for 1 yr. The primary endpoint was the change in average intimal index (plaque area divided by the vessel area) measured by intravascular ultrasonography. Coronary endothelium-dependent vasoreactivity was also assessed. During the 1-yr treatment, the intimal index increased in the placebo group by 8% but did not change significantly in the treatment group (0.8%). Coronary endothelial function remained stable in both groups. This study suggested that supplementation with vitamins C and E retards the early progression of transplant-associated coronary arteriosclerosis.

Supplementation with 500 mg of vitamins C, 400 IU of E and 12 mg β-carotene or 1000 mg of vitamin C, 800 IU of E, and 24 mg β-carotene did not significantly alter brachial reactivity in a 12-wk trial of 18 nonsmokers with established CAD but no diabetes *(51)*.

Niacin

In patients with hyperlipidemia, niacin decreases morbidity and mortality rates *(52)*. Niacin is most effective in increasing HDL C *(53,54)*. The combination of statins and low-dose niacin is effective in improving the LDL C/HDL C ratio rather than the drug alone *(55–58)*. The doses of niacin ranged from 1000 to 3000 mg/d in these studies. These doses usually have side effects, including flushing, gastrointestinal (GI) problems, and liver function test abnormalities. In a recent small study *(59)*, the addition of very low-dose niacin 50 mg administered twice daily for 3 mo, increased the mean HDL cholesterol by 2.1 mg/dL vs –0.56 mg/dL for the placebo group ($p = .0246$). In addition, no major side effects were noted and no patients stopped the study medication as a result of side effects. The dose of niacin used was similar to that found in a B-complex supplement.

There is numerous circumstantial evidence for the benefit of vitamins to prevent CVD, but there is no convincing evidence in the literature in favor of supplements of antioxidant vitamins. Vitamin E, β-carotene, and vitamin C can inhibit the oxidative modification of LDL. This action could positively influence the atherosclerotic process and the progression of CVD. However, clinical trials with β-carotene indicate that supplements should not be taken. The data for vitamin C are limited, and the data for vitamin E from the ATBC study (150 mg/d), CHAOS (400–800 mg/d), GISSI (300 mg/d), HOPE (400 mg/d), and HPS (600 mg/d) suggest the absence of relevant clinical effects of antioxidant vitamins on CVD risk. Additional concerns are that vitamins E and C can act as pro-oxidants *(60)*, and vitamin E may interfere with the benefits of cholesterol-lowering drugs by lowering HDL_2 levels and preventing HDL_2 rise with lipid-altering therapy *(61)*. Therefore, recommendation of vitamin supplements is difficult to justify at this time. A recent report on self-selected vitamins E and C or multivitamins by 83,639 US male physicians for a 5.5-yr period was not associated with a significant decrease in total CVD or CHD mortality *(62)*.

Long-term randomized placebo-controlled trials are the gold standard for establishing the benefits of treatment to prevent disease. There are ongoing primary and secondary prevention trials with vitamin E, β-carotene, and C supplementation. These studies have included healthy men and women and patients with CVD. The evidence currently available does not support any public health policy recommendations for antioxidant supplementation. Meanwhile, the American population should be encouraged to increase its fruit and vegetable consumption because of their unique antioxidant content, as well as low-fat and high-fiber properties.

Optimizing nutrient intake must be achieved by improving diet. Foods have hundreds of antioxidants and other nutrients that act in synergy to promote health. It has been difficult so far to determine which components of such diets provide the protection against CVD. Diets that are plant based, with fruits and vegetables and whole grains, have consistently shown to be cardioprotective in large prospective cohort studies. A clinically sound approach is to encourage the American population to consume a diet consisting of whole grains, legumes, several fruits and vegetables, nuts, seeds, fatty fish (such as salmon and mackerel), and nonfat or low-fat dairy foods; include physical activity on a daily basis; and maintain a healthy body weight.

REFERENCES

1. Food and Drug Administration. Dietary supplements. Available at: http://www.fda.gov. Accessed.
2. Subcommittee on the Tenth Edition of the RDAs. Food and Nutrition Board, Commission on Life Sciences, National Research Council. National Academy Press, 1989.
3. Steinberg D, Parthasarathy S, Carew TE, Khoo JD, Witztum JL. Beyond cholesterol: modifications of low density lipoproteins that increase its atherogenicity. N Engl J Med 1989;320:915–924.
4. Rong JX, Rangaswamy S, Shen L, Dave R, Chang YH, Peterson H. Arterial injury by cholesterol oxidation products causes endothelial dysfunction and arterial wall cholesterol accumulation. Arterioscl Thromb Vasc Biol 1998;18:1885–1894.
5. Bjorkhem I, Henriksson-Freyschuss A, Breuer O, Diczfalusy U, Berglund L, Henriksson P. The antioxidant butylated hydroxytoluene protects against atherosclerosis. Arterioscl Thromb 1991;11:15–22.
6. Diaz MN, Frei B, Vita JA, Keaney JF. Antioxidants and atherosclerotic heart disease. N Engl J Med 337:408–416.
7. Gey KF, Brubacher GB, Stahelin HB. Plasma levels of antioxidant vitamins in relation to ischemic heart disease and cancer. Am J Clin Nutr 1987;45:1368–1377.
8. Enstrom JE, Karim LE, Klein MA. Vitamin C intake and mortality among a sample of theunited States population. Epidemiology 1992;3:194–202.
9. Khaw KT, Bingham S, Welch A, et al. Relation between plasma ascorbic acid and mortality in men and women in EPIC-Norfolk prospective study: a prospective population study. Lancet 2001;357:657–663.
10. Kushi LH, Folsom AR, Prineas RJ, Mink PJ, Ying W, BostickW. Dietary antioxidant vitamins and death from coronary heart disease in postmenopausal women. N Engl J Med 1996;334:1156–1162.
11. Rimm EB, Stampher MJ, Ascherio A, et al. Vitamin E consumption and the risk of coronary disease in men. N Engl J Med 193;328:145–146.
12. Food and Nutrition Board, Institute of Medicine. A Report of the Panel on Dietary Antioxidants and Related Compounds. Dietary Reference Intakes for Vitamin C, Vitamin E, Vitamin C, Selenium and Carotenoids. National Academy Press, Washington, DC, 2000.
13. Stampfer MJ, Hennekens CH, Manson JE, et al. Vitamin E consumption and the risk of coronary disease in women. N Engl J Med 1993;328:1444–1449.
14. Miwa K, Miyagi Y, Igawa A, Nakagawa K, Inoue A. Vitamin E deficiency in variant angina. Circulation 1996;94:14–18
15. The Alpha-Tocopherol, Beta-Carotene Cancer Prevention Study Group. The effect of vitamin E and beta-carotene on the incidence of lung cancer and other cancers in male smokers. N Engl J Med 1994;330:1029–1035.
16. Virtamo J, Rapola JM, Ripatti S, et al. Effects of vitamin E and beta-carotene on the incidence of primary nonfatal myocardial infection and fatal coronary heart disease. Arch Intern Med 1998;158:668–675.
17. Stephens NG, Parson A, Schofield PM, Kelly F, Cheeseman K, Mitchinson MJ. Randomised controlled trial of vitamin E in patients with coronary disease. Cambridge Heart Antioxidant Study (CHAOS). Lancet 1996;347:781–786.
18. The HOPE (Heart Outcomes Prevention Evaluation) Study Investigators. Vitamin E supplementation and cardio-vascular events in high- risk patients. N Engl J Med 2000;342:154–160.
19. Lonn EM, Yusuf S, Dzavik V, et al for the SECURE Investigators. Effects of ramipril and vitamin E on atherosclerosis. Circulation 2001;103:919–925.

20. GISSI-Prevenzione Investigators (Gruppo Italiano per lo Sudio della Sopravvivenze nell'infarto Miocardico). Dietary supplementation with n-3 polyunsaturated fatty acids and vitamin E after myocardial infarction: results of the GISSI- Prevenzione trial. Lancet 1999;354:447–455.

21. MRC/BHF Heart Protection Study Collaborative Group, MRC/BHF Heart Protection Study of cholesterol-lowering therapy and of antioxidant vitamin supplementation in a wide range of patients at increased risk of coronary heart disease death: early safety and efficacy experience. Eur Heart J 1999;20:725–741. Lancet 2002;360:23–33.

22. Steinberg D. Cinical trials of antioxidants in atherosclerosis: are we doing the right things? Lancet 1995;349:36–38.

23. Collaborative group of the Primary Prevention Project. Low dose aspirin and vitamin E in people at cardiovascular risk: a randomized trial in general practice. Lancet 2001;357:89–95.

24. Jialal I, Norkus E, Cristol I, Grundy SM. Beta carotene inhibits the oxidative modifications of low-density lipoprotein. Biochem Biophys Acta 1991;1086:134–138.

25. Hennekens CH, Buning JE, Manson JE. Lack of effect of long-term supplementation with beta carotene on the incidence of malignant neoplasms and cardiovascular disease. N Engl J Med 1996;N334:1145–1149.

26. Omenn GS, Goodman E, Thornquist MD, et al. Effects of a combination of beta-carotene and vitamin A on lung cancer and cardiovascular disease. N Engl J Med 1996;334:1150–1155.

27. van Poppel G, Kardinaal A, Princen H, Kok FJ. Antioxidants and coronary heart disease. Ann Med 1994;26:429–434

28. Kuller LH, Evans RW. Homocysteine, vitamins and cardiovascular disease. Circulation 1998;98:196–199.

29. Stampfer MJ, Malinow MR, Willett WCE. A prospective study of plasma homocyt(e)ine and risk of myocardial infarction in US physicians. JAMA 1992;268:877–881.

30. Rimin EB, Willett WC, Hu FB. Folate and vitamin B6 from diet and supplement in relation to risk of coronary heart disease among women. JAMA 1998;279:359–364.

31. Voutilainen S, Rissanen TH, Virtanen J, Lakka TA, Salonen JT. Low dietary Folate intake is associated with an excess incidence of acute coronary events. Circulation 2001;103:2674–2680.

32. Food standards: amendment of standards of identity for enriched grain products to require addition of folic acid. Fed Register 1996;61:8781–8797.

33. Tucker KL, Mahnken B, Wilson PW, Jacques P, Selhub J. Folic acid fortification of the food supply. Potential benefits and risks for the elderly population. JAMA 1996;276:1879–1885.

34. Malinow MR, Duell PB, Hess DL, Anderson PH, Kruger WD, Phillipson BE, Gluckman RA, Block PC, and Upson BM. Reduction of plasma homocysteine levels by breafast cereal fortified with folic acid in patients with coronary heart disease. N. Engl. J Med. 1998;338:1009–1015.

35. Jacques PF, Selhub J, Boston AG, Wilson PW, Rosenberg IH. The effect of folic acid fortification on plasma folate and total homocysteine concentrations. N Engl J Med 1999;340:1449–1454

36. Usui M, Matsuoka H, Miyazaki H, Ueda S, Okuda S, Imaizum T. Endothelial dysfunction by acute hyperhomocysteinemia restoration by folic acid. Clin Sci 1999;96:235–239.

37. Wilmink HW, Stroes ESG, Erkelens WD, et al. Influence of folic acid on postprandial endothelial dysfunction. Arterioscl Thromb Vasc Biol 2000;20:185–188.

38. Pullin CH, Ashfield-Watt PA, Burr ML, et al. Optimization of dietary folate or low dose folic acid supplements lower homocysteine but do not enhance endothelial function in healthy adults, irrespective of the methylenetetrahydrofolate reductase (C677T) genotype. J Am Coll Cardiol 2001;38:1799–1805.

39. Nakano E, Higgins JA, Powers HJ. Short communication. Folate protects against oxidative modification of human LDL. Br J Nutr 2001;86:637–639.

40. Schnyder G, Roffi M, Pin R, et al. Decreased rate of coronary restenosis with lowering of plasma homocysteine levels. N Engl J Med 2001;345:1593–1600.

41. Schnyder G, Roffi M, Flammer Y, et al. Effect of homocysteine-lowering therapy with folic acid, vitamin B_{12} and vitamin B_6 on clinical outcome after percutaneous coronary intervention. JAMA 2002;288:973–979.

42. Genser D, Pracher H, Hauer R, et al. Relation of homocysteine, vitamin B_{12} and folate to coronary in-stent restenosis. Am J Cardiol 2002;89:495–499.

43. Brown AA, Hu FB. Dietary modulation of endothelial function: implications for cardiovascular disease. Am J Clin Nutr 2001;73:673–686.

44. Katz DL, Nawaz H, Boukhalil J, et al. Acute effects of oats and vitamin E on endothelial responses to ingested fat. Am J Prev Med 2001;20:124–129.

45. Chambers JC, McGregor A, Jean-Marie J, Obeid OA, Kooner JS. Demonstration of rapid onset vascular endothelial function after hyperhomocysteinemia: an effect reversible with vitamin C therapy. Circulation 1999;99:1156–1160.

46. Skyrme-Jones RA, O'Brien OC, Berry KL, Meredith IT. Vitamin E supplementation improves endothelial function in type 1 diabetes mellitus: a randomized, placebo-controlled study. J Am Coll Cardiol 2000;36:94–102.

47. Kugiyama K, Motoyama T, Doi H, et al. Improvement of endothelial vasomotor dysfunction by treatment with alpha-tocopherol in patients with high remnant lipoprotein levels. J Am Coll Cardiol 1999;33:1512–1518.

48. Richartz BM, Werner GS, Ferrari M, Figulla HR. Reversibility of coronary endothelial vasomotor dysfunction in idiopathic dilated cardiomyopathy; acute effects of vitamin C. Am J Cardiol 2001;88:10001–1005.

49. Rossig L, Hoffmann J, Hugel B, et al. Vitamin C inhibits endothelial cell apoptosis in congestive heart failure. Circulation 2001;104:2181–2187.

50. Fang JC, Kinlay S, Beltrame J, et al. Effect of vitamins C and E on Progression of transplant associated arteriosclerosis: a randomized trial. Lancet 2002;359:1108–1113.

51. McKechnie R, Rubenfire M, Mosca L. Antioxidant nutrient supplementation and brachial reactivity in patients with coronary artery disease. Lab Clin Med 2002;139;133–139.

52. Canner PL, Berge KG, Winger NK, et al. Fifteen year mortality in Coronary Drug Project patients: long term benefits with niacin. J Am Coll Cardiol 1986;8:1245–1255.

53. Schectman G, Hiatt A. Evaluation of the effectiveness of lipid lowering therapy (bile acid sequestrants, niacin, psyllium and lovastatin) for treating hypercholesterolemia in veterans. Am J Cardiol 1993;71:758–765.

54. Ellingworth DR, Stein EA, Mitchell YB, et al. Comparative effects of lovastatin and niacin in primary hypercholesterolemia: a prospective trial. Arch Intern Med 1994;154:1586–1595.

55. Davignon J, Raederer G, Montigny M, et al. Comparative efficacy and safety of pravastatin, nicotinic acid and the two combined in patients with hypercholesterolemia. Am J Cardiol 1994;73:339–345.

56. Jokubaitis LA. Fluvastatin in combination and other lipid-lowering agents. Br J Clin Pract 1996;77A(suppl):28–32.

57. Jacobson TA, Chin MM, Fromel GJ, Jokubaitis LA, Amorosa LF. Fluvastatin with and without niacin for hypercholesterolemia. Am J Cardiol 1994;74:149–154.

58. Vacek JL, Dittmeier G, Chiarelli T, White J, Bell JJ. Comparison of lovastatin (20mg) and nicotinic acid (1.2) with either drug for type 11 hyperlipidemia. Am J Cardiol 1995;76:182–184

59. Wink J, Giacoppe G, King J. Effect of very-low-dose niacin on high-density lipoprotein in patients undergoing long-term statin therapy. Am Heart J 2002;143:514–518.

60. Institute of Medicine Dietary Reference Intakes for Vitamin C, Vitamin E, Selenium, and Carotenoids. National Academy Press, Washington, DC, 2000.

61. Cheung MC, Zhao XQ, Chait A, Albers JJ, Brown G. Antioxidant supplements block the response of HDL to Simvastatin-Niacin therapy in patients with coronary artery disease and low HDL. Arterioscler Thromb Vasc Biol 2001;21;1320–1326.

62. Muntwyler J, Hennekens CH, Manson JE, Buring JE, Gaziano JM. Vitamin supplement use in a low risk population of US male physicians and subsequent cardiovascular mortality. Arch Intern Med 2002;162:1472–1476.

6 Oils and Fats in the Prevention and Treatment of Cardiovascular Disease

Penny M. Kris-Etherton, PhD, RD,
Kari D. Hecker PhD, RD,
Terry D. Etherton, PhD,
and Valerie K. Fishell, MS

CONTENTS

INTRODUCTION

For the first time, Dietary Reference Intakes (DRIs) for macronutrients have been established by the National Academies' Institute of Medicine for the United States and Canada *(1)*. This science-based report

From: *Contemporary Cardiology*
Complementary and Alternative Cardiovascular Medicine
Edited by: R. A. Stein and M. C. Oz © Humana Press Inc., Totowa, NJ

makes new recommendations for energy, carbohydrates, fiber, fat, fatty acids, cholesterol, protein, and amino acids. The DRI Report embraces the philosophy of making dietary recommendations that assure a nutritionally adequate diet, promote good health, prevent chronic disease, and avoid overconsumption. Recommendations suggest that adults should consume a diet that provides 45% to 65% of their calories from carbohydrates, 10% to 35% from protein, and 20% to 35% from fat. The report advises that saturated fat, *trans* fat, and cholesterol be as low as possible. Because polyunsaturated fatty acids (PUFAs) are essential nutrients, the DRI Report recommends 17 g/d for men and 12 g/d for women of linoleic acid (C18:2), an omega-6 PUFA. For α-linolenic acid (ALA), an omega-3 fatty acid, 1.6 and 1.1 g/d should be consumed by men and women, respectively. The recommendations for PUFA are based on average intakes in the United States. For simplicity, the report recommends that 5% to 10% of calories come from PUFA and 0.6% to 1.2% come from ALA. Importantly, approx 10% of omega-3 fatty acid intake can come from long-chain, highly unsaturated fatty acids, eicosapentaenoic acid (EPA) and docosahexaenoic acid (DHA). Because of the total fat recommendation and the guidance provided about saturated fat, *trans* fat, and PUFA intake, the balance will be derived from monounsaturated fatty acids (MUFAs). The range of total fat from 20% to 35% of calories recognizes that healthy diets can be planned over a reasonably broad range of fat intake, as long as saturated fat, *trans* fat, and cholesterol are kept as low as possible. This range in total fat reflects the health benefits of unsaturated fat in the context of a nutritionally adequate diet that promotes a healthy weight. The range of all macronutrients acknowledges that there are many healthy diets with respect to macronutrient profiles, as long as each diet meets the specific recommendations made in the DRI Report for saturated fat, *trans* fat, cholesterol, total fiber (38 g/d for men and 25 g/d for women), and added sugar (a maximum of 25% or fewer calories from added sugars).

Although the DRI Report for macronutrients is made for healthy populations, it is consistent with the latest guidelines from the National Cholesterol Education Program Adult Treatment Panel (ATP) III *(2)* for primary and secondary prevention of coronary heart disease (CHD). These treatment guidelines target low-density lipoprotein (LDL) cholesterol, as well as other major risk factors for CHD. ATP III recommends a diet that provides fewer than 7% of calories from saturated fat and fewer than 200 mg of cholesterol per day. In addition, up to 10% of calories from PUFA and up to 20% of calories from MUFA are allowed. A total fat recommendation of 25% to 35% of calories is also made in ATP III. Collectively, both ATP III and the DRI Report have made recommendations that acknowledge the health benefits of unsaturated fat. In addition, the *Dietary Guidelines 2000* recommend a diet low in saturated fat and cholesterol and moderate in total fat *(3)*.

The new guidelines represent a shift in philosophy about total fat content in the diet. Previous guidance highlighted the importance of reducing total fat. The message that evolved was: "consume a low fat-diet." As a result, this often was taken to an extreme, with the effect that fat was the focal point of the diet in a way that ignored calories and micronutrients. However, an abundance of recent research has shown many health benefits of unsaturated fats, which, in part, was the impetus for revising the low-fat diet message. As a result, a contemporary diet message was developed that advocates a diet moderate in total fat but low in saturated fat, *trans* fat, and cholesterol. This diet message underscores the important functions of fat in the diet and the health benefits of unsaturated fats.

This chapter reviews the scientific evidence that supports the current dietary recommendations for fat and fatty acids. These recommendations are guided by a philosophy of reducing certain nutrients that have adverse effects on risk factors for cardiovascular disease (CVD) (e.g., saturated fat, *trans* fat, and cholesterol) and replacing these with healthful nutrients, including healthy fats, as well as carbohydrates. The chapter discusses the evidence in support of replacing unhealthy fats with healthy fats, notably unsaturated fatty acids, to reduce CVD risk. In addition, important food sources of different fatty acids in the diet are presented to facilitate diet planning.

SATURATED FATTY ACIDS

The Seven Countries Study *(4)* was a landmark epidemiologic investigation that reported a significant association between serum cholesterol and increased risk of coronary disease and between diet and serum cholesterol levels. With respect to diet, saturated fat intake (as a percentage of calories) was significantly correlated with serum cholesterol levels; 80% of the variability resulted from differences in dietary saturated fat intake among the populations. Moreover, saturated fat intake was also correlated with 5-yr incidence of CHD.

The epidemiologic evidence prompted carefully controlled clinical studies to be conducted to evaluate the effects of fat classes and individual fatty acids on plasma lipids and lipoproteins.

The results from many of the well-controlled clinical studies were used to develop blood cholesterol predictive equations for estimating the changes in total cholesterol in response to changes in type of fat and amount of dietary cholesterol. The original equations developed by Keys et al. *(5)* and Hegsted et al. *(6)*, reported by both in 1965, and more recently by Mensink and Katan *(7)*, Hegsted et al. *(8)*, and Clarke et al. *(9)*, demonstrated that saturated fat was hypercholesterolemic, whereas PUFA lowered blood cholesterol levels. Saturated fat was twice as potent in raising blood cholesterol levels as PUFA was in lowering them. Specifically, the blood cholesterol predictive equations demonstrated that for each 1% increase in saturated fatty acids (SFAs), blood cholesterol increased 1.5 to 2.7 mg/dL. The investigators reported that MUFA had a neutral effect and that dietary cholesterol raised the blood cholesterol level but less so than saturated fat. A summary of the effect of SFA on LDL cholesterol is shown in Fig. 1.

TRANS FATTY ACIDS

Trans fatty acids are unsaturated fatty acids with one or more double bonds in the trans configuration. The resulting extended fatty acid chain is similar to saturated fat. Several epidemiologic studies have reported a positive relationship between *trans* fatty acid intake and both incidence of CHD and risk factors for CHD, notably lipids and lipoproteins *(10–12)*.

Numerous early controlled feeding studies reported that hydrogenated fats elicited a blood cholesterol response that was intermediate to that observed for unhydrogenated oils and saturated fats (reviewed in ref. *13*). More recently, studies have been conducted to evaluate the plasma lipid and lipoprotein effects of *trans* fatty acids. These studies have consistently shown that *trans* fatty acids increase plasma total and LDL cholesterol relative to unsaturated fatty acids *(14–16)*. *Trans* fatty acids elicit comparable cholesterol-raising effects vs SFA. In addition, *trans* fatty acids do not increase high-density lipoprotein (HDL) cholesterol as does SFA *(17)*, resulting in a lower HDL cholesterol and a worsening of the LDL:HDL ratio which, in turn, increases CHD risk (*see* Fig. 2) *(18)*.

DIETARY CHOLESTEROL

Numerous controlled clinical studies have shown a positive linear association between dietary cholesterol and LDL cholesterol. Consequently, because of an increase in LDL cholesterol, there is an increase in CHD risk. However, the LDL cholesterol-raising effect of dietary cholesterol is less than that of SFA. An increase of 100 mg/d of dietary cholesterol is predicted to result in a 0.5 to 1 mmol/L increase in total serum cholesterol, resulting in a 1% to 2% increase in CHD risk (*see* Fig. 3) *(1)*.

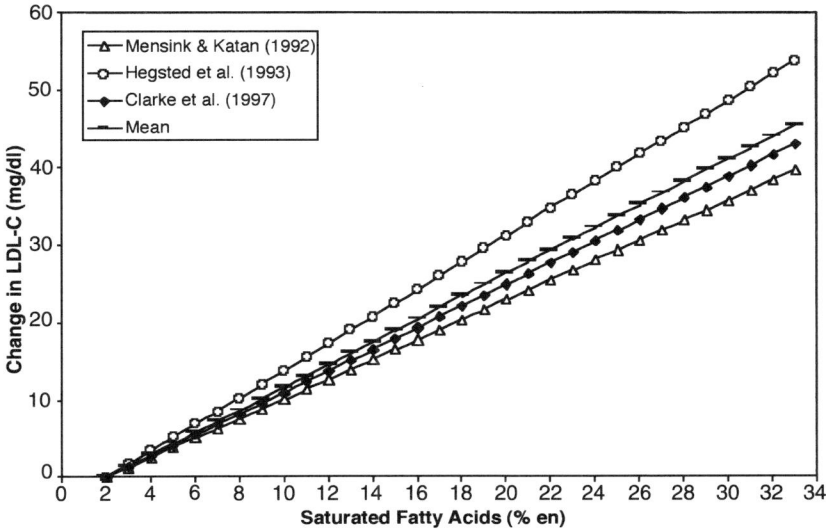

Fig. 1. Predicted changes in LDL cholesterol in response to increase in SAF (from 2% to 33% energy). *Source:* Institute of Medicine of the National Academies. Dietary Reference Intakes for Energy, Carbohydrate, Fiber, Fat, Fatty Acids, Cholesterol, Protein and Amino Acids. Washington, DC, National Academies Press, 2002.

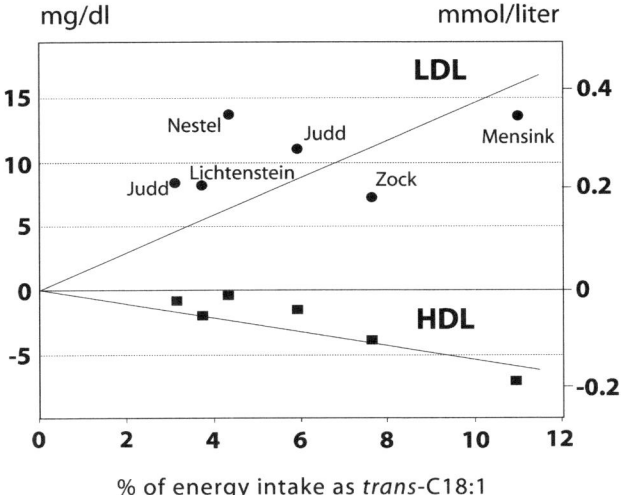

Fig. 2. Effects of exchange of *trans* monounsaturated fatty acids for oleic acid on lipoprotein cholesterol levels. *Source*: Katan MB, Zock PL, Mensink RP. *Trans* fatty acids and their effects on lipoproteins in humans. Annu Rev Nutr 1995;15:473–493.

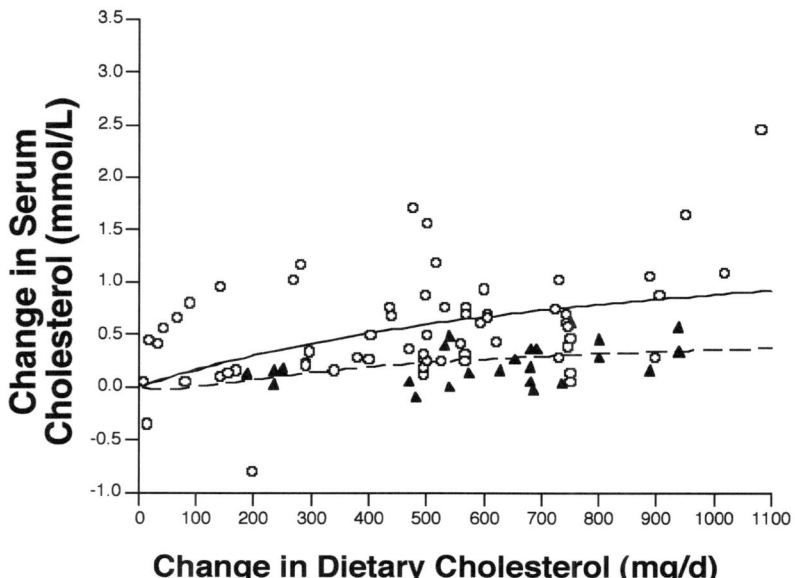

Fig. 3. Relationship between change in dietary cholesterol (0–1100 mg/d) and change in cholesterol concentration. *Source:* Institute of Medicine of the National Academies. Dietary Reference Intakes for Energy, Carbohydrate, Fiber, Fat, Fatty Acids, Cholesterol, Protein, and Amino Acids. Washington DC, National Academies Press, 2002.

UNSATURATED FATTY ACIDS

The evidence is convincing to support the recommendation to decrease saturated fat, *trans* fat, and cholesterol to reduce CVD risk. There is provocative and compelling new evidence that shows beneficial effects of unsaturated fatty acids. The emergence of this new appreciation that unsaturated fatty acids decrease CVD risk has been an impetus for revising our dietary messages regarding unsaturated fat, and, in turn, total fat. Critical to this new approach is that unsaturated fats be included in a nutritionally adequate diet at a level that meets energy needs and elicits the expected health effects. Consequently, the diet message has transitioned from a low-fat to a moderate-fat recommendation to ensure adequate intake of unsaturated fatty acids.

MONOUNSATURATED FATTY ACIDS

MUFAs decrease total cholesterol and LDL cholesterol when substituted for SFA. When MUFAs replace SFA calories, plasma triglycerides decrease and HDL cholesterol levels are maintained. In contrast, a low-fat, high-carbohydrate, cholesterol-lowering diet increases triglycerides and lowers HDL cholesterol *(19)*. Thus, a diet moderate in total fat from MUFA and low in SFA calories results in a more favorable CHD risk profile than does a low-fat diet. Both diets would be expected to lower total and LDL cholesterol similarly, however, a moderate-fat, high-MUFA diet elicits a more favorable LDL cholesterol/HDL cholesterol ratio, as well as plasma triglyceride level. The advice to consume a moderate-fat diet with emphasis on MUFA must be done so in the context of keeping SFA low, because all fats carry SFA and ensure that energy balance is maintained, because all fats are energy dense.

The message that unsaturated fats can be part of a healthy diet must be translated sensibly to prevent overconsumption. For example, some populations living in the Mediterranean region safely consume diets containing greater than 20% energy from MUFA. However, there is, some preliminary and limited evidence that excessive MUFA intake may be problematic. One study showed that flow-mediated dilation (an indicator of vascular health) decreased in human subjects in response to a 50-g fat load from olive oil compared with canola oil *(20)*. Interestingly, this response was attenuated when antioxidants were included in the fat load. Balsamic vinegar also had the same effect. Another study has shown that MUFAs induce atherosclerosis in monkeys fed an atherogenic diet *(21)*. These are isolated reports of adverse effects of MUFA on CVD risk status that should be further studied. In contrast, there is convincing evidence that MUFAs have important health effects in the context of current dietary guidance.

POLYUNSATURATED FATTY ACIDS

PUFAs are mainly comprised of omega-6 and omega-3 fatty acids. The distinction between the two fatty acid classes is made on the basis of the position of the first double bond from the CH_3 terminus (yielding the designations omega-6 or omega-3). PUFAs contribute approx 7% of total energy intake from fat in the diet of adults in the United States *(22)*. Linoleic acid (18:2n-6) is the major PUFA, comprising 84–89% of the total PUFA energy, whereas ALA (18:3n-3) contributes 9–11% of the total PUFA energy in the diet of the adult population. Intake of n-3 fatty acids is approx 1.6 g/d (approx 0.7% of energy), of which 1.4 g is ALA and 0.1–0.2 g is EPA (20:5) and DHA (22:6).

Omega-6 Fatty Acids

Prospective epidemiologic studies have reported an inverse association between linoleic acid intake and risk of coronary death *(23,24)*. In addition, a cross-sectional study reported an inverse association between linoleic acid intake and CHD prevalence *(25)*. The epidemiologic studies showing a beneficial effect of omega-6 PUFA are supportive of earlier clinical trials conducted to assess the effects of diets high in PUFA but low in SFA and cholesterol on the risk of coronary morbidity and mortality. Several major primary and secondary prevention trials *(26–29)* were conducted to assess the effects of diets that provided 35–39% of calories from total fat, 13–21% of calories from PUFA, and approx 9% of calories from SFA and were low in cholesterol. The studies were the first to show that a high-PUFA diet decreased serum cholesterol levels markedly (13–16%), which was associated with a concurrent decrease in CVD events. Although initially these findings sparked much interest in the use of a high-PUFA diet to decrease CVD risk, enthusiasm diminished because of limited data from long-term studies and the scarcity of data from population groups who followed this diet habitually. Questions were also raised about the role of PUFA in oxidation reactions, risk of cancer, and some evidence that high intakes of PUFA can inhibit formation of long-chain omega-3 PUFA from ALA *(1)*.

Because of the lack of population data about the safety of high-PUFA diets, interest was sparked in assessing the role of MUFA in a blood cholesterol-lowering diet (i.e., low in SFA and cholesterol) as a substitute for SFA calories. Based on a significant database of experimental studies with diets that can be consumed habitually, although PUFA do have a greater total and LDL cholesterol-lowering effect vs MUFA, the differences are small. Thus, for practical purposes, MUFA or PUFA elicit blood cholesterol-lowering effects that are quite similar when incorporated in a diet that meets current recommendations *(30)*.

There are emerging CVD risk factors that play a role in atherogenesis and inflammation. One area of great interest relates to the regulatory effects that fatty acids have on expression of genes involved in leukocyte adhesion molecule synthesis. Omega-3 fatty acids inhibit endothelial activation, and omega-6 fatty acids have a less potent inhibitory effect, albeit more so than MUFA *(31)*. In summary, PUFAs have cardioprotective effects that are mediated by multiple mechanisms that extend beyond the risk reduction conferred by decreases in total and LDL cholesterol.

Omega-3 Fatty Acids

The primary plant-derived omega-3 fatty acid is ALA and the marine-derived omega-3 fatty acids are EPA, C20:5n-3 and DHA C22:6n-3. There is an impressive database from epidemiologic studies and randomized controlled clinical trials that omega-3 fatty acids have cardioprotective effects. These effects have been demonstrated for EPA and DHA, as well as ALA.

Numerous epidemiologic studies have shown that fish consumption beneficially affects several coronary endpoints and, notably, sudden death. In the US Physicians' Health Study, men who consumed fish at least once weekly had a relative risk of sudden death of 0.48 ($p = 0.04$) vs men who consumed fish less than once per month *(32)*. More recently, the Physicians' Health Study reported an inverse relationship between blood levels of long-chain omega-3 fatty acids and risk of sudden death in men without a CVD history *(33)*. The relative risk of sudden death was significantly lower in men with levels in the third quartile (RR = 0.28) and the fourth quartile (RR = 0.19), compared with men whose blood levels were in the first quartile. The Nurses' Health Study reported an inverse association between fish intake and omega-3 fatty acids and CHD death *(34)*. Compared with women who rarely ate fish (<1/mo), the risk for CHD death was 21%, 29%, 31%, and 34% lower for fish consumption 1–3 times/mo, 1/wk, 2–4 times/wk, and more than 5 times/wk, respectively (p for trend = 0.001).

Consistent with the epidemiologic data for EPA and DHA, based on fish consumption, population studies have shown beneficial effects of ALA on coronary endpoints. In the Nurses' Health Study, Hu et al. reported a dose–response relationship between ALA intake and relative risk of fatal ischemic heart disease, which was decreased by 45% in the highest quintile (p for trend = 0.01) *(35)*. Likewise, in the Health Professionals' Study conducted with men, a 1% increase in ALA intake was associated with a 0.41 relative risk for acute MI (p for trend = 0.01) *(36)*. ALA intake in these two studies was 0.7–0.8 g/d, and highest quintile intakes were 1.4–1.5 g/d.

Randomized controlled clinical trials with both EPA and DHA and ALA have confirmed the epidemiologic findings. In the Diet and Reinfarction Trial (DART), male survivors of a myocardial infarction (MI) were advised to increase their intake of oily fish to 200 to 400 g/wk *(37)*. After 2 yr, there was a significant reduction in total mortality, especially for fatal MI. A subgroup of subjects in the DART Trial ingested 1.5 g/d of fish oil in place of consuming fish. In this group, there was a significant reduction in CHD death and all-cause mortality *(38)*. In the GISSI-Prevenzione Trial, subjects with a recent MI were randomized to one of four treatment groups: 850 mg/d of EPA + DHA, 300 mg/d vitamin E, both, or neither *(39)*. After 3.5 yr of follow up, the group given the omega-3 fatty acids alone experienced a 15% reduction in the primary endpoint of death, nonfatal MI, and nonfatal stroke ($p < 0.02$).

There was a 20% reduction in all-cause mortality ($p = 0.01$), and a 45% reduction in sudden death ($p < 0.001$) compared to the control group; vitamin E provided no additional benefit.

Beneficial effects of ALA on CVD endpoints have also been shown in a widely cited randomized controlled clinical trial. The Lyon Heart Trial was a secondary prevention trial designed to test whether a Mediterranean-type diet, including increased amounts of ALA, would reduce reoccurrence rates of cardiac events, compared with a prudent Western diet *(40)*. Subjects in the experimental group were instructed to adopt a Mediterranean-type diet that contained more bread, more root and green vegetables, more fish, fruit at least once daily, less red meat (replaced with poultry), and margarine high in ALA supplied by the study to replace butter and cream. This diet provided 30% of calories from fat, 8% from saturated fat, 13% from monounsaturated fat, 4.6% from polyunsaturated fat (0.84% ALA), and 203 mg/d of cholesterol. Despite a similar coronary risk factor profile (plasma lipids and lipoproteins, systolic and diastolic blood pressure, body mass index [BMI], and smoking status), subjects following the Mediterranean-type diet had a 50–70% lower risk of recurrent heart disease. There were marked reductions in cardiac death and nonfatal MI, major secondary endpoints, and minor events. Although the difference in ALA intakes between groups was 0.5 vs 1.5 g/d, it is impossible to ascribe the benefit unambiguously to ALA, because there were many other dietary variables: saturated fat and cholesterol decreased and monounsaturated fat increased, as did the fruit and vegetable consumption. Nonetheless, this study has provided exciting, suggestive evidence that ALA has a cardioprotective effect. Further studies are needed to definitively establish the role of ALA.

CONJUGATED LINOLEIC ACID

Conjugated linoleic acid (CLA) comprises nine different positional and geometric isomers of linoleic acid in which the double bonds are conjugated instead of being in the typical methylene-interrupted configuration *(41)*. Only two of the isomers, *cis*-9, *trans*-11 and *trans*-10, *cis*-12, are biologically active *(1)*. They are formed from the microbial isomerization of dietary linoleic acid. CLA levels are higher in animal products than in plant products. Foods from ruminants, such as milk and meat, are the major dietary sources of CLA.

CLA beneficially affects plasma lipids and lipoproteins, as well as atherosclerosis in rabbits *(42)* and hamsters *(43)*. In both studies, the CLA treatment groups had markedly lower (approx 20%) total and LDL cholesterol levels and triglyceride levels. HDL cholesterol levels were unaffected by CLA. CLA had more potent effects than linoleic acid *(43)*. CLA also has antioxidant effects *(41)* and, consequently, may protect LDL from oxidative modification in vivo. However, another study reported that CLA induces lipid peroxidation in humans *(44)*. Additional studies are needed to clarify the relationship between CLA and CVD.

Another important biological effect of CLA is that it reduces body fat in humans. Blankson et al. *(45)* fed overweight subjects 3.4, 5.1, or 6.8 g of CLA/d for 12 wk and found that body fat decreased only in the groups receiving 3.4 g or 6.8 g/d of CLA. Likewise, Riserus et al. *(46)* reported that middle-aged men with abdominal obesity had a significant decrease in abdominal adipose tissue mass after consuming 4.2 g of CLA/d for 4 wk. Additional information is needed to establish the role of CLA in regulating adipose tissue mass in humans. Collectively, CLA has some effects on important risk factors for CVD that would be expected to favorably affect coronary risk.

TOTAL FAT

Fats are mixtures of different fatty acids and all contain SFAs, MUFAs, and PUFAs (*see* Fig. 4). Whereas all contain linoleic acid, not all fats contain ALA. It is apparent that diets can be developed that are high in certain fatty acid classes by emphasizing specific fats. However, there are limits to the amount of total fat that can be included in the diet, because all fats are energy dense and contain SFAs. Population studies in Western societies have shown that total fat tracks with both calories and saturated fat because of prevailing dietary patterns that include certain fats and oils *(1)*. In addition, there is a limit to the amount of total fat in the diet because numerous foods must be incorporated to meet nutrient needs within the context of meeting (and not exceeding) energy needs. Thus, to achieve a healthy fatty acid profile in the diet, fats that are good sources of unsaturated fats can be substituted for saturated fat. Alternatively, total fat (and saturated fat) can be reduced in the diet in conjunction with some fat source modifications.

NUTRIENTS AND BIOACTIVE COMPOUNDS IN FATS AND OILS

Vegetable oils are a rich source of vitamin E, which is a potent antioxidant nutrient. Both epidemiologic and in vitro studies show beneficial effects of vitamin E, especially of α-tocopherol, on both incidence of CVD and important markers, including decreased oxidized LDL, reduced platelet adhesion and aggregation, and inhibition of smooth muscle cell proliferation, for CVD *(47)*. To date, results from clinical

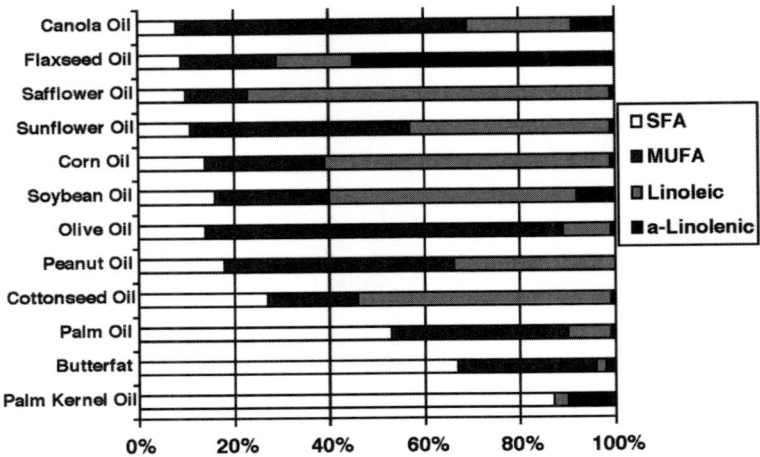

Fig. 4. Typical fatty acid compositions. *Source*: Fatty acid content normalized to 100%. USDA Nutrient Database for Standard Reference (Release 15).

trials with α-tocopherol have yielded mixed results concerning CVD endpoints *(48)*. As expected, studies have reported that adults *(49)* and children 2 to 8 yr of age *(50)* who consume a low-fat diet have inadequate vitamin E intakes.

Vegetable oils are also a source of plant sterols, commonly referred to as phytosterols, and are structurally similar to cholesterol. The primary plant sterols in the diet are sitosterol, stigmasterol, and campesterol. They are not synthesized in humans, as is cholesterol, and are poorly absorbed. Plant sterols are naturally present in vegetable oils and significantly reduce cholesterol absorption *(51)*. Studies show sitosterol or mixtures of plant sterols (approx 1 g/d) reduce blood cholesterol levels in humans by approx 10% *(52,53)*.

Margarines that deliver plant sterol mixtures have been developed for blood cholesterol lowering (reviewed in ref. *54*). The plant sterol mixtures are derived from different oil sources, including pine tree woodpulp (tall oil), soybean oil, ricebran oil, and sheanut oil. Plant sterol/stanol ester margarines have a cholesterol-lowering effect. Collectively, the stanol/stanol ester margarine studies have fed approx 2–3 g of stanols as either the free or the esterified form in full-fat or lower fat margarines or mayonnaise. Two grams per day, which the ATP III recommends as part of the Therapeutic Lifestyle Changes (TLC) diet *(2)*, can lower LDL cholesterol from 9% to 20% beyond that attainable by a diet low in SFA and cholesterol and drug therapy *(55)*. These margarines have hydrogenated soybean oil listed on the ingredient label but, importantly, they are low in *trans* fatty acids (0 to <0.5 g/serving; 1 serving = 1 tbsp).

Olive oil, particularly the first pressed or better known "extra virgin" type, has phenolic components that are powerful antioxidants *(56)* and have greater antioxidative properties than more highly refined olive oil *(57)*. Studies have shown a protective effect of the phenolic compounds in extra virgin olive oil on LDL oxidative susceptibility in the fasted state *(58)* and after consumption of a meal *(59)*. Canola oil has similar antioxidative effects compared with olive oil *(60)*. In addition, peanut oil is a source of resveratrol. Resveratrol inhibits LDL oxidative suscepti-bility in vitro *(61)*, platelet aggregation, and eicosanoid synthesis *(62)*. Rice bran oil is a source of tocotrienols. Tocotrienols have important antioxidant properties *(63)*.

Unsaturated fat food sources include nuts, as well as legumes, pea-nuts, seeds, and avocados. Epidemiologic and clinical studies have reported that nuts have cardioprotective effects *(64)*, which may be explained, in part, by their unsaturated fat content. However, nuts also contain arginine, dietary fiber, folate, vitamin B_6, niacin, magnesium, copper, zinc, calcium, potassium, and a range of bioactive compounds, such as ellagic acid, flavonoids, phenolic compounds, and isoflavones. Thus, they are a rich source of many nutrients that could elicit beneficial effects on CVD risk. Avocados, in addition to being a rich source of monounsaturated fat, are a good source of vitamin A, folate, and potas-sium, which could benefit heart health via multiple mechanisms.

It is evident that fat is more than a source of fatty acids and provides several nutrients and bioactive compounds that have cardioprotective effects. Thus, inclusion of healthy fats and oils in the diet to replace saturated fat provides a strategy for delivering an array of nutritional factors that can reduce CVD risk. Inherent to this approach is to add unsaturated fats to the diet in a way that strikes a balance between too little and levels that provide excessive calories and displace other nutrients.

PRACTICAL APPLICATIONS

The recommended diet to decrease CVD risk is low in saturated fat, *trans* fat, and cholesterol and adequate in unsaturated fatty acids. In addition, it should be nutritionally adequate and meet energy needs. This section provides practical tips for planning a heart-healthy diet that meets current recommendations for type and amount of total fat (20% to 35% of calories). Figure 4 shows the fatty acid profile of common dietary fats and oils. Fats are mixtures of fatty acids. Thus, it is important to empha-size fats that are lower in saturated fat and include those that are higher in MUFA and both classes of PUFA. Table 1 presents a summary of major food fatty acid sources; fats frequently are incorporated into foods and not consumed in isolation. Additional information about the fatty acid profile and cholesterol and energy content of different fat-containing foods is shown in Table 2, which provides more detailed information about the type and quantity of fat found in popular fat-containing foods. Notable differences are evident, including the amount of total fat, all fatty acid classes, cholesterol, and energy. Tables 3 to 5 present information about the *trans* fat, cholesterol, and CLA content of certain foods that are high in these constituents. Note that the *trans* fat content of certain margarines, commercial peanut butter, and special cholesterol-lowering margarines is low. Table 6 shows the fatty acid profile of nuts and seeds, all of which are good sources of unsaturated fat. The American Heart Association *2000 Dietary Guidelines* recommend achieving a desirable cholesterol profile by limiting foods high in saturated fat and cholesterol and substituting unsaturated fat from vegetables, fish, legumes, and nuts. The ATP III report provides some examples of how to achieve a higher fat level with the guidelines of the TLC diet. Some strategies include using peanuts and almonds to replace carbohydrate calories. Two menus are presented in Table 7 that show the range in fat recommendations (from 20% to 35% of calories) that can be implemented to promote heart health. They demonstrate how simple substitutions in a low-fat diet can result in a moderate fat diet that is low in saturated fat, *trans* fat, and cholesterol. Moreover, both dietary patterns are representative of those that can be implemented readily in the United States.

SUMMARY

There has been a shift in the recommendation about total fat that has redirected the emphasis from a low-fat to a moderate-fat message. It is clear that healthy fats have benefits that result from their unsaturated fatty acid profile, as well as other bioactive constituents. There is a range of recommended levels of fat that can be incorporated in a heart-healthy diet. The new recommendations for total fat provide flexibility in diet planning. The option of varying fat level in a diet on an individual basis should promote adherence to a healthy diet. To effectively individualize implementation of the total fat recommendation requires a good understanding of how to incorporate different amounts of total fat into a heart-healthy diet that meets nutrient and energy needs.

Table 1
Major Food Source of Different Fatty Acids

Fats that raise cholesterol	Sources	Examples
Saturated fats	Foods from animal sources	Whole milk, cream, ice cream, whole-milk cheeses, butter, lard, and fatty meats*
	Certain plant oils	Palm, palm kernel and coconut oils, and cocoa butter
Trans fats	Partially hydrogenated vegetable oils	Cookies, crackers, cakes, shortening, margarine, fried foods (i.e., French fries and donuts)

*Lean cuts of meat (beef, pork, lamb, and veal) contain fewer than 5 g saturated fat per 3-oz serving.†

Fats that lower cholesterol	Sources	Examples
Monounsaturated fats	Certain plant oils	Olive, canola and peanut oils, nuts, and avocados
Polyunsaturated fats	Certain plant oils	Safflower, sesame, soybean, corn and sunflower-seed oils, nuts, and seeds
N-3 fatty acids	Certain plant oils	Canola, flaxseed, soybean oils, walnuts, and walnut oil
	Fish oils	Salmon, tuna, mackerel, trout, sardines, and various shellfish

Sources: American Heart Association: http://www.americanheart.org.
†USDA Nutrient Database for Standard Reference (Release 15).

Table 2
Type and Quantity of Dietary Fat in Selected Foods

Sources (3-oz portion and cooked, unless noted otherwise)	Total fat* (g)	Saturated fat (g)	MUFA (g)	PUFA (g)	Omega-3 (g)	Cholesterol (mg)	Total calories (kcal)
Meats							
Beef							
Loin (T-bone)	8.5	3.1	4.2	0.3	—	50	174
Ground beef, 20% fat	14.8	5.7	6.5	0.4	—	76	231
Ground beef, 5% fat	6.4	2.8	2.7	0.4	—	76	164
Pork							
Loin (chop)	8.2	3.0	3.7	0.65	—	69	178
Ham, cured	7.7	2.7	3.8	1.2	—	50	151
Lamb							
Loin (chop)	8.3	3.2	3.4	0.7	—	74	172
Leg	6.6	2.3	2.9	0.4	—	76	162
Veal							
Loin (chop)	5.9	2.2	2.1	0.5	—	90	149
Top round	2.9	1.0	1.0	0.25	—	88	128
Poultry							
Chicken (without skin)							
Light	3.9	1.1	1.3	0.8	—	73	148
Dark	8.3	2.3	3.0	1.9	—	80	175

(continued)

88

Table 2 (Continued)

Sources (3-oz portion and cooked, unless noted otherwise)	Total fat* (g)	Saturated fat (g)	MUFA (g)	PUFA (g)	Omega-3 (g)	Cholesterol (mg)	Total calories (kcal)
Chicken (with skin)							
Light	9.5	2.7	3.7	2.0	–	74	195
Dark	13.2	3.6	5.2	2.9	–	76	211
Turkey (without skin)							
Light	2.8	0.9	0.5	0.7	–	59	134
Dark	6.2	2.1	1.4	1.8	–	73	160
Fish							
Salmon, Atlantic	10.5	2.1	3.8	3.8	1.9	54	175
Tuna, yellow fin	1.0	0.3	0.2	0.3	0.25	49	118
Flounder	1.3	0.3	0.2	0.5	0.5	58	99
Shellfish and mollusks							
Lobster	0.5	0.1	0.1	0.1	0.1	64	83
Shrimp	0.9	0.2	0.2	0.4	0.2	166	84
Clams	1.7	0.2	0.1	0.5	–	57	126
Oysters	4.2	1.3	0.5	1.6	0.6	89	116
Dairy							
Milk (8 oz, 1 cup)							
Whole, 3.3% fat	8.2	5.1	2.4	0.3	–	35	149
Skim, <1% fat	0.4	0.3	0.1	0.02	–	5	86

(continued)

Table 2 (Continued)
Type and Quantity of Dietary Fat in Selected Foods

Sources (3-oz portion and cooked, unless noted otherwise)	Total fat* (g)	Saturated fat (g)	MUFA (g)	PUFA (g)	Omega-3 (g)	Cholesterol (mg)	Total calories (kcal)
Cheese (1 oz)							
Cheddar	9.4	6.0	2.7	0.3	–	30	114
Cheddar, low-fat	2.0	1.2	0.6	0.06	–	6	49
Mozzarella, part-skim	4.9	3.1	1.4	0.1	–	15	80
Fats (oils) and nuts							
Oils (1 tbsp)							
Canola	14	1.0	8.2	4.1	1.3	–	124
Olive	14	1.8	10	1.1	–	–	119
Soybean	14	2.0	3.2	7.9	0.9	–	120
Nuts (1 oz)							
Walnuts, English	18.5	1.7	2.5	13.4	2.5	–	185
Almonds, dry roasted	15	1.1	9.5	3.6	–	–	169
Peanuts, dry roasted	14	2.0	7.0	4.4	–	–	166
Mixed, dry roasted	14.6	2.0	9.0	3.1	–	–	168
Peanut Butter (2 tbsp)	16	3.3	7.8	4.4	–	–	190

MUFA, monounsaturated fat; PUFA, polyunsaturated fat.
*The sum of the fat classes does not always equal the total fat content because some fatty acids are not accounted for and/or are not included.
Source: USDA Nutrient Database for Standard Reference (Release 15): http://www.nal.usda.gov/fnic/foodcomp.

Table 3
Trans Fat Content of Processed Foods

Portion size	Food	Trans *fat, g*
Dairy products		
8 oz	Milk, nonfat, skim	0
8 oz	Milk, whole	0.16–0.22
1 oz	Cheese, cheddar	0.24
1 oz	Cheese, American	0.01–0.22
Oils/fats/dressings		
1 tbsp	Margarine, hard stick	1.95–3.76
1 tbsp	Margarine, soft tub	0.46–1.70
1 tbsp	Shortening	1.60–4.88
1 tbsp	Mayonnaise	0.35–0.51
1 tbsp	Salad dressing	0.03–0.56
1 tbsp	Lard	0.06–0.23
Snack foods		
1 oz	Crackers, snack	1.64–2.35
1 oz	Crackers, cheese	2.08
1 oz	Crackers, saltine	0.42–1.11
1 oz	Potato chips	0–2.98
1 oz	Popcorn, microwave	0.88–2.14
Fried foods		
Small	French fries, fast food	1.46–2.87
Medium	French fries, fast food	2.30–4.52
Large	French fries, fast food	2.91–5.71
Baked goods		
1 slice	Bread, white	0.03–0.35
1 slice	Cake, pound	1.6
1 oz	Cookies, chocolate chip	1.12–2.53
1 oz	Cookies, chocolate sandwich	1.36–1.76
1 oz	Doughnut, cake type	0.15–1.93
1 oz	Dinner roll	0.07–0.09
Sweets		
1 oz	Frosting	0.96–1.13
1 oz	Candy, chocolate	0.03
1/2 cup	Ice cream	0.29–0.33
Other		
1 oz	Breakfast cereal, ready to eat	0.04–0.35
3 oz	Ground beef, cooked	0.59
2 tbsp	Peanut butter	<0.5

Source: USDA Nutrient Database, Special Purpose Table No. 1, Fat and Fatty Acid Content of Selected Foods Containing Trans-Fatty Acids.

Table 4
Food Sources That Are High in Cholesterol

Food	Cholesterol (mg/serving)	Total fat (g/serving)
Eggs		
Jumbo	276	8.1
Extra large	246	7.2
Large	213	6.2
Medium	187	5.5
Small	157	4.6
Seafood and meats		
Shrimp, 3 oz	166	0.9
Beef liver, 3 oz	330	4.2
Beef heart, 3 oz	164	4.8
Beef kidney, 3 oz	330	2.9
Pork chitterlings, 3 oz	122	24.4
Dairy foods		
Butter, 1 tbsp	33	12.2
Half-and-half cream, 2 tbsp	11	3.5
Sour cream, 2 tbsp	11	5
Milk		
Whole, 3.25% milk fat, 1 cup	34	8.2
Reduced fat, 2% milk fat, 1 cup	20	4.7
Lowfat, 1% milk fat, 1 cup	10	2.6
Skim, 0% milk fat, 1 cup	5	0.5
Vanilla ice cream		
Premium brand, 1 cup	90	24
Low-fat, 1 cup	20	4
Fat-free, 1 cup	0	0

Source: USDA Nutrient Database for Standard Reference (Release 15).

Table 5
Conjugated Linoleic Acid (CLA) Content of Uncooked Foods

Food	Total CLA, mg/g fat
Meat	
Fresh ground beef	4.3
Beef, round	2.9
Veal	2.7
Lamb	5.6
Pork	0.6
Poultry	
Chicken	0.9
Ground turkey	2.5
Seafood	
Salmon	0.3
Trout, freshwater	0.5
Shrimp	0.6
Dairy products	
Milk, whole, homogenized	5.5
Butter	4.7
Sour cream	4.6
Plain yogurt	4.8
Ice cream	3.6
Cheddar cheese, sharp	3.6
Mozzarella cheese	4.9
Colby cheese	6.1
Cottage cheese	4.5
Swiss, reduced fat	6.7
Processed cheese, American	5.0
Vegetable oils	
Safflower	0.7
Sunflower	0.4
Canola	0.5
Corn	0.2

Source: Chin et al. (65).

Table 6
Foods That Are Rich Source of Unsaturated Fats, per 100 g

Food	Calories (kcal)	Total fat (g)	SFA (g)	MUFA (g)	PUFA (g)	Linoleic acid (g)	Linolenic acid (g)
Nuts							
Almond	578	51	4	32	12	12	0
Brazil	656	66	16	23	24	24	0
Cashew	574	46	9	27	8	8	0
Hazelnut	628	61	4	46	8	8	0
Macadamia	716	76	12	59	1	1	0
Pecan	691	72	6	41	22	21	1
Pistachio	567	46	4	25	14	14	0
Walnut	654	65	6	9	47	38	9
Mixed nut	594	52	7	31	11	11	0
Legumes							
Peanuts	585	50	7	25	16	16	0
Soybeans, dry roasted	450	22	3	5	12	11	2
Seeds							
Flax	500	34	3	7	22	5	19
Pumpkin	541	46	9	14	21	21	0
Sunflower	582	50	5	10	33	33	0
Avocado	119	14	0	10	2	2	0

SAF, saturated fatty acid; MUFA, monounsaturated fatty acid, PUFA, polyunsaturated fatty acid. *Source:* USDA Nutrient Database for Standard Reference (Release 15).

Table 7
2400 kcal Sample Menus

Food	20% of kcal from fat	35% of kcal from fat
Breakfast		
Shredded wheat cereal	1 cup	1 cup
Skim milk	1 cup	1 cup
Blueberries	1/2 cup	1/2 cup
Orange juice	1 cup	3/4 cup
Coffee	1 cup	1 cup
Skim milk for coffee	2 tbsp	2 tbsp
Lunch		
Roast beef, lean	2 oz	2 oz
Cheddar cheese, reduced fat	1 oz slice	1 oz slice
Whole wheat bread	2 slices	2 slices
Tomato, sliced	2 slices	2 slices
Lettuce	2 leaves	2 leaves
Mayonnaise, low-calorie	1 tbsp	1 tbsp
Baby carrots	10 pieces	10 pieces
Apple, medium	1 item	1 item
Dinner		
Salmon, cooked, dry heat	3 oz	3 oz
Parmesan cheese	1 tbsp	1 tbsp
Safflower oil	1 tbsp	1 tbsp
Almonds		2 tbsp
Brown rice	1 cup	1/2 cup
Mixed vegetables	1/2 cup	1/2 cup
Dinner roll	1 item	1 item
Margarine, soft tub		2 tsp
Strawberries	1 cup	1 cup
Vanilla low-fat frozen yogurt	1/2 cup	1/2 cup
Snack		
Skim milk	1 cup	
Fig Newton cookies, fat-free	3 items	
Mixed nuts		1/4 cup

(continued)

Table 7 (Continued)
2400 kcal Sample Menus

Food	20% of kcal from fat	35% of kcal from fat
Nutrient analysis		
Calories	2004	2003
Protein, % of kcal	18	18
Carbohydrate, % of kcal	63	51
Fat, % of kcal	20	35
Saturated fat, % of kcal	6	8
Monunsaturated fat, % of kcal	5	14
Polyunsaturated fat, % of kcal	9	13
Linoleic, g		
Linolenic, g	0.4	0.6
EPA + DHA, g 1.1	1.1	
Trans fat, g	0	0.4
Cholesterol, mg	130	126
Fiber, total, g 34	36	
Soluble, g	8	6.3
Sodium, mg	2300	2200
Calcium, mg	1300	1000

Source: Nutr V, First DataBank, Inc., San Bruno, CA.

REFERENCES

1. Institute of Medicine of the National Academies. Dietary Reference Intakes for Energy, Carbohydrate, Fiber, Fat, Fatty Acids, Cholesterol, Protein and Amino Acids. Washington, DC, National Academies Press, 2002.
2. National Institutes of Health. Third Report of the Expert Panel on Detection, Evaluation, and Treatment of High Blood Cholesterol in Adults (Adult Treatment Panel III). NIH Publication No. 01-3670, 2001.
3. US Department of Agriculture. Dietary Guidelines for Americans. 5th ed. Washington, DC.
4. Keys A. Coronary heart disease in Seven Countries. Circulation 1970;41:I1I–211.
5. Keys A, Anderson JT, Grande F. Serum cholesterol response to changes in the diet. II. The effect of cholesterol in the diet. Metabolism 1965;14:759–765.
6. Hegsted DM, McGandy RB, Myers ML, Stare FJ. Quantitative effects of dietary fat on serum cholesterol in man. Am J Clin Nutr 1965;17:281–295.
7. Mensink RP, Katan MB. Effect of dietary fatty acids on serum lipids and lipoproteins. A meta-analysis of 27 trials. Arterioscler Thromb 1992;129:911–919.
8. Hegsted DM, Ausman LM, Johnson JA, Dallal GE. Dietary fat and serum lipids: an evaluation of the experimental data. Am J Clin Nutr 1993;57:875–883. [Erratum, Am J Clin Nutr 1993;58:245.]
9. Clarke R, Frost C, Collins R, Appleby P, Peto R. Dietary lipids and blood cholesterol: Quantitative meta-analysis of metabolic ward studies. Br Med J 1997;314:112–117.
10. Oomen CM, Ockem MC, Feskensm EJ, van Erp-Baartm MA, Kokm FJ, Kromhout D. Association between trans fatty acid intake and 10-year risk of coronary heart disease in the Zutphen Elderly Study: a prospective population-based study. Lancet 2001;357:746–751.
11. Kromhout, D., Menotti, A., Bloemberg, B., et al. Dietary saturated and trans fatty acids and cholesterol and 25-year mortality from coronary heart disease: the Seven Countries Study. Prev Med 1995;24:308–315.
12. Willett WC, Stampfer MJ, Manson JE, et al. Intake of trans fatty acids and risk of coronary heart disease among women. Lancet 1993;341:581–585.
13. Trans fatty acids and coronary heart disease risk. Report of the expert panel on trans fatty acids and coronary heart disease. Am J Clin Nutr 1995;62,:655S–708S.
14. Lichtenstein AH, Ausman LM, Jalbert SM, Schaefer EJ. Effects of different forms of dietary hydrogenated fats on serum lipoprotein cholesterol levels. N Engl J Med 1999;340:1933–1940.
15. Mensink RP, Zock PL, Katan MB, Hornstra G. Effect of dietary cis and trans fatty acids on serum lipoprotein[a] levels in humans. J Lipid Res 1992;33:1493–1501.
16. Mensink RP, Katan MB. Effect of dietary trans fatty acids on high-density and low-density lipoprotein cholesterol levels in healthy subjects. N Engl J Med 1990;323:439–445.
17. Judd JT, Baer DJ, Clevidence BA, Kris-Etherton P, Muesing RA, Iwane M. Dietary cis and trans monounsaturated and saturated FA and plasma lipids and lipoproteins in men. Lipids 2002;37:123–131.
18. Katan MB, Zock PL, Mensink RP. Trans fatty acids and their effects on lipoproteins in humans. Ann Rev Nutr 1995;15:473–493.
19. Kris-Etherton PM. AHA Science Advisory. Monounsaturated fatty acids and risk of cardiovascular disease. American Heart Association. Nutrition Committee. Circulation 1999;100:1253–1258.
20. Vogel RA, Corretti MC, Plotnick GD. The postprandial effect of components of the Mediterranean diet on endothelial function. J Am Coll Cardiol 2000;36:1455–1460.

21. Rudel LL, Parks JS, Sawyer JK. Compared with dietary monounsaturated and saturated fat, polyunsaturated fat protects African green monkeys from coronary artery atherosclerosis. Arterioscler Thromb Vasc Biol 1995;15:2101–2110.
22. Kris-Etherton PM, Taylor-Shaffer D, et al. Polyunsaturated fatty acids in the food chain in the United States. Am J Clin Nutr 2000;71:179S–188S.
23. Gartside PS, Glueck CJ. Relationship of dietary intake to hospital admission for coronary heart and vascular disease: the NHANES II national probability study. J Am Coll Nutr 1993;12:676–684.
24. Arntzenius AC, Kromhout D, Barth JD, et al. Diet, lipoproteins, and the progression of coronary atherosclerosis. The Leiden Intervention Trial. N Engl J Med 1985;312:805–811.
25. Djousse L, Pankow JS, Eckfeldt JH, et al. Relation between dietary linolenic acid and coronary artery disease in the National Heart, Lung, and Blood Institute Family Heart Study. Am J Clin Nutr 2001;74:612–619.
26. Frantz ID Jr, Dawson EA, Ashman PL, et al. Test of effect of lipid lowering by diet on cardiovascular risk. The Minnesota Coronary Survey. Arteriosclerosis 1989;9:129–135.
27. Miettinen M, Turpeinen O, Karvonen MJ, Elosuo R, Paavilainen E. Effect of cholesterol-lowering diet on mortality from coronary heart-disease and other causes. A twelve-year clinical trial in men and women. Lancet 1972;2:835–838.
28. Leren P. The Oslo diet-heart study. Eleven-year report. Circulation 1970;42:935–942.
29. Dayton S, Pearce ML, Hashimoto S, Dixon WJ, Tomiyasu U. A controlled clinical trial of a diet high in unsaturated fat in preventing complications of atherosclerosis (American Heart Association Monograph No. 25). Circulation 1969;39–40:(Suppl II):1–63.
30. Krauss, R. M., Eckel, R. H., Howard, B., et al. AHA Dietary Guidelines: revision 2000: A statement for healthcare professionals from the Nutrition Committee of the American Heart Association. Circulation 2000;102:2284–2299.
31. De Caterina R, Liao JK, Libby P. (2000) Fatty acid modulation of endothelial activation. Am J Clin Nutr 2000;71(Suppl 1):213S–223S.
32. Albert CM, Hennekens CH, O'Donnell CJ, et al. Fish consumption and risk of sudden cardiac death. JAMA 1998;279:23–28.
33. Albert CM, Campos H, Stampfer MJ, et al. Blood levels of long-chain n-3 fatty acids and the risk of sudden death. N Engl J Med 2002;346:1113–1118.
34. Hu FB, Bronner L, Willett WC, et al. Fish and omega-3 fatty acid intake and risk of coronary heart disease in women. JAMA 2002;287:1815–1821.
35. Hu FB, Stampfer MJ, Manson JE, et al. Dietary intake of α-linolenic acid and risk of fatal ischemic heart disease among women. Am J Clin Nutr 1999;69:890–897.
36. Ascherio A, Rimm EB, Giovannucci EL, et al. Dietary fat and risk of coronary heart disease in men: cohort follow up study in the United States. Br Med J 1996;313:84–90.
37. Burr ML, Fehily AM, Gilbert JF, et al. Effects of changes in fat, fish and fibre intakes on death and myocardial reinfarction: diet and reinfarction trial (DART). Lancet 1989;2:757–761.
38. Burr ML, Sweetham PM, Fehily AM. Diet and Reinfarction. Eur Heart J 1994;15:1152–1153.
39. GISSI-Prevenzione Investigators. Dietary supplementation with n-3 polyunsaturated fatty acids and vitamin E after myocardial infarction: results of the GISSI-Prevenzione trial. Lancet 1999;354:447–455.
40. De Lorgeril M, Salen P, Martin JL, Monjaud I, Delaye J, Mamelle N. Mediterranean diet, traditional risk factors, and the rate of cardiovascular complications after

myocardial infarction: Final report of the Lyon Diet Heart Study. Circulation 1999;99:779–785.

41. Decker EA. The role of phenolics, conjugated linoleic acid, carnosine, and pyrroloquinoline quinone as nonessential dietary antioxidants. Nutr Rev 1995;53:49–58.

42. Kritchevsky D, Tepper SA, Wright S, Tso P, Czarnecki SK. Influence of conjugated linoleic acid (CLA) on establishment and progression of atherosclerosis in rabbits. J Am Coll Nutr 2000;19:472S–477S.

43. Nicolosi RJ, Rogers EJ, Kritchevsky D, Sameca JA, Huth PJ. Dietary conjugated linoleic acid reduces plasma lipoproteins and early aortic atherosclerosis in hyercholesterolaemic hamsters. Artery 1997;22:266–277.

44. Basu S, Smedman A, Vessby B. Conjugated linoleic acid induces lipid peroxidation in humans. FEBS Lett 2000;468:33–36.

45. Blankson H, Stakkestad JA, Fagertun H, Thom E, Wadstein J, Gudmundsen O. Conjugated linoleic acid reduces body fat mass in overweight and obese humans. J Nutr 2000;130:2943–2948.

46. Riserus U, Berglund L, Vessby B. Conjugated linoleic acid (CLA) reduced abdominal adipose tissue in obese middle-aged men with signs of the metabolic syndrome: a randomised controlled trial. Int J Obes Relat Metab Disord 2001;25:1129–1135.

47. Kaul N, Devaraj S, Jialal I. Alpha-tocopherol and atherosclerosis. Exp Biol Med 2001;226:5–12.

48. Jialal I, Traber M, Devaraj S. Is there a vitamin E paradox? Curr Opin Lipidol 2001;12:49–53.

49. Peterson S, Sigman-Grant M, Eissenstat B, Kris-Etherton P. Impact of adopting lower-fat food choices on energy and nutrient intakes of American adults. J Am Diet Assoc 1999;99:177–183.

50. Ballew C, Kuester S, Serdula M, Bowman B, Dietz W. Nutrient intakes and dietary patterns of young children by dietary fat intakes. J Pediatr 2000;136:143–145.

51. Ostlund RE Jr, Racette SB, Okeke A, Stenson WF. Phytosterols that are naturally present in commercial corn oil significantly reduce cholesterol absorption in humans. Am J Clin Nutr 2002;75:1000–1004.

52. Howard BV, Kritchevsky D. Phytochemicals and cardiovascular disease. Circulation 1997;95:2591–2593.

53. Vahouny GV, Kritchevsky D. Plant and marine sterols and cholesterol metabolism. In: Spiller GA, ed. Nutritional Pharmacology. New York, Alan R Liss Inc, 1981, pp. 31–72.

54. Jones PJ, Ntanios F. Comparable efficacy of hydrogenated versus nonhydrogenated plant sterol esters on circulating cholesterol levels in humans. Nutr Rev 1998;56:245–252.

55. Lichtenstein AH, Deckelbaum RJ. Stanol/sterol ester-containing foods and blood cholesterol levels. Circulation 2001;103:1177–1179.

56. Gutfinger T. Polyphenols in olive oils. J Am Oil Chem Soc 1981;58:966–968.

57. Fito M, Covas MI, Lamuela-Raventos RM, et al. Protective effect of olive oil and its phenolic compounds against low density lipoprotein oxidation. Lipids 2000;35:633–638.

58. Masella R, Giovannini C, Vari R, et al. Effects of dietary virgin olive oil phenols on low density lipoprotein oxidation in hyperlipidemic patients. Lipids 2001;36:1195–1202.

59. Vissers MN, Zock PL, Leenen R, Roodenburg AJ, van Putte KP, Katan MB. Effect of consumption of phenols from olives and extra virgin oil on LDL oxidizability in healthy humans. Free Radic Res 2001;35:619–629.

60. Nielsen NS, Pedersen A, Sandstrom B, Marckmann P, Hoy CE. Different effects of diets rich in olive oil, rapeseed oil and sunflower-seed oil on postprandial lipid and lipoprotein concentrations and on lipoprotein oxidation susceptibility. Br J Nutr 2002;87:489–499.
61. Fremont L, Belguendouz L, Delpal S. Antioxidant activity of resveratrol and alcohol-free wine polyphenols related to LDL oxidation and polyunsaturated fatty acids. Life Sci 1999;64:2511–2521.
62. Pace-Asciak CR, Hahn S, Diamandis EP, Soleas G, Goldberg DM. The red wine phenolics trans-resveratrol and quercetin block human platelet aggregation and eicosanoid synthesis: implications for protection against coronary heart disease. Clin Chim Acta 1995;235:207–219.
63. Tomeo AC, Geller M, Watkins TR, Gapor A, Bierenbaum ML. Antioxidant effects of tocotrienols in patients with hyperlipidemia and carotid stenosis. Lipids 1995;30:1179–1183.
64. Kris-Etherton PM, Zhao G, Binkoski AE, Coval SM, Etherton TD. The effects of nuts on coronary heart disease risk. Nutr Rev 2001;59:103–111.
65. Chin SF, Liu W, Storkson JM, Ha YL, Pariza MW. Dietary sources of conjugated dienoic isomers of linoleic acid, a newly recognized class of anticarcinogens. J Food Comp Anal 1992;5:185–197.

7

Nutrachemicals in the Prevention and Treatment of Cardiovascular Disease

Arshad M. Safi, MD,
Cynthia A. Samala, RD,
and Richard A. Stein, MD

CONTENTS

INTRODUCTION

Cardiovascular disease (CVD) remains the most common cause of mortality in the United States. The emphasis on prevention, early detection, and recent advents in pharmacological and interventional approaches has resulted in significant reduction in the associated mortality and mor-

From: *Contemporary Cardiology*
Complementary and Alternative Cardiovascular Medicine
Edited by: R. A. Stein and M. C. Oz © Humana Press Inc., Totowa, NJ

bidity. There is widespread public interest in the use of alternative medicine to prevent and treat these diseases. The cardiovascular system is more susceptible to free radical oxidative stress and premature aging than any other body system. Certain herbal and dietary factors have antioxidant, anti-inflammatory, and antiproliferative properties. Therefore, select supplements may play a preventive and therapeutic role in CVD. Conflicting reports in the biomedical literature and lack of information from health care professionals have led to the misunderstanding about supplements' roles in patients with CVDs. This chapter reviews the most commonly used nutrachemicals.

L-ARGININE

L-arginine is an essential amino acid and is required for protein synthesis. It is found in red meat, fish, poultry, and dairy products. Nitric oxide synthase (NOS) converts L-arginine to nitric oxide (NO) in vascular endothelial cells. NO is also known as the endothelial-derived relaxation factor (EDRF). NO is a potent vasodilator and modulates a significant portion of endothelial function in coronary and peripheral circulations. These beneficial effects can be jeopardized if there is impaired NO production. It is postulated that a reduction in available L-arginine, in part because of the presence of endogenous inhibitors, will result in impaired NO production and endothelial dysfunction. Therefore, L-arginine administration could enhance endogenous NO production, which could result in favorable clinical outcomes.

Role in CVD

Studies have shown beneficial effects of L-arginine supplementation in a relatively small number of patients with coronary artery disease (CAD). Lerman et al. *(1)* reported the beneficial effects of oral supplementation of L-arginine in 26 patients with small-vessel CAD. Coronary blood flow (CBF) reserve in response to acetylcholine was assessed at baseline and at 6-mo intervals. In this small, blinded, controlled trial, the L-arginine group demonstrated a significant increase in CBF compared with placebo (149 ± 20% vs 6 + 9%, $p < 0.05$). This finding was also associated with decreased plasma endothelin level, which is a potent vasoconstrictor. It has been postulated that increased NO production may inhibit the endothelin production through a cyclic guanosine monophosphate (cGMP) dependent pathway. Blum et al. *(2)* illustrated the benefits of oral L-arginine therapy (9 g/d for 3 mo) in a crossover, double-blind study of 10 patients with intractable class IV angina, despite treatment with aspirin, calcium channel blockers, nitrates, and high-dose beta-blockers. L-arginine therapy resulted in clinical improvement in seven patients (from angina pectoris class IV to class II). These patients also showed reduction in proinflammatory cytokines (interleukin [IL]-1-β, IL-6) and downregulation of cell adhesion molecules (P-selectin, E-selectin, and intercellular adhesion molecule [ICAM]). In another prospective, double-blind, randomized crossover study (3) of 10 young men with CAD, the endothelial-dependent vasodilation and reduction in monocyte adhesion to endothelial cells were evident by the third week of supplementation with L-arginine (7 g three times/d). Bednarz et al. (4) assessed the effects of L-arginine on electrocardiographic changes in 25 patients with CAD. Oral supplementation of L-arginine had no effect on QT intervals, QT dispersion, or ST depression. There was a significant increase in exercise tolerance ($p < 0.03$), which was attributed to enhanced peripheral vasodiltation and improved skeletal muscle perfusion.

"Negative" studies to date include that of Blum et al. (5) who studied the effect of 1-mo of oral L-arginine therapy in 30 patients with CAD on adequate medical therapy. Although plasma arginine levels were increased, there was no improvement in NO bioavailability. A double-blind study by Quyyumi (6) also failed to produce any improvement in myocardial ischemia in 22 stable patients with CAD with L-arginine supplementation. Differences in outcomes in these studies may result from study design, duration of therapy, different dosages for supplementation, and other factors.

NO also plays an important role in the peripheral circulation. Boger et al. (7) demonstrated reduced urinary excretion of nitrates (a measure that correlates well with the amount of NO produced by endothelial cells) and cGMP in 77 patients with peripheral arterial occlusive disease (PAOD), suggesting reduced NO formation. This study also found high levels of asymmetrical dimethyl arginine (ADMA), the endogenous NO synthase inhibitor. The same author (8) also studied the effect of L-arginine supplementation in 39 patients with PAOD manifested by intermittent claudication in a noncontrolled trial. The walking distances were assessed on a treadmill and flow-induced vasodilation of femoral artery was periodically assessed by ultrasonography. L-arginine was associated with significant increase in pain-free walking and absolute walking distances. There was also elevation of plasma L-arginine/ADMA ratio, increased urinary nitrate, and cGMP excretion rates, suggesting restoration of endogenous NO production.

Vasodilators, such as angiotensin-converting enzyme (ACE) inhibitors, hydralazine, and nitrates, improve the functional class and survival in patients with congestive heart failure (CHF). A study documented an impaired endothelium-dependent vasodilation of peripheral vasculature in 16 patients with heart failure *(9)*. This may suggest a role for L-arginine therapy as a potential NO substrate donor. Bocchi et al. *(10)* demonstrated the effect of L-arginine on hemodynamics in seven patients with CHF. L-arginine did not improve the left ventricular contractility. However, cardiac performance was improved by reduction in blood pressure and systemic vascular resistance, with concomitant increases in the right atrial pressure, stroke volume, and cardiac output. In another group of 15 patients with heart failure, oral L-arginine supplementation resulted in improved functional status, which was indicated by increased walking distance and lower score on the living with heart failure questionnaire *(11)*. Koifman et al. *(12)* reported the same hemodynamic responses in 12 patients with CHF (ejection fraction [EF] <35%) by iv infusion L-arginine. Hambrecht et al. *(13)* studied the effect of combined L-arginine supplementation and local exercise training on endothelium-dependent vasodilation in a randomized controlled trial of 40 patients. This combination resulted in an additive improvement in endothelial function, when compared to L-arginine supplementation or exercise alone. It is well known that skeletal muscle metabolism, which is impaired in heart failure because of poor perfusion and exercise intolerance, has been correlated with poor outcome in patients with heart failure. Hence, combining these interventions may be more prudent in improving the outcome in patients with heart failure.

Neointimal proliferation remains the most important factor causing in-stent restenosis after PTCA and is caused by smooth muscle cell (SMCs) proliferation. NO inhibits key processes, such as monocyte adhesion, platelet aggregation, and SMC proliferation. NO may also promote apoptosis of vascular SMCs. Suzuki et al. *(14)* analyzed the effect of intramural administration of L-arginine, via a Dispatch catheter (Scimed) over 15 min, after optimal stent placement in 50 patients who were randomized to an L-arginine group or a saline group. Serial angiography and intravascular ultrasonography were performed to measure stent area, lumen area, and neointimal area. The L-arginine group demonstrated a lower neointimal volume (25 vs 39 mm^3, $p = 0.049$). This study suggested a novel role of local delivery of L-arginine to reduce in-stent restenosis.

Hypercholesteremia is associated with endothelial dysfunction at an early stage, even when there is no evident atheromatous lesion. L-arginine infusion in patients with hypercholesteremia has resulted in improved endothelial-dependent vasodilation in a controlled study by Creager et al. *(15)*. L-arginine has also been reported to reduce the endothelial adhesiveness of monocytes and platelet aggregation in patients with hypercholesteremia, compared with healthy individuals. Boger et al. *(16)* studied aortic atherosclerosis after a high-fat–cholesterol diet in rabbits. Rabbits given L-arginine with the diet developed fewer lesions than those without L-arginine (control group) and fewer lesions than a third group of rabbits who were given lovastatin with a high-fat–high-cholesterol diet.

Endothelial dysfunction is present in individuals with hypertension and studies have failed to show any beneficial effects of L-arginine in this patient group *(17)*. The postulated mechanism of endothelial dysfunction in hypertension is an imbalance between vasodilator and vasoconstrictor factors rather than NO substrate deficiency. Patients with hypertension and associated left ventricular hypertrophy (LVH) may complain of angina, despite angiographically normal epicardial coronary arteries. In a cohort of 12 patients, Mohri et al. *(18)* demonstrated that inhibition of endogenous NO production, with intracoronary N^G-monomethyl-L-arginine (L-NMMA), unmasked myocardial ischemia (evident by decreased lactate uptake and increased lactate production in coronary sinus sampling) during pacing-induced tachycardia. This myocardial ischemia was reversed by intracoronary L-arginine. Therefore, L-arginine may have a potential role as an antianginal agent in patients with hypertension with angina, LVH, and normal epicardial coronary arteries.

In conclusion, multiple small studies of L-arginine supplementation have yielded favorable responses in patients with CAD and CHF. L-arginine-modulated enhancement of endothelial function has been noted in patients with hypercholesteremia. Vascular dysfunction in patients with diabetes and hypertension may reflect endothelial-independent mechanisms; hence, the role for L-arginine is not clearly evident. Of interest is a study by Houghton and colleagues *(19)* that demonstrated an L-arginine-mediated augumentation of CBF in African American men and women when compared with matched Caucasian, suggesting a possible target group that may benefit more than the others.

These findings must be confirmed by larger studies of longer duration that address the effects of L-arginine in myocardial ischemia, cardiac transplant patients, and in patients undergoing percutaneous coronary interventions (PCI).

> *Trade name*: R-Gene 10 (Pharmacia Corp.), L-Arginine (Twin Labs)
> *Adverse reactions*: Nausea, abdominal cramps, and diarrhea. Additionally, there are few anecdotal reports of recurrence of oral herpes lesion with its supplementation.
> *Contraindications*: Hypersensitivity, genetic disorder argininemia
> *Usual study dosage*: 8–21 g/d

TAURINE

Taurine is a conditionally essential sulfonic amino acid and found as free and in small peptides forms. It is present in high amounts in the retina, the brain, platelets, neutrophils, myocardium, skeletal, and smooth muscles. Taurine is important in the development of normal central and visual systems. Major dietary sources of taurine are animal food and seaweed, with low levels found in plant foods. The metabolic effects of taurine include modulation of intracellular calcium levels, detoxification, membrane stabilization, and osmoregulation. It has antioxidant activity, and some investigators believe it has hypocholesteremic, hypotensive, antiatherogenic, and ionotropic properties.

Role in CVD

Taurine is abundantly present as a free amino acid in the myocardium. Taurine-mediated increase in myocardial contractility is not mediated via the cyclic adenosine monophosphate (cAMP). It modulates the activity of low-voltage-dependent Ca^{2+} channels in addition to its effect on other channels. This resulting increased intracellular calcium during the action potential is believed to be the underlying mechanism for its ionotropic properties. Taurine deficiency has been associated with cardiomyopathy, and simple taurine replacement often leads to complete recovery.

Azuma et al. *(20)* studied the effect of adding taurine to conventional treatment in 14 patients with CHF in a double-blind, randomized, crossover, and placebo-controlled study. The taurine group ($n = 7$) showed marked improvement in New York Heart Association (NYHA) functional class, pulmonary crackles, and chest film abnormalities ($p < 0.02$). These results corresponded with reduction in preejection period index on noninvasive testing, suggesting a positive ionotropic effect. In another controlled study, Azuma et al. *(21)* demonstrated the beneficial effect on the indexes of cardiac performance in 17 patients who received taurine (3 g/d). There was no effect on the heart rate or blood pressure. However, left ventricular systolic function improved (mean EF from 39% to 47%, $p < 0.01$) and there was a significant increase in stroke volume and cardiac output ($p < 0.05$). In a double-blind trial of supplement or placebo, Jeejeebhoy et al. *(22)* reported a significant reduction in the left ventricular end-diastolic volume (LVEDV), with a combined supplement (containing taurine, CoQ_{10}, and carnitine) in 41 patients with CHF (EF ≤ 40%). These studies suggest the need for an appropriate clinical trial to define the role of taurine supplementation in patients with CHF.

There are limited data regarding the role of taurine in atherosclerosis prevention. A proposed role is based on a recent report by Nonaka et al. *(23)*, who demonstrated that taurine ingestion restored the secretion and expression of extracellular-superoxide dismutase (EC-SOD). It has been reported that homocysteine reduces the secretion and expression of EC-SOD in vascular SMCs, causing premature atherosclerosis. This effect at the cellular level may play an important role in preventing atherosclerosis. Yamori et al. *(24)* reported an inverse relationship between taurine intake and the incidence of coronary heart disease (CHD).

Trade name: Mega Taurine (Twin Lab)
Adverse reactions: None reported
Contraindications: Hypersensitivity
Usual study dosage: 500 mg–3 g/d

COENZYME Q_{10} (COQ_{10})

Since its identification in 1957, CoQ_{10} has been widely used in patients in Japan, Russia, and Europe as part of their CVD treatment. CoQ_{10} belongs to a family of substances called ubiquinones, which are lipophilic, water-insoluble substances involved in electron transport and energy production in the mitochondria. It is an essential cofactor in many of the metabolic pathways, particularly in the production of adenosine triphosphate (ATP) in oxidative respiration. The supplemental form is typically derived from tobacco leaf extracts, fermented sugarcane, and beets.

Role in CVD

Supplemental CoQ_{10} has been reported in diverse studies to have cardioprotective, cytoprotective, and neuroprotective activities. CoQ_{10} has been studied in patients with systolic and/or diastolic dysfunction CHF.

Langsjoen et al. *(25)* evaluated the effect of daily 100 mg of CoQ_{10} for 5 yr in a noncontrolled study of 126 patients with mean ejection fraction of 41%. The authors reported an overall improvement of EF in 87% of patients, 71% of whom achieved a significant improvement after 3 mo of therapy and 16% in 6 mo. Furhtermore, this study also demonstrated the absence of any adverse effects of CoQ_{10} supplementation for 6 yr. The same authors *(26)* also reported the beneficial effects of CoQ_{10} in 109 patients with hypertension and isolated diastolic dysfunction. CoQ_{10} supplementation resulted in improved diastolic function, clinical improvement, and lowering of blood pressure, with resultant regression of left ventricular hypertrophy. Another controlled study by Hoffman-Bang et al. *(27)* showed significant improvement in terms of exercise capacity and quality of life (QOL) in patients with heart failure with additional therapy with CoQ_{10}, when compared with patients on conventional therapy. Folkers et al. *(28)* reported the safety of CoQ_{10} in patients awaiting cardiac transplantation with improvement in their functional class and proposed that this would allow a longer waiting period for a donor heart. Baggio et al. *(29)* did the largest, multicenter, noncontrolled study in 2664 patients with NYHA class II and III CHF. There was a significant improvement in clinical signs and symptoms of heart failure at the end of 3 mo of CoQ_{10} therapy. In a Scandinavian multicenter study of 79 patients *(30)*, CoQ_{10} resulted in slight improvement in EF, increased maximal exercise capacity, and a decrease in scoring for leg fatigue and dyspnea. It also significantly improved the QOL ($p = 0.016$).

Several studies have demonstrated no beneficial effects of CoQ_{10} supplementation. Khatta et al. *(31)* performed a small (55 patient) randomized clinical trial on the effect of CoQ_{10}. There was no increase in ejection fraction, oxygen consumption, or exercise duration. Watson et al. *(32)* also failed to demonstrate any improvement in resting left ventricular systolic function or QOL with oral CoQ_{10} in 27 patients with CHF.

Kamikawa et al. *(33)* reported the beneficial effect of CoQ_{10} in 12 patients with chronic stable angina. In this small double-blinded, placebo-controlled, randomized crossover study, oral CoQ_{10} administration was associated with reduced frequency of angina and lesser use of nitroglycerine. There was also a significant increase in exercise time ($p < 0.05$), with delay in the onset of ST-segment depression ($p < 0.01$), when compared with the placebo group.

Being an essential cofactor for oxidative metabolism in heart, CoQ_{10} plays a role in myocardial preservation during heart surgery. Judy et al. *(34)* studied the effect of CoQ_{10} supplementation in 10 high-risk patients 14 d before and 30 d after heart surgery. Beneficial effects of CoQ_{10} supplementation were evident, as measured by myocardial ATP, cardiac function, postoperative recovery time, and course. Chen et al. *(35)* also noted a presevatory role of preoperative CoQ_{10} in 11 patients who were undergoing heart surgery.

In summary, CoQ_{10} supplementation may have a potential beneficial role in patients with CHF, angina, and myocardial preservation during cardiac surgery. However, the conflicting outcomes from a small group of well-designed studies leave the significance of its effect uncertain.

Trade names: Lynae CoQ10 (Boscogen), Natures Blend Coenzyme Q10 (National Vitamin Company), and Ultra CoQ10 (Twinlab)
Adverse reactions: Nausea, epigastric distress, and diarrhea
Contraindications: None known
Usual dosage: 30–300 mg/d

CARNITINE

Carnitine is an amino acid derivative that is found in all body cells, especially striated muscles. It is synthesized in the liver, kidneys, and brain from the amino acids lysine and methionine. Two analogs of carnitine, acetyl-L-carnitine (ALC) and propionyl-L-carnitine (PLC), have been used. Carnitine plays an important role in the transport of free fatty acids (FFA) across the inner mitochondrial membranes for ATP production. As a cofactor, carnitine enhances carbohydrate metabolism and reduces toxic metabolites produced during ischemic conditions. Although its approved indications are primary/secondary carnitine deficiencies, it is widely used in multiple cardiovascular conditions.

Role in CVD

L-carnitine may beneficially affect cardiac function and also may have cardioprotective activity resulting from its antioxidant effects. It may also lower, to a variable extent, the plasma triglycerides and elevate high-density lipoprotein (HDL)-cholesterol levels.

Both free and total myocardial carnitine levels are reduced during periods of prolonged acute ischemia. This is noted significantly in the ischemic zone, and mild reductions are noted in the adjacent nonischemic areas. This reduction is associated with a significant elevation in FFAs and toxic ester levels, with a reduction in ATP and creatine phosphate. These intracellular changes in the ischemic myocardium can result in a poor outcome after acute myocardial infarction (AMI). It has been suggested that carnitine supplementation may mitigate ischemic injury. The beneficial effects may include enhanced glucose oxidation, preservation of myocardial carnitine, reduction in loss of high-energy phosphates, and reduction in the accumulation of toxic esters. These metabolic changes could translate into better clinical outcomes, such as reduction in cardiac arrhythmias, preservation of myocardial function, and ST elevation *(36)*.

There are few trials suggesting the beneficial role of carnitine in patients with acute myocardial infarction. Rebuzzi et al. *(37)* found that L-carnitine reduced the extent of myocardial infarction if given within 8 h of symptom onset. The CEDIM (L-Carnitine Ecocardiografia Digitalizzata Infarto Miocardico) trial *(38)* studied patients after their first anterior wall myocardial infarction. In this double-blind, randomized controlled trial, 472 patients were treated with either L-carnitine (iv for 5 d, followed by orally) or a placebo for 12 mo. Although there was no change in overall ejection fractions, there were significant reductions in left ventricular diastolic and systolic dimension in the active group. The incidence of death or CHF was 6% with carnitine vs 9.6% with placebo [p = ns]. L-carnitine has been also studied in post-myocardial infarction (MI) patients. Davini et al. *(39)* showed a significant decrease in mortality with carnitine (1.2% vs 12.5%, $p < 0.005$) at 1-yr follow-up. However, this was an open trial. Lack of blinding and higher number of hypertensive patients in the control arm may make the results unreliable. Carnitine also plays a protective role in patients with ischemic heart disease. Corbucci et al. *(40)* demonstrated the absence of ischemic changes in the carnitine group vs the control group in 120 patients undergoing extracorporeal circulation (ECC) during aortopulmonary bypass surgery. Levels of lactate, pyruvate, and succinate/fumarate ratio, reflective of glycolytic cellular metabolism, were measured before and after ECC. These levels remained in the normal range in patients with supplemental carnitine when compared to the placebo group.

Several small, uncontrolled studies have noted a lower systemic vascular resistance, an augmented ionotropic state, and enhanced lactate extraction as a consequence of carnitine treatment *(36)*. If confirmed, these reported hemodynamic effects would suggest a role in CHF treatment. It is well documented that carnitine deficiency causes dilated cardiomyopathy, along with skeletal myopathy. In selected studies, supplementation has led to significant responses. Mancini et al. *(41)* studied 60 patients with CHF (EF < 50%, NYHA class II or III) for 180 d. Patients received 500 mg/3 times a day of PLC or placebo. The only other medications included digoxin and diuretics. There was significant improvement in exercise times (increased by 26%) and ejection fractions (increased by 14%). In an other larger study of 574 patients with heart failure and EF < 40%, exercise tolerance was significantly improved in the carnitine group when compared with placebo *(42)*. However, the carnitine group demonstrated a slightly higher mortality (3.0% vs 1.9%) and a higher admission rate (6.3% vs 5.3%). Romagnoli et al. *(43)* studied the effects of L-carnitine in patients undergoing dialysis. Their observational study showed that L-carnitine addition to conventional therapy resulted in overall improved clinical status, with increased mean ejection fraction from 32% to 41.8 % ($p < 0.05$) and reduction in erythropoietin dosage.

Carnitine supplementation has also been noted to reduce the levels of free FFA and triglycerides in clinical studies *(44)*. However, the mechanism is not clear. Larger clinical trails are needed to verify the lipid-lowering effects of carnitine.

Lower carnitine levels have been found in the muscle biopsies of patients undergoing revascularization procedure for severe peripheral vascular disease (PVD). In a double-blind, placebo-controlled, dose-titration, multicenter trial, Brevetti et al. *(45)* have shown that active treatment with PLC significantly improved maximum walking distance and time to onset of symptoms with minimal adverse side effects in 245 patients with PVD.

Palazuoli et al. *(46)* have also shown that L-carnitine reduced anti-arrhythmic activity of the ischemic myocardium in 30 patients with ischemic heart disease. Patients were divided into three groups (carnitine group, propafenone group, and carnitine + propafenone group). The carnitine group showed significant reduction in arrhythmic activity, measured by extrasystolic ventricular multifocal beats. This response was further substantiated in the combination group.

The results of clinical studies of carnitine and its derivatives in ischemic heart disease (IHD) and PVD therapy should be the subject of a large, randomized, controlled clinical trial. The role in CHF is equivocal, and the report of an increased mortality and admission rate associated with an improved ejection fraction should limit its use pending further studies.

> *Trade names*: Carnitor, Proxeed (Sigma-Tau), Carni Fuel, Mega L-Car
> nitine (Twin Lab), and Maximal Burner Carnitine (Bricker Labs)
> *Adverse reactions*: Nausea, vomiting, abdominal cramps, diarrhea,
> myasthenia, and seizure activity
> *Contraindications*: None known
> *Usual study dosage*: 20 mg–2 g/d

N-ACETYLCYSTEINE

N-Acetylcysteine (NAC) is the *N*-acetyl derivative of the protein amino acid L-cysteine. It is available as a nutritional supplement and as a drug. It is an excellent source of sulfhydryl (SH) group. NAC is a reducing agent and acts directly as free radical scavengers. It is also a mucolytic and hepatoprotectant and may have antiapoptotic activity. NAC has been mainly used as an effective antidote for acetaminophen poisoning.

Role in CVD

Gavish et al. *(47)* suggested that NAC could cause the reduction of lipoprotein(a), a complex of low-density lipoproteins (LDLs) that is associated with increased risk for atherosclerosis and thrombosis. In their report of two patients, there was a 70% reduction in Lp(a) levels. Two studies have also suggested the lowering of serum homocysteine levels with NAC administration of NAC *(48,49)*.

Horowitz et al. *(50)* have also demonstrated that NAC potentiated the hemodynamic responsiveness to nitroglycerine in 10 patients. The proposed mechanism is that guanylate cyclase activation by nitroglycerine is modulated by SH availability. NAC is a potential SH group donor and hence can enhance the intracellular concentration of cGMP. This leads to smooth muscle relaxation and vasodilation. This may suggest a role for NAC in patients who are refractory to NTG or for potentiation of NTG effects. Ardissino et al. *(51)* studied the effect of NTG in combination with NAC in 200 patients. End-point events included death, myocardial infarction, and refractory angina requiring revascularization. When used in combination with NAC, NTG was associated with 13% end-point events, as compared to 31% when used alone or 39% in those receiving placebo ($p = 0.0052$). There was higher incidence of side effects, especially headache (31% of patients) in the combination group.

In a small randomized trial *(52)* of 83 patients with chronic renal insufficiency (creatinine > 2.5 mg/dL), acetylcysteine resulted in a 10-fold reduction in contrast induced nephropathy (CIN) compared to placebo (2% vs 21%, $p = 0.01$). Postulated beneficial effects have been attributed to the vasodilatory and antioxidant properties of acetylcysteine, resulting in improved renal hemodynamics and preventing direct damage to tubules.

In summary, NAC may have a potential use in combination with NTG to potentiate its effects and reverse the nitrate tolerance. It is now used in patients with creatine more than 2.5 mg/dL who are undergoing cardiac catheterization or PCI to reduce nephrotoxicity.

> *Trade names*: NAC fuel (Twin Lab), N-A-C Sustain (Jarrow Formula), and Mucomyst (Apothecon)
> *Adverse reactions*: Nausea, vomiting, diarrhea, rashes, and headache with oral NAC; iv NAC could cause bronchospasm, stomatitis, rhinorrhea, tinnitus, chills, and fever in addition to gastrointestinal (GI) symptoms with oral dose
> *Contraindications*: None known
> *Usual dosage*: 600 mg, 3 times/d

CREATINE

Creatine is an amino acid, with 95% of its body concentration present in the skeletal muscles. It is mainly synthesized in the liver and kidneys from arginine and glycine. It plays an important role in the rapid phosphorylation of adenosine 5'-diphosphate (ADP) to adenosine triphosphate (ADT). Higher skeletal muscle levels are associated with improved muscle performance.

Role in CVD

Studies have reported reduced levels of creatine contents in the skeletal muscles of patients with CHF. In a study of 17 patients, Gordon et al. *(53)* reported a significant improvement in exercise performance (strength and endurance) in patients with CHF. There was no reported change in the ejection fractions. Andrews et al. *(54)* studied the effects of creatine supplementation (20 g/d) in patients with CHF ($n = 10$), compared with the placebo group ($n = 10$). The creatine group showed a significant increase in skeletal muscle endurance and an improvement in the metabolic responses to exercise in muscle groups, which were impaired because of CHF.

> *Trade names*: Creatine Fuel (Twin Lab), Muscle Power (Mason Vitamins), Creatine Booster (Champion Nutrition), Power Creatine (Champion Nutrition), Crea-Tek (Iron Tek), Creavescent (GEN), Phosphagen (GNC), Creatigen (Bricker Labs), Perfect Creatine (Nature's Best), and Xtra Advantage Creatine Serum (Muscle Marketing USA)
>
> *Adverse reactions*: Nausea, vomiting, diarrhea, rashes, fatigue, seizure, migraine, polymyositis, anxiety, nervousness, myopathy, and atrial fibrillation
>
> *Contraindications*: Renal failure or renal disorders, such as nephritic syndrome
>
> *Usual dosage*: Loading dose of 20 g followed by 2 g/d

GLUTATHIONE

Glutathione is typically used as a collective term to refer to the tripeptide L-γ-glutamyl-L-cysteinylglycine in both its reduced and its dimeric forms. It is primarily synthesized in the liver. Glutathione is involved in DNA synthesis and repair, protein and prostaglandin synthesis, amino acid transport, prevention of oxidative cell damage, and enzyme activation. It is present in fruits, vegetables, and meat products, but body levels do not correlate with dietary intake.

Role in CVD

Glutathione is a potent antioxidant agent that reduces inactivation of endothelial-derived NO and enhances NO activity *(55)*. Atherosclerosis of coronary and peripheral circulation is associated with reduced NO basal and stimulated activity. Low total serum glutathione (tGSH) levels have been reported in male offspring of parents with premature CHD, suggesting that it as a significant independent predictor of parental CHD *(56)*. Prasad et al. *(57)* have demonstrated that glutathione supplementation resulted in improved human endothelial function. Its infusion also suppresses the vasoconstrictor response of epicardial vessels to acetylcholine of patients with spastic angina. This phenomenon of enhanced NO bioavailability by glutathione or related thiol substances suggests a potential role for this nutrachemical supplement.

S-nitrosoglutathione is an NO donor with preferential action on platelets. Langford et al. *(58)* demonstrated a significant inhibition in the coronary angioplasty-induced increase in platelet surface expression of P-selectin and glycoprotein IIb/IIIa with glutathione administration resulting in platelet inhibition in seven patients undergoing angioplasty. In a subsequent report, the same authors *(59)* verified these results in 40 patients presenting with AMI (*n* = 20) and unstable angina (*n* = 20).

Platelet inhibition and improved endothelial-mediated vasomotion of atherosclerotic vessels by glutathione suggest a role in acute coronary syndromes or PCI. However, there have, been no appropriate studies in that regard.

Adverse reactions: None reported
Contraindications: Hypersensitivity
Usual dosage: 50–60 mg/d

SELENIUM

Selenium is an essential trace element. It enters the food chain through incorporation into plant protein via the soil. It has structural and enzymic roles, and it is a powerful antioxidant, regulating the activity of the glutathione peroxidase enzymes, which catalyze the detoxification of peroxide and organic hydroperoxides. It has been mostly used to reduce cancer-related mortality.

Role in CVD

Selenium deficiency is a rare cause of dilated, congestive cardiomyopathy. In Asia and Africa, cardiomyopathy resulting from dietary selenium deficiency is known as Keshan disease *(60)*. It is usually seen in patients with malabsorption or long-term selenium-deficient parenteral alimentation. Selenium deficiency leads to depletion of the enzymes that protect cell membranes from free radicals. Once fully developed, cardiomyopathy is irreversible. Prophylactic administration of sodium selenite tablets prevents new cases of cardiomyopathy in selenium-deficient geographic areas.

Selenium deficiency has also been reported to promote platelet aggregation *(61)*. This deficiency inhibits prostacyclin synthetase, causing reduced prostacyclin and increased thromboxane activity, which is a vasoconstrictor and platelet aggregator. Correlation between low selenium levels and increased MI has been reported *(62)*, and some reports have suggested the protective role of high serum selenium levels. However, in the Physicians' Health Study, Salvini et al. *(63)* failed to reveal any association between high plasma selenium levels and reduced risk of MI in 251 patients.

A clinical role of selenium supplementation, other than in selenium-deficient cardiomyopathy, is not currently supported by existing studies.

> *Trade names*: Sele-Pak (Solopak Laboratories), Selepen (American Pharmaceutical Parners), Selenium Oceanic (Freeda Vitamins), and Selenomax (Mason Vitamins)
> *Adverse reactions*: Hair and nail brittleness and loss, skin rash, fatigue, irritability, nausea, and garlic-like breath
> *Contraindications*: Hypersensitivity
> *Usual dosage*: 50–200 mg/d

RESVERATROL

Resveratrol is a phytoalexin. It is produced by plants that are responding to injury or fungal infection. It is present in vines, seeds, roots, and stalks, with higher concentration in grape skins. Resveratrol is mainly found in red vine, purple grape juice, mulberries, and peanuts. White vine contains a small amount of resveratrol.

Role in CVD

Resveratrol may have cardioprotective effects; some studies have suggested its antioxidant, antiinflammatory, and antiplatelet aggregation effects. Wang et al. *(64)* demonstrated the inhibition of ADP-induced platelet aggregation in rabbits and normal subjects by resveratrol. Moderate consumption of red vine is reported to be associated with reduced morbidity and mortality from CHD. The potential cardioprotective effect of red wine is attributed to resveratrol. Better controlled randomized studies are needed to evaluate the efficacy of resveratrol in preventing and ameliorating atherosclerosis.

> *Trade name*: Protykin Resveratrol (Natrol) and Resveratrol Antioxidant Protection (Source Naturals)
> *Adverse reactions*: None reported
> *Contraindications*: Hypersensitivity
> *Usual dosage*: 16 mg/d

PANTETHINE

Pantethine is a more active metabolic form of the vitamin B_5, commonly known as pantothenic acid. Pantethine constitutes the active part of the coenzyme A molecule and acyl carrier proteins (ACP).

Role in CVD

Although pantethine has no direct cardiovascular effects, it is believed to be a potent hypolipidemic agent. Gaddi et al. *(65)* studied the effect of pantethine (300 mg/3 times a day) in 29 patients with type IIb and IV hyperlipidemia for 8 wk in a double-blind protocol. Pantethine caused significant reduction in total cholesterol and low-density lipoprotein (LDL) cholesterol. It also elevated HDL cholesterol. Eto et al. *(66)* reported the effects of 9-mo therapy with pantethine in 16 patients with diabetes. The therapy group showed a significant reduction in plasma β-thromboglobulin, triglycerides, total cholesterol, LDL cholesterol, apo-E, and apo-CII levels. It also reduced platelets aggregability.

CONCLUSION

Some evidence discussed in this chapter suggests a favorable effect of nutrachemical supplementation in the prevention and treatment of certain cardiovascular disorders. Large, long-term controlled randomized studies are needed to evaluate their effect on patients and their interaction with conventional therapy before clinical use. To date, potential safety issues have been noted with carnitine in a small clinical trial. The long-term safety of other nutraceuticals is uncertain, given the absence of large long-term clinical trials.

REFERENCES

1. Lerman A, Burnett JC, Higano ST, McKinley LJ, Holmes DR, Jr. Long-term L-arginine supplementation improves small-vessel coronary endothelial function in humans. Circulation 1998;97:2123–2128.
2. Blum A, Porat R, Rosenchein U, et al. Clinical and inflammatory effects of dietary L-arginine in patients with intractable angina pectoris. Am J Cardiol 1999;15:1488–1490.
3. Adams MR, McCredie R, Jessup W, Robinson J, Sullivan D, Celermajer DS. Oral L-arginine improves endothelium-dependent dilatation and reduces monocyte adhesion to endothelial cells in young men with coronary artery disease. Atherosclerosis 1997;129:261–269.
4. Bednarz B, Wolk R, Chamiec T, Herbaczynska-Cedro K, Winek D, Ceremuzynski L. Effects of oral L-arginine supplementation on exercise-induced QT dispersion and exercise tolerance in stable angina pectoris. Int J Cardiol 2000;75:205–210.
5. Blum A, Hathaway L, Mincemoyer R, et al. Oral L-arginine in patients with coronary artery disease on medical management. Circulation 2000;101:2160–2164.
6. Quyyumi AA. Does acute improvement of endothelial dysfunction in coronary artery disease improve myocardial ischemia? A double-blind comparison of parenteral D- and L-arginine. J Am Coll Cardiol 1998;32:904–911.
7. Boger RH, Bode-Boger SM, Thiele W, Alexander K, Frolich JC. Biochemical evidence for impaired nitric oxide synthesis in patients with peripheral arterial occlusive disease. Circulation 1997;95:2068–2074.

8. Boger RH, Bode-Boger SM, Thiele W, Creutzig A, Alexander K, Frolich JC. Restoring vascular nitric oxide formation by L-arginine improves the symptoms of intermittent claudication in patients with peripheral arterial occlusive disease. J Am Coll Cardiol 1998;32:1336–1344.
9. Katz AD, Khan T, Zeballos GA, et al. Decreased activity of the L-arginine-nitric oxide metabolic pathway in patients with congestive heart failure. Circulation 1999;99:2113–2117.
10. Bocchi EA, Moraes AV, Esteves-Filho A, et al. L-arginine reduces heart rate and improves hemodynamics in severe congestive heart failure. Clin Cardiol 2000;23:205–210.
11. Rector TS, Bank AJ, Mullen KA, et al. Randomized, double-blind, placebo-controlled study of supplemental oral L-arginine in patients with heart failure. Circulation 1996;93:2135–2141.
12. Koifman B, Wollman Y, Bogomolny N, et al. Improvement of cardiac performance by intravenous infusion of L-arginine in patients with moderate congestive heart failure. J Am Coll Cardiol 1995;26:1251–1256.
13. Hambrecht R, Hilbrich L, Erbs S, et al. Correction of endothelial dysfunction in chronic heart failure: additional effects of exercise training and oral L-arginine supplementation. J Am Coll Cardiol 2000;35:706–713.
14. Suzuki T, Hayase M, Hibi K, et al. Effect of local delivery of L-arginine on in-stent restenosis in humans. Am J Cardiol 2002;89:363–367.
15. Creager MA, Gallagher SJ, Girerd XJ, Coleman SM, Dzau VJ, Cook JP. L-arginine improves endothelial dependent vasodilation in hypercholesterolemic humans. J Clin Invest 1992;90:1248–1253.
16. Boger RH, Bode-Boger SM, Brandes RP, et al. Dietary L-arginine reduces the progression of atherosclerosis in cholesterol-fed rabbits. Circulation 1997;96:1282–1290.
17. Toutouzas PC, Tousoulis D, Davies GJ. Nitric oxide synthesis in atherosclerosis. Eur Heart J 1998;19:1504–1511.
18. Mohri M, Ichiki T, Hirooka Y, Takeshita A. Endogenous nitric oxide prevents myocardial ischemia in patients with hypertension and left ventricular hypertrophy. Am Heart J 2002;143:684–689.
19. Houghton JL, Philbin EF, Strogatz DS, et al. The presence of African American race predicts improvement in coronary endothelial function after supplementary L-arginine. J Am Coll Cardiol 2002;39:1314–1322.
20. Azuma J, Sawamura A, Awata N, et al. Therapeutic effect of taurine in congestive heart failure: a double-blind cross over trial. Clin Cardiol 1985;8:276–282.
21. Azuma J, Sawamura A, Awata N. Usefulness of taurine in chronic heart failure and its prospective application. Jap Circ J 1992;56:95–99.
22. Jeejeebhoy F, Keith M, Freeman M, et al. Nutritional supplementation with MyoVive repletes essential cardiac myocyte nutrients and reduces left ventricular size in patients with left ventricular dysfunction. Am Heart J 2002;143:1092–1100.
23. Nonaka H, Tsujino T, Watari Y, Emoto N, Yokoyama M. Taurine prevents the decrease in expression and secretion of extracellular superoxide dismutase induced by homocysteine. Amelioration of homocysteine-induced endoplasmic reticulum stress by taurine. Circulation 2001;104:1165–1170.
24. Yamori Y, Nara Y, Ikeda K, Mizushima S. Is taurine a preventive nutritional factor of cardiovascular diseases or just a biological marker of nutrition? Adv Exp Med Biol 1996;403:623–629.
25. Langsjoen PH, Langsjoen PH, Folkers K. Long-term efficacy and safety of coenzyme Q10 therapy for idiopathic dilated cardiomyopathy. Am J Cardiol 1990;65:512–523.

26. Langsjoen PH, Langsjoen PH, Folkers K. Isolated diastolic dysfunction of the myocardium and its response to CoQ10 treatment. Clin Invest 1993;71:S140–144.

27. Hoffman-Bang C, Rehnqvist N, Swedberg K, Astrom H. Coenzyme Q_{10} as an adjunctive in treatment of congestive heart failure. Am J Cardiol 1992;19(Suppl):216A.

28. Folkers K, Langsjoen PH, Langsjoen PH. Therapy with coenzyme Q_{10} of patients in heart failure who are eligible or ineligible for a transplant. Biochem Biophys Res Comm 1992;182:247–253.

29. Baggio E, Gandini R, Placher AC, Passeri M, Carmosino G. Italian multicenter study on safety and efficacy of coenzyme Q_{10}. Mol Aspect Med 1994;15:S287–S294.

30. Hoffman-Bang C, Rehnqvist N, Swedberg K, Wiklund I, Astrom H for the CoQ$_{10}$ study group. Coenzyme Q10 as an adjunctive in the treatment of chronic congestive heart failure. J Card Fail 1995;1:101–107.

31. Khatta M, Alexander BS, Krichten CM, et al. The effect of coenzyme Q_{10} in patients with congestive heart failure. Ann Intern Med 2000;132:636–640.

32. Watson PS, Scalia GM, Galbraith A, Burstow DJ, Bett N, Aroney CN. Lack of effect of coenzyme Q_{10} on left ventricular function in patients with congestive heart failure. J Am Coll Cardiol 1999;33:1549–1552.

33. Kamikawa T, Kobayashi A, Yamashita T, Hayashi H, Yamazaki N. Effects of coenzyme Q10 on exercise tolerance in chronic stable angina pectoris. Am J Cardiol 1985;56:247–251.

34. Judy WV, Stogsdill WW, Folkers K. Myocardial preservation by therapy with coenzyme Q_{10} during heart surgery. Clin Investig 1993;71:S155–161.

35. Chen YF, Lin YT, Wu SC. Effectiveness of coenzyme Q_{10} on myocardial preservation during hypothermic cardioplegic arrest. J Thorac Cardiovasc Surg 1994;107:242–247.

36. Arsenian MA. Carnitine and its derivatives in cardiovascular disease. Prog Cardiovasc Dis 1997;40:265–286.

37. Rebuzzi AG, Schiavoni G, Amico CM, et al. Beneficial effect of L-carnitine in the reduction of nectrotic area in acute myocardial infarction. Drugs Exp Clin Res 1984;10:219–223.

38. Iliceto S, Scrutinio D, Bruzzi P, et al. Effect of L-carnitine administration on left ventricular remodeling after acute anterior myocardial infarction: the L-Carnitine Ecocardiografia Digitalizzata Infarto Miocardico (CEDIM) trial. J Am Coll Cardiol 1995;26:380–387.

39. Davini P, Bigalli A, Lamanna F, Boem A. Controlled study on L-carnitine therapeutic efficacy in post-infarction. Drugs Exp Clin Res 1992;18:335–365.

40. Corbucci GG, Menichetti A, Cogliatti A, Nicoli P, Ruvolo C. Metabolic aspects of acute tissue hypoxia during extracorporeal circulation and their modification induced by L-carnitine treatment. Int J Clin Pharmacol Res 1992;12:149–157.

41. Mancini M, Rengo F, Lingetti M, Sorrentino GP, Nolfe G. Controlled study on the therapeutic efficacy of propionyl-L-carnitine in patients with congestive heart failure. Arzneimittel-Forschung 1992;42:1101–1104.

42. De Giuli F, Pasini E, Opasich C, Mazzoletti A, Ferrari R. Effects of propionyl-L-carnitine in patients with heart failure (abstract). J Mol Cell Cardiol 1995;27:V44.

43. Romagnoli GF, Naso A, Carraro G, Lidestri V. Beneficial effects of L-carnitine in dialysis patients with impaired left ventricular function; an observational study. Curr Med Res Opin 2002;18:172–175.

44. Ghidini O, Azzuro M, Vita G, Sartori G. Evaluation of therapeutic efficacy of L-carnitine in congestive heart failure. Int J Clin Pharmacol Ther Toxicol 1988;26:217–220.

45. Brevetti G, Perna S, Sabba C, Martone VD, Condorelli M. Propionyl-L-carnitine in intermittent claudication: double-blind, placebo-controlled, dose titration, multicenter study. J Am Coll Cardiol 1995;26:1411–1416.
46. Palazzuli V, Mondillo S, Faglia S, D'Aprile N, Camporeale A, Gennari C. The evaluation of antiarrhythmic activity of L-carnitine and propafenone in ischemic cardiomyopathy. Clinica Therapeutica 1993;142:155–159.
47. Gavish D, Breslow JL. Lipoprotein(a) reduction by N-acetylcysteine. Lancet 1991;337:203–204.
48. Wiklund O, Fager G, Andersson A, Lundstam U, Masson P, Hultberg B. N-acetylcysteine treatment lowers plasma homocysteine but not serum lipoprotein(a) levels. Atherosclerosis 1996;119:99–106.
49. Bostom AG, Shemin D, Yoburn D, Fisher DH, Nadeau MR, Selhub J. Lack of effect of oral N-acetylcysteine on the acute dialysis-related lowering of total plasma homocysteine in hemodialysis patients. Atherosclerosis 1996;120:241–244.
50. Horowitz JD, Antman EM, Lorell BH, Barry WH, Smith TW. Potentiation of cardio-vascular effect of nitroglycerine by N-acetylcysteine. Circulation 1983;68:1247–1253.
51. Ardissino D, Merlini PA, Savonitto S, et al. Effect of transdermal nitroglycerine or N-acetylcysteine, or both, in the long-term treatment of unstable angina pectoris. J Am Coll Cardiol 1997;29:941–947.
52. Tepel M, Giet M, Schwarzfeld C, Laufer U, Liermann D, Zidek W. Prevention of radiographic-contrast-agent-induced reductions in renal function by acetylcysteine. N Engl J Med 2000;343:180–184.
53. Gordon A, Hultman E, Kaijser L, et al. Creatine supplementation in chronic heart failure increases skeletal muscle creatine phosphate and muscle performance. Cardiovasc Res 1995;30:413–418.
54. Andrews R, Greenhaff P, Curtis S, Perry A, Cowley AJ. The effect of dietary creatine supplementation on skeletal muscle metabolism in congestive heart failure. Eur Heart J 1998;19:617-622.
55. Stamler JS, Slivka A. Biological chemistry of thiols in vasculature and in vascular-related diseases. Nutr Rev 1996;54:1–30.
56. Morrison JA, Jacobsen DW, Sprecher DL, Robinson K, Khoury P, Daniels SR. Serum glutathione in adolescent males predicts parental coronary heart disease. Circulation 1999;100(22):2244–2247.
57. Prasad A, Andrews NP, Padder FA, Husain M, Quyyumi AA. Glutathione reverses endothelial dysfunction and improves nitric oxide bioavailability. J Am Coll Cardiol 1999;34:507–514.
58. Langford EJ, Brown AS, Wainwright RJ, et al. Inhibition of platelet activity by S-nitrosoglutathione during coronary angioplasty. Lancet 1994;344:1458–1460.
59. Langford EJ, Wainwright RJ, Martin JF. Platelet activation in acute myocardial infarction and unstable angina is inhibited by nitric oxide donors. Arterioscl Thromb Vasc Biol 1996;16:51–55.
60. Burke MP, Opeskin K. Fulminant heart failure due to selenium deficiency cardi-omyopathy (Keshan disease). Med Sci Law 2002;42:10–13.
61. Neve J. Selenium as a risk factor for cardiovascular diseases. J Cardiovasc Risk 1996;3:42–47.
62. Kok FJ, Hofman A, Witteman JC, et al.Decreased selenium levels in acute myocar-dial infarction. JAMA 1989;263:949–950.
63. Salvini S, Hennekens CH, Morris S, Willett WC, Stampfer MJ. Plasma levels of the antioxidant selenium and risk of myocardial infarction among U.S. Physicians. Am J Cardiol 1995;76:1218–1221.

64. Wang Z, Zou J, Huang Y, Cao K, Xu Y, Wu JM. Effect of resveratrol on platelet aggregation in vivo and in vitro. Chin Med J 2002;115:378–380.
65. Gaddi A, Descovich GC, Noseda G, et al. Controlled evaluation of pantethine, a natural hypolipidemic compound, in patients with different forms of hyperlipoproteinemia. Atherosclerosis 1984;50:73–83.
66. Eto M, Watanabe K, Chonan N. Lowering effect of pantethine on plasma B-thromboglobulin and lipids in diabetes mellitus. Artery 1987;15:1–12.
67. *PDR* for Nutritional Supplements (Hendler SS, Rorvik D, eds.). Montvale, NJ, Economics Company Inc., 2001.

8 Meditation and Cardiovascular Disease

Erin L. Olivo, *PhD*

THE MIND–BODY CONNECTION

The connection between the mind and body is a concept that is increasingly being accepted in mainstream Western culture. Technological advances have made it possible to understand and map the connection among emotion, mood, and biology. As a result, we now have a mounting body of evidence that supports the link between psychological state, autonomic activity, and the development of coronary heart disease (CHD) *(1–6)*. This basic mind–brain–body paradigm has been diagrammatically represented by Sloan et al. *(7)*, as seen in Fig. 1 below. In this model, the autonomic nervous system is seen as a factor linking psychology and chronic stress to CHD development and outcome.

Paralleling the advances in our understanding of the role of stress and psychology in disease processes is the research conducted to find potential interventions in this mind–brain–body paradigm. Scientific evidence supports the use of various mind–body techniques to favorably alter various physiologic and psychological aspects of health, particularly

From: *Contemporary Cardiology*
Complementary and Alternative Cardiovascular Medicine
Edited by: R. A. Stein and M. C. Oz © Humana Press Inc., Totowa, NJ

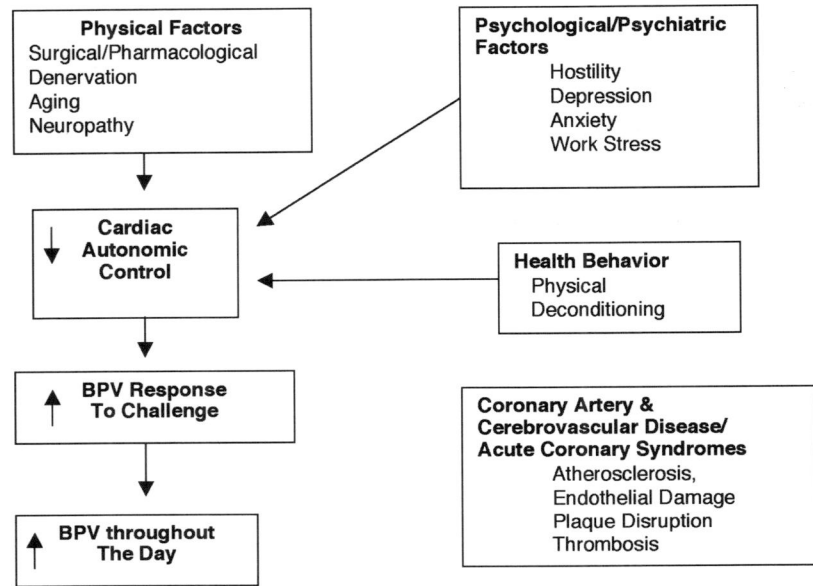

Fig. 1. The mind–brain–body paradigm *(7)*.

regarding cardiovascular risk factors and stress *(8,9)*. The medical use
of these interventions, which can be generally categorized under the
label of complementary and alternative medicine (CAM), has increased
significantly during the last decade *(10,11)*. This interest is reflected in
the active use of such therapies by the general public. A study of trends
in the use of CAM approaches in the United States in the past decade
indicate that an approx 42% of the public reported use of CAM therapies
in 1997 *(12)*. This same trend can be found in cardiac surgery patients.
Of the cardiac surgery patients surveyed at Columbia Presbyterian
Medical Center (New York) in 1998, 75% reported having used at least
one form of alternative treatment in the previous 12 mo *(13)*. In addition,
it is likely that these rates of usage are on the rise, because CAM therapies are increasingly being popularized by mainstream media.

MEDITATION AS A MIND–BODY INTERVENTION

One of the most widely used and well-studied CAM therapies is
meditation. Although there are many variations of meditative practice,
meditation can be broadly defined as any activity that involves the controlled regulation of attention. One of the primary benefits of meditation
is the achievement of a "relaxation response," a term coined by Herbert
Benson to describe the hypometabolic changes, such as reduction in

oxygen consumption, increased galvanic skin resistance, and decreased heart rate, respiration rate, and blood pressure, associated with a state of decreased sympathetic nervous system activity (8,9).

Meditative practice dates back centuries and its origin is in several largely Eastern spiritual traditions. Regardless of its religious origin, meditation's primary goal is to achieve a state of consciousness described as "restful alertness," which in the various traditions is known as "jhana," "samadhi," "nirvana," or "enlightenment" (14,15). Although religious in origin, the basic principles of meditative practice need not be practiced in a spiritual context. Indeed, healthcare professionals who are currently applying meditation as a mind–body intervention for their patients are doing so independently of their spiritual or religious origins.

There are two general forms of meditation, and each has slightly different methods and goals: concentration meditation, exemplified by transcendental meditation (TM) and mindfulness meditation (MM).

Transcendental Meditation

TM is the principal approach for stress reduction and self-development of the traditional comprehensive prevention-oriented natural system of healing know as Maharishi Ayur-Veda. This approach was initially introduced to the West by Maharishi Mahesh Yogi (14,16,17). TM practice requires no changes in lifestyle, personal beliefs, philosophy, diet, or physical activity (16). TM is typically taught either individually or in a group by an instructor who has been trained by Maharishi Mahesh Yogi. This approach focuses on one object: the sensation of breath entering and leaving the body, or a mantra (a sound or phrase that is repeated silently). This is known as the concentration, or "one-pointed," method of meditation, which Buddhists call shamatha or samadhi practices (14). Maharishi describes the nature of this narrowing of attention and the process of TM as "turning the attention inward toward the subtler levels of a thought until the mind transcends the experience of the subtlest state of the thought and arrives at the source of the thought" (18, p. 470).

Students are instructed to maintain a passive attitude throughout the meditation practice. If distracting thoughts or images arise, they are to be disregarded and the meditator's attention should be redirected to the mantra or the breath. The student is also instructed to sit in a comfortable position to minimize the amount of muscular work required during meditation. TM students are typically instructed to practice the technique twice daily for 20-min periods. The overall results of this meditation practice have been described as the development of a distinct psychophysiological state of restful alertness (18,19).

Mindfulness Meditation

Mindfulness is the other major classification of meditation practice, which is also known as *vipassana*, or insight meditation *(14)*. The practice of mindfulness begins with the cultivation of one-pointed attention, as in TM, but then progresses to include a wider scope of observation. Events that arise in the meditator's field of awareness, such as thoughts, feelings, or sensations, are not ignored or suppressed but rather simply noted and observed. This observation is done without judging or analyzing. Mindfulness involves intentional, nonjudgmental, moment-to-moment awareness *(15,20,21)*. Observing events in this way allows the meditator to create some distance between himself or herself and the thought or emotion being experienced. This helps the meditator feel less involved with an emotion or thought and allows for a deeper perspective so that thoughts and feelings are recognized as mental events rather than as necessarily accurate reflections of reality. By observing thoughts and emotions in this more distanced, mindful, and accepting way, an individual can approach a stressful situation with a mindful response rather than automatically reacting to it or engaging in worry or negative thinking that might escalate the stressful situation and lead to increased distress *(15,20–23)*.

One of the most standardized methods of mindfulness training is the Mindfulness-Based Stress Reduction (MBSR) program developed by Jon Kabat-Zinn *(20)*. The first MSBR program was, and still is, conducted through the Stress Reduction Clinic at the University of Massachusetts Medical Center *(20)*. MBSR is a clinical behavioral medicine program that provides systematic mindfulness training to a population with a range of chronic medical and stress related disorders. The program is conducted in a group format. Mixed groups of approx 30 participants meet weekly for 8–10 wk. Group sessions last 2–2.5 h and consist of instruction and practice of MM skills, as well as psychoeducational discussions of stress and coping. The last week is usually conducted as a full-day "retreat." Specific homework assignments are given each week to incorporate and generalize mindfulness practice into everyday life. Mindfulness practice outside of the group usually consists of at least 45 min of practice each day, 6 d/wk. Early in the treatment program participants are given audiotapes that they may use to guide their practice. Participants are instructed in the practice of sitting meditation, meditation using Hatha yoga postures, walking meditation, and the practice of mindfulness during everyday activities, such as eating, washing dishes, or standing *(20–23)*. There are currently an estimated 240 MBSR programs in North America and Europe, and the University of Massachusetts Medical Center is now offering professional training programs for clinicians who are interested in using such interventions with their patients *(23,24)*.

When Kabat-Zinn trains his health care professionals, he cautions them to remember that MM has in both its techniques and its objectives a "non-doing orientation" *(24,* p. 768). There is no objective other than simple awareness of the present moment, which might include pleasant states of relaxation but may also include unpleasant feeling states. Both are to be observed with the same attitude of acceptance and nonjudgment. The goals and attitudes that professionals and patients might have related to the practice and its ability to generate relaxation or relief from suffering are intentionally observed as a part of the practice itself and are also to be regarded with an attitude of nonattachment. Kabat-Zinn highlights that MM in the medical setting contains a paradoxical element. Patients are often referred for mindfulness training for specific reasons and with hopes of achieving specific health related goals, yet, paradoxically, patients are told early in their mindfulness training that "the best way to get somewhere is to try not to get anywhere at all but to simply be where they are already, with awareness" *(24,* p. 769). Kabat-Zinn suggests that progress in MM is best measured by the level of acceptance of the mindfulness process itself and in the patient's increasing ability to face his or her life experience *(24)*.

RESEARCH ON MEDITATION PRACTICE

The scientific research on meditation is extensive. However, much of the research conducted to date has methodological limitations. There are few controlled studies, and, overall, sample sizes have been small. In addition, there is a lack of standardization of what constitutes meditation practice. The lack of clear operational definitions of the various types of meditation leads to ambiguity and difficulty comparing studies. There is often confusion between TM, MM, and relaxation. The ambiguity and overlap of these interventions has made it difficult to isolate the mechanism of change in these practices. Finally, there is a lack of consensus of the training requirements for practitioners delivering the interventions. None of the studies to date has included information about the training of the clinicians, nor does it use clinical adherence or competence measures. Despite these methodological weaknesses, there is mounting evidence to support the use of meditative practice in a medical setting. What is clear is that further, more rigorous research is required. What follows is an overall review of the research in this area. Studies of both TM and MM are included in this review.

Physiologic Impact of Meditation (Nonclinical Samples)

Perhaps the most researched area in meditation has been the physiologic impact of meditative practice. This research represents the earliest studied aspect of meditative practice, dating back to as early as 1935, when French cardiologist Theresa Brosse, traveled to India to study the physiology of meditation *(25)*. Now, more than 50 yr later, there is a strong body of evidence describing both acute and lasting physiologic changes that occur as a result of meditation. Nearly exclusively focused on TM, these studies, as a whole, describe a distinct pattern of physiologic response. The most significant of these results will be reviewed below. For ease of discussion, results have been divided into major physiologic systems or areas. A more complete review of research in this area has been published by Jevning and colleagues *(19)*.

OXYGEN CONSUMPTION AND RESPIRATION

In the early studies of the impact of meditation on respiration, Wallace and colleagues reported a marked decrease in O_2 consumption and CO_2 elimination during a 30-min TM practice, with no change in respiratory quotient (subjects acted as their own controls). A decrease in respiration rate and minute ventilation was also found *(8,26–29)*. As the availability of long-term meditators has increased over time, there have been several more sophisticated studies that have replicated and furthered these findings *(29–32)*. Some researchers found even more marked decreases in respiration and also noted several episodes of respiratory suspension that were linked to a subjective report of an experience of what has been termed "transcendental consciousness" *(30,31)*. These findings sparked further study investigations of the other physiologic changes present in these respiratory suspensions to define and describe this state of "transcendental consciousness" *(31,32)*. These autonomic and biochemical findings will be reviewed below. In addition, several studies compared the respiratory changes found in TM with those found during ordinary rest or relaxed states. These studies found a significant difference in mean declines in respiration between TM and rest or relaxation in nonmeditators *(29,30)*.

ENDOCRINE AND NEUROTRANSMITTER EFFECTS

The overall results of research on the endocrinologic impact of meditation show acute declines in hormones that are implicated in the stress response. Cortisol, thyroid-stimulating hormone (TSH), and growth hormone (GH) all decline during TM practice *(33)*. Several longitudinal studies confirm that these effects are long lasting in subjects who regularly practice meditation *(33–35)*. Several other hormones remained unchanged in either longitudinal or acute TM studies. These include testosterone, insulin, T3, T4, and luteinizing hormone (LH) *(33,35)*.

Studies investigating the impact of meditation on neurotransmitters suggest that the regular practice of meditation has a significant impact on the sympathetic-adrenal medulla system. Michaels and colleagues first reported a nonsignificant acute decrease in catecholamine levels during TM *(36)*. Subsequently, in an advancement of this research, Infante and colleagues conducted a controlled study of catecholamine plasma levels, which considered the impact of circadian cycles and time of day. Infante and colleagues found significantly lower morning and evening norepinephrine levels and morning epinephrine levels in the TM group than in the control subjects *(37)*. Another controlled study investigating the urinary metabolite of serotonin, 5-hydroxyindoleaceatic acid (5-HIAA) found significant increases after 30 min of practicing TM. In addition, throughout the experiment, 5-HIAA levels were higher in meditators than they were in rest subjects *(38)*.

AUTONOMIC EFFECTS

There have been numerous studies investigating the acute and long-term impact of meditation on autonomic activity. The overall results indicate decreased activation and include such findings as increased galvanic skin resistance (GSR), decreased spontaneous electrodermal response (EDR), and decreased heart rate *(8,9,27,28)*. A meta-analysis of 31 studies comparing physiological differences between TM and rest control groups indicated that those subjects who had been practicing TM for a long time exhibited significantly lower baseline levels of spontaneous skin resistance responses, respiration rate, heart rate, and plasma lactate before meditation than comparison subjects did before rest *(39)*.

Yet another group of studies investigated the impact of meditation on recovery from stressful stimulation. Several researchers have reported significantly faster habituation or return to baseline (as measured by GSR, EDR, and heart rate) after exposure to stressful stimuli in meditators as compared to controls *(40,41)*.

HEMODYNAMIC EFFECTS

Hemodynamic variables, such as systolic and diastolic blood pressures cardiac output, and total peripheral resistance (TPR) have also been a focus of study regarding how they are affected by the practice of meditation. Individuals who practice TM have lower resting systolic and diastolic blood pressures than matched controls *(42–44)*. Because blood pressure is the product of cardiac output and TPR, changes in these variables have also been studied during meditation. An investigation of circulation that used dye-dilution and radioactive clearance methods yielded results that demonstrated a small but significant increase in cardiac output (15%) during TM. In perhaps the only controlled study investigating the impact of meditation on TPR, subjects in the TM group exhibited significantly decreased TPR and systolic blood pressure, compared with increases in the eyes-closed relaxation control group *(43)*.

ELECTROENCEPHALOGRAM DURING MEDITATION

Studies of electroencephalogram (EEG) during meditation demonstrate an increase in intensity of slow alpha waves and occasional theta wave activity. Beta and delta waves either decrease or remain constant during meditation *(26,27)*. This pattern has been very well replicated in numerous studies and has been distinguished as different from relaxation *(31,45,46)*. In fact, one study investigated the difference between EEG activity in TM and MM and compared both with relaxation *(46)*. These findings demonstrated significant mean amplitude frequency differences between the two meditation conditions and relaxation at all bandwidths and at numerous cortical sites, as well as significant differences between concentration and mindfulness at all bandwidths. The authors interpreted their results as indicating that TM and MM represent unique forms of consciousness and are not merely varying degrees of a state of relaxation *(46)*.

Impact of Meditation on Cardiac Disease Process and Risk Factors (Clinical)

Clinical research on the health-related outcomes of meditation practice is still in its early development, and there is a need for more controlled studies *(23)*. However, the mounting evidence discussed earlier in this chapter, which indicates that a meditation program can result in the sustained lowering of BP, heart rate, cardiac output, and TPR in nonclinical samples *(8,9,27,28,39,42,43)*, suggests the need for further clinical research .

Schneider and colleagues conducted one of the more rigorous clinical studies on health-related outcome *(47)*. This randomized, controlled, single-blind trial, with 3-mo follow-up, tested the efficacy of two stress-education approaches to the treatment of mild hypertension in older African Americans. Subjects were randomly assigned to one of three study groups: the TM program, progressive muscle relaxation (PMR), or a lifestyle modification education control (EC) program. TM significantly reduced both systolic and diastolic pressures, as did PMR. However, the reductions in systolic and diastolic blood pressures were significantly greater in the TM group than in the PMR group. TM was approximately twice as effective as PMR in reducing blood pressure.

Castillo-Richmond *(48)* studied the same patient population and evaluated the effects of the TM meditation program on carotid intimamedia thickness (IMT), a valid surrogate measure for coronary atherosclerosis. IMT is a predictor of coronary outcomes and stroke and is associated with psychosocial stress factors *(48)*. This randomized controlled clinical trial evaluated the comparison of TM vs an education control program on IMT during a 6–9-mo period. After controlling for age and pretest IMT values, analyses showed a statistically significant decrease in posttest IMT values for subjects in the TM group, compared with an increase in the values of the control group. These results suggest that stress reduction with the TM program is associated with reduced carotid atherosclerosis in African Americans with hypertension, compared to health education *(48)*.

Zamarra and colleagues investigated the effects of TM on the incidence of exercise-induced myocardial ischemia in patients with known coronary artery disease (CAD) *(49)*. In this small (21-subject) randomized, controlled, single-blind, pilot study, subjects were assigned to the TM program group or to a wait-list control group. At baseline and at the completion of the intervention (8 mo later), patients underwent symptom-limited exercise tolerance tests. Compared with the control group participants, the patients who participated in the TM program demonstrated significantly greater exercise tolerance, higher maximal workload, and delayed onset of ST-segment depression *(49)*.

Psychological Impact of Meditation

In addition to the well-documented physiologic effects of meditation, researchers have begun to measure the impact such practice may have on psychological variables. Numerous studies have shown that depression and anxiety are associated with increased risk of CAD and adverse cardiac events *(50–54)*. Symptoms such as subjective feelings of stress, depression, anxiety, panic attacks, and chronic pain have all been the focus of meditation research. Again, the research in this area suffers from small sample sizes and few controlled studies. Additional methodological problems, such as the use of unvalidated measures and failure to control for concurrent treatments limit the ability to confidently draw conclusive evidence from these studies. However, overall, the preliminary evidence supports some usefulness of meditation in decreasing these symptoms. Research in this area has been predominantly conducted using the MM technique. For excellent reviews of the treatment literature, more extensive than is possible here, *see* refs. *22* and *23*.

The results of three randomized, controlled studies of MBSR in nonclinical samples suggest that this intervention may be effective in decreasing stress, anxiety, and depressive symptoms in the general population (55–57).

Astin (55) compared university undergraduates engaged in an 8-wk MBSR program with peer controls not engaged in MM on a well-validated measure of general, physical, and psychological well-being. The MBSR group demonstrated statistically significant lower postintervention scores on the Global Severity Index (GSI) of the SCL-90, with a 65% average reduction in scores. Scores on the subscales for depression, anxiety, obsessive-compulsive symptoms, interpersonal sensitivity, psychoticism, and paranoid ideation were also significantly lower postintervention when compared with controls.

Shapiro and colleagues (56) used the same measure of general psychological well-being in their controlled study that compared premedical and medical students engaged in the 8-wk MSBR program with a gender-matched waiting-list control group. Findings were similar to previous studies, with the MBSR group exhibiting significantly lower postintervention scores on the GSI and on the depression and state anxiety subscales than on waiting-list controls. In addition, the MBSR participants also demonstrated significantly greater scores on the empathy subscale. Change in scores from preintervention to postintervention for the waiting-list controls who subsequently received the MM training also supported these findings. These participants demonstrated significant reductions in GSI and the depression subscale, as well as lower state anxiety and greater empathy after the MBSR program (56).

Williams et al. (57) conducted a randomized controlled trial of an MBSR program offered to self-identified "stressed" volunteers from the local West Virginia community. The MBSR group received the 8-wk standard MBSR intervention, and the control group received educational materials and community referrals. Intervention subjects reported significant decreases from baseline on measures of the effect of daily hassles, psychological distress as measured by the SCL-90, and medical symptoms, as compared to control subjects. These results were maintained at the 3-mo follow-up assessment (57).

In clinical samples, two randomized, controlled studies have been conducted (58,59). Speca et al. (58) studied the impact of an MSBR program with a mixed group of patients with cancer. Findings showed the significant reductions in total mood disturbance and stress symptoms of 65% and 35%, respectively. In addition, amount of time spent meditating was significantly correlated with reduction in mood disturbance (58). Teasdale et al. (59) conducted a randomized controlled trial of an MBSR-based treatment for recently recovered depressed patients after medication therapy. The intervention in this study was a combined modality using cognitive therapy and MBSR called mindfulness-based cognitive therapy (MBCT). MBCT patients who had three or more previous depressive episodes showed a much lower relapse rate (37%) than the treatment as usual (TAU) group (66%) during the 1-yr study period. Relapse rates for the MBCT and TAU groups did not differ for patients who had only one or two previous depressive episodes *(59)*.

There have been numerous uncontrolled studies of the impact of meditation on psychological symptoms. Kabat-Zinn *(60–62)* reports findings from several studies of his MBSR program with patients with chronic pain that indicate reductions on self-report measures of present-moment pain, negative body image, inhibition of activity by pain symptoms, mood disturbance, and psychological symptomatology, including depression and anxiety *(60–62)*. These results were maintained for up to 4 yr after the meditation training, with the exception of the measure of present-moment pain *(62)*. The subjects in this study had received previous treatment for their chronic pain, with little or no results, making the positive findings even more impressive in this treatment-resistant group *(60–62)*.

Kabat-Zinn's research studying the impact of MBSR programs on anxiety and panic disorder *(63,64)* has demonstrated significant reductions in the severity of symptoms from baseline to postintervention. Subjects were rigorously assessed using *Diagnostic and Statistical Manual (DSM)-III-R* criteria for generalized anxiety disorder or panic disorder with or without agoraphobia. Clinically and statistically significant posttreatment reductions were found in both subjective and objective symptoms of anxiety and depression, and these results were maintained at the 3-yr follow-up. Unfortunately, 50% of the patients in the study were also being treated with psychotropic medications during the MBSR program and approx 50% received additional treatment for their anxiety disorder after the MBSR treatment, making it difficult to establish the relative therapeutic contribution of each intervention *(63,64)*.

Despite the methodological flaws, the preponderance of evidence regarding the impact of MBSR programs on psychological symptoms does suggest that it may be a useful intervention. However, what is clear from this research is the need for additional, more rigorous research investigating this promising clinical tool.

Adverse Impact of Meditation

Although the clinical use of meditation strategies has shown several positive effects in decreasing autonomic arousal and mediating psychological and stress symptoms, there is a small body of literature that suggests there may be some potential adverse meditation effects *(65–69)*.

Studies of adverse impact were predominantly conducted on meditators using a TM approach, and the sample sizes were small *(65–68)*. Examples of adverse effects reported include such difficulties as precipitation of psychiatric illness (namely psychosis), impaired reality testing, increased anxiety and panic, increased sense of isolation, and increased negative emotions *(65–69)*. In two studies investigating differences among novice and long-term meditators, length of practice was positively correlated with higher frequency of report of adverse impact *(68,69)*. One of the most recent studies of adverse impact, conducted by Shapiro *(69)*, attempted to replicate earlier findings of TM in an MM population of meditators. Although Shapiro did, in fact, replicate the findings of significant adverse events reported by meditators surveyed (62.9%), he points out that these same meditators reported significantly more positive effects than negative ones. He also points out that many of the individuals who reported adverse effects characterized this impact as "a part of positive personal transformation" *(69,* p. 66). Although much of this research has methodological flaws, such as small sample size and low response rates, it is a useful reminder to clinicians of the need to maintain an awareness of the potential harmful impact of the interventions we use.

MEDITATION FOR HEALTH CARE PROFESSIONALS

Although in the current discussion meditation has been considered solely as an intervention for patients, several mindfulness researchers have suggested that it may also be a useful tool for health care professionals to use as a personal strategy for enhancing their own health care practice *(70,71)*. There is no doubt that the practice of medicine is a stressful and demanding endeavor. The stress-reduction benefits discussed in detail are as beneficial to health providers as they are to the patients they treat. In addition, health care professionals are uniquely positioned to encounter, face to face, the suffering of the patients they treat each day. Often providers respond to this suffering with one of two extreme unmindful responses. They either become lost in sympathy for the other, or, as happens all too often, maintain a safe distance, remaining aloof and uninvolved. Perhaps if health providers could cultivate an attitude of mindfulness (moment-to-moment awareness, nonjudgment, and nonattachment to outcome) and apply this practice to their encounters with patients, they would not only be better able to be present and effective for their patients but also be more deeply in touch with their own life experiences *(71)*.

REFERENCES

1. Miller TQ, Smith TW, Turner CW, Giuijarro ML, Hallet AJ. A meta-analytic review of research on hostility and physical health. Psychol Bull 1996;119:322–348.
2. Rosenman RH, Brand RJ, Jenkins CD, Freidman M, Strauss R, Wurm M. Coronary heart disease in the Western Collaborative Group Study. Final follow-up experience of 8-1/2 years. JAMA 1975;233:872–877.
3. Matthews KA, Haynes SG. Type A behavior pattern and coronary disease risk: update and critical evaluation. Am J Epidemiol 1986;123:923–960.
4. Barefoot JC, Larsen S, Von der Lieth L, Schroll M. Hostility, incidence of acute myocardial infarction, and mortality in a sample of older Danish men and women. Am J Epidemiol 1995;142:477–484.
5. Mittleman MA, Maclure M, Sherwood JB, et al. Triggering of acute myocardial infarction onset by episodes of anger. Circulation 1995;92:1720–1725.
6. Everson SA, Kauhanen J, Kaplan GA, et al. Hostility and increased risk of mortality and acute myocardial infarction: The mediating role of behavioral risk factors. Am J Epidemiol 1997;146:142–152.
7. Sloan RP, Shapiro PA, Bagiella E, Myers M, Gorman JM. Cardiac autonomic control buffers blood pressure variability responses to challenge: a psychophysiologic model of coronary artery disease. Psychosom Med 1999;61:58–68.
8. Beary JF, Benson H. A simple psychophysiologic technique which elicits the hypometabolic changes of the relaxation response. Psychosom Med 1974;36:115–120.
9. Hoffman JW, Benson H, Arns PA, et al. Reduced sympathetic nervous system responsivity associated with the relaxation response. Science 1982;215:190–192.
10. Gordon NP, Sobel DS, Tarazona, EZ. Use of and interest in alternative therapies among adult primary care clinicians and adult members in a large health maintenance organization. West J Med 1998;169:153–161.
11. Hopper I, Cohen M. Complementary therapies and the medical profession, a study of medical students' attitudes. Alt Ther Health Med 1998;4:68–73.
12. Eisenberg DM, Davis RB, Ettner SL, et al. Trends in alternative medicine use in the United States, 1990–1997: results of a follow-up national survey. JAMA 1998;280:1569–1575.
13. Liu EH, Turner LM, Lin SX, et al. Use of alternative medicine by patients undergoing cardiac surgery. J Thorac Cardiovasc Surg 2000;120:335–341.
14. Goleman D. The Meditative Mind. Putnam, New York, 1988.
15. Kabat-Zinn J. Wherever You Go There You Are: Mindfulness Meditation In Everyday Life. Hyperion, New York, 1994.
16. Roth R. Maharishi Maresh Yogi's transcendental meditation. Primus, Washington DC, 1994.
17. Yogi MM. Maharishi's Vedic approach to health. Maharishi Vedic University Press, Vlodrop, Holland, 1995.
18. Yogi MM. On the Bhagavad Gita. Penguin, Baltimore, MD, 1969.
19. Jevning R, Wallace RK, Biedebach M. The physiology of meditation: a review. A wakeful hypometabolic integrated response. Neurosci Biobehav Rev 1992;16:415–424.
20. Kabat-Zinn J. Full Catastrophe Living. Using the Wisdom of Your Body and Mind to Face Stress, Pain and Illness. Bantam Doubleday Dell Publishing, New York, 1990.
21. Hahn TN. The Miracle of Mindfulness. Beacon Press, Boston, 1976.
22. Baer RA. Mindfulness training as a clinical intervention: a conceptual and empirical review. Clin Psychol Sci Pract 2003;10:125–143.

23. Bishop SR. What do we really know about mindfulness-based stress reduction? Psychosom Med 2002;64:71–84.
24. Kabat-Zinn J. Meditation. In: Holland JC, ed. Psycho-oncology. Oxford University Press, New York, 1998, pp.767–779.
25. Brose T. A psychophysiological study. Main Curr Mod Thought 1946;4:77–84.
26. Wallace RK. Physiological effects of transcendental meditation. Science 1970;167:1251–1254.
27. Wallace RK, Benson H, Wilson AF. A wakeful hypometabolic physiologic state. Am J Physiol 1971;221:795–799.
28. Wallace RK, Benson H. The physiology of meditation. Sci Amer 1972;262:84–90.
29. Wolkove N, Kreisman H, Darragh D, Cohen C, Frank H. Effect of transcendental meditation on breathing and respiratory control. J Appl Physiol 1984;56:607–612.
30. Farrow JT, Hebert R. Breath suspension during the transcendental meditation technique. Psychosom Med 1982;44:133–153.
31. Badawi K, Wallace RK, Orme-Johnson D, Rouzere AM. Electrophysiological characteristics of respiratory suspension periods occurring during the practice of the Transcendental Meditation program. Psychosom Med 1984;46:267–276.
32. Travis F, Wallace RK. Autonomic patterns during respiratory suspensions: possible markers of transcendental consciousness. Psychophysiology 1997;34:39–46.
33. Jevning R, Wilson AF, Davidson MJ. Adrenocortical activity during meditation. Horm Behav 1978;10:54–60.
34. MacLean CRK, Walton KG, Wenneberg SR, et al. Effects of the Transcendental Meditation program on adaptive mechanisms: changes in hormone levels and responses to stress after 4 months of practice. Psychoneuroendocrinology 1997;22:277–295.
35. Werner OR, Wallace RK, Charles B, Janssen G, Stryker T, Chalmers RA. Long term endocrinologic changes in subjects practicing the Transcendental Meditation and TM-Sidhi program. Psychosom Med 1986;48:59–66.
36. Michaels RR, Huber MJ, McCann DS. Evaluation of transcendental meditation as a method of reducing stress. Science 1976;192:1242–1244.
37. Infante JR, Torres-Avisbal M, Pinel P, et al. Catecholamine levels in practitioners of the transcendental meditation technique. Phys Behav 2001;72:141–146.
38. Wallace RK, Simon B, Guich S, et al. Rise in urinary 5-hydroxyindoleaceatic acid (5-HIAA) associated with practice of the transcendental meditation program. Soc Neurosci Abs 1980;6:725.
39. Dillbeck MC, Orme-Johnson DW. Physiological differences between transcendental meditation and rest. Am Psychol 1987;42:879–881.
40. Goleman D, Schwartz G. Meditation as an intervention in stress-reactivity. J Consult Clin Psychol 1976;44:456–466.
41. Michaels RR, Pano J, McCann DS, Vander AJ. Renin, cortisol and aldosterone during transcendental meditation. Psychosom Med 1979;41:50–54.
42. Wallace RK, Silver J, Mills PJ, Dillbeck MC, Wagoner DE. Systolic blood pressure and long term practice of the Transcendental Meditation and TM-Sidhi programs: effects of TM on systolic blood pressure. Psychosom Med 1983;45:451–456.
43. Barnes VA, Treiber FA, Turner JR, Davis H. Acute effects of transcendental meditation on hemodynamic functioning in middle-aged adults. Psychosom Med 1999;61:525–531.
44. Wenneberg SR, Schneider RH, Walton KG, et al. A controlled study of the effects of the transcendental meditation program on cardiovascular reactivity and ambulatory blood pressure. Int J Neurosci 1997;89:15–28.

45. Khare KC, Nigam SK. A study of electroencephalogram in meditators. Indian J Physiol Pharmacol 2000;44:173–178.
46. Dunn BR, Hartigan JA, Mikulas WL. Concentration and mindfulness meditations: unique forms of consciousness? Appl Psychophysiol Biofeed 1999;24:147–165.
47. Schneider RH, Staggers F, Alexander CN, et al. A randomized controlled trial of stress reduction for hypertension in older African Americans. Hypertension 1995;26:820–827.
48. Castillo-Richmond A, Schneider RH, Alexander CN, et al. Effects of stress reduction on carotid artherosclerosis in hypertensive African Americans. Stroke 2000;31:568–573.
49. Zamarra JW, Schneider RH, Besseghini I, Robinson DK, Salerno W. Usefulness of the transcendental meditation program in the treatment of patients with coronary artery disease. Am J Cardiol 1996;77:867–870.
50. Connerey I, Shapiro PA, McLaughlin JS, Bagiella E, Sloan RP. Relation between depression after coronary artery bypass surgery and 12-month outcome: a prospective study. Lancet 2001;358:1766–1771.
51. Booth-Kewley S, Friedman HS. Psychological predictors of heart disease: a quantitative review. Psychol Bull 1987;101:343–362.
52. Weissman MM, Markowitz JS, Oullette R, Greenwald S, Kahn JP. Panic disorder and cardiovascular/cerebrovascular problems: results from a community survey. Am J Psychiatry 1990;147:1504–1508.
53. Kawachi I, Sparrow D, Vokonos PS, Weiss ST. Symptoms of anxiety and risk of coronary heart disease. Circulation 1994;90:2225–2229.
54. Gullette EC, Blumenthal JA, Babyak M, et al. Effects of mental stress on myocardial ischemia during daily life. JAMA 1997;227:1521–1526.
55. Astin J. Stress reduction through mindfulness meditation: effects on psychological symptomatology, sense of control, and spiritual experiences. Psyhcother Psychosom 1997;66:97–106.
56. Shapiro SL, Schwartz GE, Bonner G. Effects of mindfulness-based stress reduction on medical and premedical students. J Behav Med 1998;8:163–190.
57. Williams KA, Kolar MM, Reger BE, Pearson JC. Evaluation of a wellness-based mindfulness stress reduction intervention: a controlled trial. Am J Health Promot 2001;15:422–432.
58. Speca M, Carlson L, Goodey E, Angen M. A randomized wait-list controlled trial: the effects of a mindfulness-based stress reduction program on mood and symptoms of stress in cancer outpatients. Psychosom Med 2000;62:613–622.
59. Teasdale JD, Segal ZV, Williams JMG, Ridgeway VA, Soulsby JM, Lau MA. Prevention of relapse/recurrence in major depression by mindfulness-based cognitive therapy. J Consult Clin Psychol 2000;68:615–623.
60. Kabat-Zinn J. An outpatient program in behavioral medicine for chronic pain patients based on the practice of mindfulness meditation: theoretical considerations and preliminary results. Gen Hosp Psychiatry 1982;4:33–47.
61. Kabat-Zinn J, Lipworth L, Burney R. The clinical use of mindfulness meditation for the self regulation of chronic pain. J Behav Med 1985;8:163–190.
62. Kabat-Zinn J, Lipworth L, Burney R, Sellers W. Four-year follow-up of a meditation based program for the self regulation of chronic pain: treatment outcome and compliance. Clin J Pain 1987;2:159–173.
63. Kabat-Zinn J, Massion AO, Kristellar J, et al. Effectiveness of a meditation-based stress reduction program in the treatment of anxiety disorders. Am J Psychiatry 1992;149:936–943.

64. Miller JJ, Fletcher K, Kabat-Zinn J. Three-year follow-up and clinical implications of a mindfulness meditation-based stress reduction intervention in the treatment of anxiety disorders. Gen Hosp Psychiatry 1995;17:192–200.
65. Walsh R, Rauche L. The precipitation of acute psychoses by intensive meditation in individuals with a history of schizophrenia. Am J Psychiatry 1979;138:185–186.
66. Lazarus AA. Pyschiatric problems precipitated by transcendental meditation. Psych Reports 1975;10:39–74.
67. French AP, Smid AC, Ingalls E. Transcendental meditation, altered reality testing and behavioral change: a case report. J Nerv Mental Dis 1975;161:55–58.
68. Otis LS. Adverse effects of transcendental meditation. In: Shapiro DH, Walsh RN, eds. Meditation: Classic and Contemporary Perspectives. Aldine, New York, 1984, pp. 201–208.
69. Shapiro DH. Adverse effects of meditation: a preliminary investigation of long-term meditators. Int J Psychosom 1992;39:62–66.
70. Epstein RM. Mindful practice. JAMA 1999;282:833–839.
71. Santorelli S. Heal thy self. Lessons on mindfulness in medicine. Bell Tower, New York, 1999.

9 Prayer and Cardiovascular Disease

Jonathan E. E. Yager, MD,
Suzanne W. Crater, RN, ANP-C,
and Mitchell W. Krucoff, MD, FACC

CONTENTS

INTRODUCTION

Prayer has been an important part of human existence for thousands of years. People turn to a prayer in times of reflection, gratitude, and crisis, including physical illness. Surveys have shown that more than

From: *Contemporary Cardiology*
Complementary and Alternative Cardiovascular Medicine
Edited by: R. A. Stein and M. C. Oz © Humana Press Inc., Totowa, NJ

90% of people believe in a Higher Being *(1,2)*. In a recent survey of complementary and alternative medicine (CAM) in the United States, 35% of people reported that they had used prayer as a therapy for their personal health concerns *(3)*. A study conducted in 1996 demonstrated that 96% of Americans believe in God, at least 90% pray, and more than 40% had attended organized religious services during the past week *(4)*. This chapter explores the relationship between prayer and cardiovascular disease (CVD) by providing terms for evaluating prayer and spirituality in a modern medical setting, by discussing the literature to date and by considering implications for future research.

CVD, particularly heart disease, raises spiritual issues. Patients with cardiac disease often undergo invasive tests and procedures and major surgery and experience troubling or even disabling symptoms. Furthermore, patients with heart disease are invariably confronted with the prospects of their own mortality. Many patients, families, and communities turn to spirituality or religious practices to help cope with the stress and uncertainty that surrounds cardiac disease and treatment, to seek a source of hope and comfort, and even potentially to influence outcome. Hospital and health care staff involved in patient care in the cardiovascular setting may also incorporate prayer formally or informally into their practice patterns. As much as prayer is a part of the fabric of care patterns, little systematic study or information about the importance of it in cardiac care has been collected to date.

DEFINITIONS AND NOMENCLATURE

Although diverse and even colorful language may be interesting for cultural, philosophical, or theological discourse, the indistinct and potentially redundant health care terminology and nomenclature confound systematic applications. To study prayer's healing effects, certain aspects of religion, spirituality, and prayer must reach at least the level of consensus definition.

Koenig defines religion as "an organized system of beliefs, practices, rituals, and symbols designed (1) to facilitate closeness to the sacred or transcendent (God, higher power, or ultimate truth/reality) and (2) to foster an understanding of one's relationship and responsibility to others in living together in a community" *(5)*. Spirituality is defined as "the personal quest for understanding answers to ultimate questions about life, about meaning, and about relationship to the sacred or transcendent, which may (or may not) lead to or arise from the development of religious rituals and the formation of community" *(5)*.

Many measurement tools exist to gauge a person's religiousness and spirituality. The Duke University Religion Index (DUREL) specifically addresses the dimensions of religion associated with health outcome, including organizational religiousness, nonorganizational religiousness, and intrinsic religiousness (5). Spirituality scales include the Index of Spiritual Orientation, INSPIRIT (Index of Core Spiritual Experiences), and the FACIT Spiritual Well-Being Scale. Numerous other scales exist and are discussed in depth in Koenig's book (5).

Prayer, particularly "healing prayer," can also be characterized in many ways or practiced in a range of prayer "models," from prayer that petitions for a specific response to prayer seeking the achievement of harmony with higher purposes, which may surpass human understanding. In the patient's world, self-prayer and the prayers of loved ones may be ascendant as a component of spiritual consciousness. In clinical trials, specific petitionary or "intercessory prayer" is the most researched prayer model to date, presumably because it lends itself to the conceptual paradigms of "therapy." Intercessory prayer has been defined as prayer calling "for aid to others" (6). "Distant healing," referring to intercessory prayer "strategies that purport to heal through some exchange or channeling of supraphysical energy" (7) independent of proximity to the patient, is a model of prayer with a structure that supports the conduct of double-blind clinical trial designs. Many other descriptors, such as the language of prayer, and the content of prayer, the number of individuals or congregations praying, the timing and duration of prayer, and the intensity, passion, faith, and concentration of the intercessors, all constitute what can currently only be considered a range of qualitative descriptors of prayer methods and models.

Prayer has the potential to exert effects on not only the intended recipient of the prayer but also the individual performing it, as well as possibly other unknown recipients. Patients and their families often pray for healing and recovery, for physicians and other care providers to perform their procedures successfully and without complications, for God or another Divine Being to "watch over" the patient during the illness, and with many other intentions and goals. In the absence of mechanistic insight or knowledge, it must be recognized that all of these qualitative descriptors incorporate an enormous influence of intuitive metaphor, with almost no definitive scientific evidence to support any prayer model in particular.

Independent of the mechanism or mechanisms, ample evidence exists that emotional and spiritual states affect health outcomes. Studies have been conducted on the association between religion and depression, anxiety, hypertension, and cancer, as well as heart disease. Although not all studies show a positive effect of religion, the overall majority show that religiousness is "protective" *(5)*.

In considering nomenclature in the context of prayer and cardiovascular health care, another important distinction must be drawn between spiritual "support" and spiritual "therapy." Spiritual support represents the health care system's ability to respond to needs defined by the patient, family, and community—is there a chapel on site, or a chaplain on site, with the ability to foster comfort and coping during the time of illness. On the other hand, spiritual therapy is a prayer, an intention, or energy that is specifically used as a therapeutic intervention, with the goal of affecting clinical outcome. To improve spiritual support, the health care system uses a process of iterative quality improvement as a component of facilities integration. On the other hand, to optimize spiritual therapy is research, which requires the review of institutional ethics committees and protection of human subjects measures, such as the informed consent process.

SPIRITUALITY AND SPIRITUALITY TRIALS IN CARDIOVASCULAR CARE

Epidemiologic studies have consistently indicated that people who are involved with a religion or religious community have fewer heart attacks, lower blood pressure, and better overall cardiovascular survival than individuals who are not involved with a religion *(5)*. Fundamental to these observations is the understanding that there is no causal implication to these data. Community involvement may lead to better health, or individuals with better health may be more involved with their communities. However, correlations with epidemiologic descriptors may suggest important directions for causal research.

Numerous prayer and spiritual intervention studies, with the intention of improving measurable clinical outcomes, have been published and have been summarized in several notable compendia by Dossey *(8)*, Koenig *(5)*, and Benor *(9)*. Published studies have examined the role of spirituality and post-CABG survival, hypertension, coronary artery disease (CAD), and cardiovascular survival. In an attempt at meta-analysis of this literature, Astin and colleagues found such association so heterogeneous and so generally composed of small, flawed observational studies that a classical meta-analysis could not be conducted *(7)*. Narrowing their focus to the best published studies available using widely accepted standards for evaluation of clinical trial designs and creating an index for therapeutic effect to combine the numerous end points measured in these studies, Astin et al. found a consistent and statistically robust suggestion that healing prayer was associated with some degree of therapeutic benefit. The conclusion that these findings supported was that more and better designs of prayer studies were indicated based on the literature available to date.

PROSPECTIVE RANDOMIZED TRIALS
OF INTERCESSORY PRAYER IN CARDIOLOGY

Only four prospective randomized, controlled clinical trials of intercessory prayer have been reported in cardiology populations (10–13). Two additional multicenter prospective randomized trials have completed enrollment of patients after bypass surgery and in patients underoing percutaneous coronary intervention. Neither of these studies has yet been reported.

The first reported study investigated the role of distant prayer in the coronary care unit (CCU) and was published in 1988 (10). In this study, all patients admitted to the CCU of San Francisco General Hospital were approached to enter the study. Patients who consented (393 of 450 approached) were randomized to receive standard care or standard care plus intercessory prayer. Each patient in the intervention group was prayed for by three to seven intercessors, who were all "born-again Christians (according to the Gospel of John 3:3)." The intercessors were told the patient's first name, general condition, diagnosis, and updates on their condition. The intercessors prayed daily for the patients until they were discharged from the hospital. Multiple clinical outcomes were measured, and each patient's hospital course was graded as "good," "intermediate," or "bad," depending on morbidity. This was done in a blinded fashion regarding patient group assignment.

Of the patients receiving prayer, 85% had a "good" hospital course, as compared to 73% in the control group. Fourteen percent of the prayer treatment group had a "bad" hospital course, as compared to 22% of the control group. These comparisons reached statistical significance with a p value of <0.01. However, the overall clinical significance of this statistical finding remains indeterminate. The prayer treatment group had fewer episodes of congestive heart failure (CHF), required fewer diuretics, had less cardiac arrest, had fewer instances of pneumonia, and required intubation and ventilation less than the control group. However, with the large number of variables examined in such a small population, these individual outcome differences were not statistically significant.

Because this the was first report of a prospective randomized trial of intercessory prayer, the provocative nature of the study findings were accompanied by insightful discussion. Byrd acknowledged that a limitation of the study design was that it did not control for other prayer not associated with the study. In other words, patients in both groups, their friends, and family likely prayed for them during the course of the study, and there was no attempt to prevent such activity or even account for it. As such, the study was essentially examining only the role of "supplementary" intercessory prayer. With this important observation, Byrd defined the landscape of clinical trials of prayer where scientific study could never expect to absolutely test the healing power of prayer. With so much "ambient" and unaccounted-for prayer in cultures in the world, the only appropriate query for a scientifically based hypothesis would be as an assessment of incremental benefit from systematically added spiritual interventions, with uncontrolled prayer activity adjusted for by the use of prospectively designed, randomized treatment assignments.

The next trial that sought to define the effect of prayer on CCU patients was published in 1999 (11). One thousand thirteen patients were randomized to receive standard CCU care, with or without teams of intercessors praying for them. Extending Byrd's observations about the landscape of clinical trials of healing prayer, Harris and colleagues were concerned that the spiritual terrain of an intensive care unit would change if staff and patients even knew a study was ongoing. That consideration was taken to the institutional ethics board/review board at the Mid-America Heart Institute, which granted permission for the study to go forward without getting informed consent from patients and without the awareness of staff.

In this study by Harris et al., teams of intercessors were given the first name of the patient only, without knowledge of the type of illness or severity of disease. They were instructed to pray for 28 d for "a speedy recovery with no complications" and "anything else that seemed appropriate to them" (11). The primary end point in this study was a predefined CCU score that sought to quantify the severity of the illness, the hospital course, and the procedures used.

The authors found an 11% reduction in the weighted CCU score (indicating better outcome) in the 484 patients in the prayer treatment group, as compared to the 529 in the control group. In an unweighted score, which merely totaled the number of events, procedures, and prescriptions, the prayer treatment group had 10% fewer elements. For both of these comparisons the p value was 0.04, indicating a statistically significant intervention benefit. Length of stay between the two groups was not statistically different. Attempts to replicate the Byrd study's findings in CCU patients by using the "good" vs "bad" hospital score showed no difference between the treatment and the control group. Like the Byrd scale, the differences seen with the Mid-America CCU severity score were of unclear clinical importance, which currently remains unreplicated and unvalidated.

Although this study further advanced the possibility that distant healing prayer might play a beneficial role in a CCU population, the cumulative weight of evidence from the two studies remained marginal. Far more significant was the approval by the institutional review board (IRB) of the protocol design to allow the study to go forward without obtaining patients' informed consent. As presented in the discussion of the final manuscript, this decision was based on the assumption that there was no known risk to receiving intercessory prayer and, similarly, no known risk for the patients *not* receiving the intervention. As opposed to the Byrd study in which the patients knew that a study was being conducted and gave informed consent, the investigators also mention that they did not want to create extra anxiety in patients who might worry that they were placed in the control group and therefore *not* receiving extra prayer.

With this study, Harris and colleagues uniquely opened the dialogue on the balance of optimal trial design for demonstration of prayer efficacy vs the protection of human subjects, which is essentially a safety concern. On the one hand, study designers were concerned that awareness that a prayer study was ongoing might itself stimulate an increase in prayer by both patients and staff in the CCU, lessening the uniqueness measurable in the prayer therapy arm. They were also concerned that awareness of the study and the randomized design might stimulate anxiety or enhance suffering.

However, in the balance, the decision that the study could be ethically conducted without the informed consent of participating subjects centered on the assumption that healing prayers could not possibly do harm. In the absence of mechanistic knowledge, it is this assumption that prayer with healing intention is intrinsically safe that remains most controversial.

A third study was published in 2001 from the Mayo Clinic, which sought to determine the effects of remote, intercessory prayer on long-term cardiovascular outcomes of CCU patients *(12)*. In this double-blind study, informed consent was obtained and patients who gave consent were randomized at hospital discharge to receive 28 d of intercessory prayer in addition to standard medical therapy or standard therapy alone. Four hundred patients were randomized to intercessory prayer, and 399 were assigned to the control group. Patients were stratified according to risk of disease progression. The primary end point was a composite of death, cardiac arrest, coronary revascularization, rehospitalization for CVD, or an emergency department visit for cardiac disease at 26 wk. No differences were seen between the two groups. Also, there were no differences between the groups in a quality-of-life score.

As the most recent of the published trials of prayer in CCU patients, the Aviles Mayo Clinic study brought clearer focus to several new areas of study design. Rather than a single all-comer's CCU population, the Aviles study risk stratified the patient cohort into high-risk and low-risk groups. Instead of derived indices, the Mayo Clinic study used well-accepted clinical outcome measures as end points and powered the study to observe a therapeutic benefit based on expected outcomes rates in the control population. In fact, the morbidity and mortality rates in the control population were lower than those used for the power calculations, reducing the power of the study to detect a treatment benefit in the population size studied.

Another issue crystalized by the Mayo Clinic report is the timing of therapy. Although the patients studied were CCU patients, therapy with prayer was begun only after discharge, whereas in both the Byrd and Harris studies, prayer therapy was initiated shortly after enrollment, when patients were still in the acute phase of CCU care. Also, whereas Byrd and Harris had set out specific content for the prayer, this was not the case with Aviles. Intercessors were allowed to pray however they wanted. They were asked to pray at least once a week, and it is certainly possible that some prayed more. Therefore, the authors comment that a potential limitation of their study is that the "dose" of prayer was not regulated.

The fourth prospective randomized controlled clinical trial in cardiology patients was the Monitoring & Actualization of Noetic TRAinings (MANTRA) Pilot study, also published in 2001 *(13)*. This study was conducted in an all-male population in the CCU at the Durham Veterans Affairs Medical Center. All patients in this study had unstable coronary syndromes and were scheduled for acute cardiac catheterization and angioplasty or coronary stenting. Outcomes measured were short-term (procedural and in-hospital) and long-term (6-mo postdischarge) standard cardiovascular complications, compiled as major adverse cardiovascular end-points. The study was a feasibility pilot to evaluate standard therapy vs four noetic therapies: stress relaxation, imagery, touch therapy, and double-blind off-site intercessory prayer. A total of 150 patients were enrolled, with 30 patients randomized to each treatment group. There were no safety or feasibility concerns. Absolute reductions in the number of patients suffering major adverse cardiac events (MACE), as well as a reduction in postangioplasty evidence of ischemia on continuous electrocardiogram monitoring, were observed in patients receiving noetic interventions, although these differences had wide confidence intervals and were not statistically significant. The greatest magnitude of absolute reduction in MACE was seen in the patients who were treated with prayer.

The MANTRA Pilot studied the most homogeneous group of patients among these reported cardiac randomized trials, with a focus on patients with acute coronary disease undergoing invasive catheter-based procedures. In addition to this more focused patient cohort, the study systematically followed nonstudy related patient, family, and chaplain prayer said before the angioplasty, reporting the presence of chaplain and/or family in the room in 66% of patients and the awareness of nonprotocol prayer by patients on their own behalf in just fewer than 50% of the patients in the control group.

The MANTRA Pilot study design was also unique for its "high-dose" prayer model. In the Byrd, Harris, and Aviles studies, between one and six intercessors were used for each patient, and all intercessors were Christians. In the MANTRA Pilot, every patient randomized to the prayer therapy treatment assignment had his or her name, age, and illness sent to nine congregations of intercessors, including several Christian, Jewish, and Buddhist denominations, who all prayed on each patient's behalf. Although not statistically significant in the small pilot population studied, the absolute reduction in complication rates of standard clinical endpoints represents one of the largest apparent treatment effects reported over the four published randomized cardiology trials.

AMERICAN COLLEGE OF CARDIOLOGY CONSENSUS STATEMENT

The American College of Cardiology (ACC) is currently preparing a consensus statement on CAM, which includes a section on spirituality (14). This consensus document states that given the current literature, no recommendations can be made regarding the application of spiritual therapy in cardiovascular medical practice. It also recommends that for the purpose of clinical studies, spirituality must be considered an investigational therapeutic agent, like any other, and that safety and efficacy trials must be conducted with full informed consent for patients. The document recommends the development of a common nomenclature for terms and standardized measures for outcomes in terms of these trials and suggests that endpoints should go beyond morbidity and mortality to include quality of life, end-of-life care issues, and cost effectiveness. That the ACC has accepted to create such a consensus document adds validity to the need for further investigation in this area.

INTERCESSORY PRAYER
AND NONCARDIOVASCULAR DISEASES

In addition to clinical trials of cardiac patients, studies evaluating intercessory prayer and distant healing have been undertaken in several patient groups, including those with HIV, blood-borne infections, infertility concerns, rheumatologic diseases, and more. A recent review *(15)* examined the relationship between religion and spirituality with mental and physical health, as well as with health-related quality of life. The authors reviewed studies concerning mortality, CVD, hypertension, depression, anxiety, substance abuse, and suicide. As noted earlier, the majority of these studies show a correlation between religious involvement or spirituality and a better health outcome, including quality of life.

Prayer has been tested in a group of patients with rheumatoid arthritis *(16)*. Forty-four patients with clinically stable disease and on stable medications received a 3-d intervention, including 6 h of educational sessions and 6 h of direct-contact intercessory prayer (face-to-face prayer with a healer). This included the healer's laying his or her hands for prolonged periods of time on the patient's affected joints. All prayers were conducted by Christian ministers. The first 29 patients received regular 3-mo follow-up. The next 15 participants received the 3-d intervention 6 mo into the study. Twenty-three of the 44 participants were then randomized to receive additional distant intercessory prayer from two ministers who prayed for the participant for at least 10 min daily for 6 mo. The distant prayer component of the study was blinded; neither the clinician responsible for the patient evaluations nor the patients knew whether they were receiving distant prayer.

The authors found that the direct prayer and hands-on intervention led to improvement in both groups; however, the blinded portion of the study with distant healing did not show any change in outcome. Because the patients were not blinded to the application of direct and hands-on prayer and there was no control group, the authors acknowledge that a placebo effect could not be excluded.

Distant healing was also studied in 20 patients with AIDS who were randomized with matched controls to receive distant healing in an outpatient setting *(17)*. As opposed to the previous study in which healers prayed for particular individuals, the prayer group received distant healing from different healers on a rotating schedule to reduce the possibility that certain healers were more efficacious than others. Each patient was treated by a total of 10 different healers, and the healers were asked to pray for their patients for 6 consecutive days, for 1 h per day. They were instructed to "direct an intention for health and well-being." The healers who rotated the patients in this study were Jewish, Christian, Buddhist, Native American, and of shamanic traditions and also included "graduates of secular schools of bioenergetic and meditative healing." The patients and their physicians did not know whether they received the interventions. The group receiving distant healing experienced fewer hospitalizations with fewer days spent in the hospital, fewer outpatient doctor visits, fewer new AIDS-defining diseases, and a lower illness severity level. This group also had significantly improved mood compared with the control group. There was no difference found in CD4 counts.

Perhaps one of the most intriguing trials of intercessory prayer occurred in a clinic for women undergoing in vitro fertilization *(18)*. In this study conducted in Korea, 219 women in a fertility clinic receiving in vitro fertilization-embryo transfer were randomly assigned to receive either distant intercessory prayer or no outside prayer in addition to standard care. In this trial, neither the patients nor their providers were aware that a trial was being conducted; therfore, informed consent was not obtained. As with the Harris study noted above, the hospital's IRB agreed to the protocol, given the apparent lack of potential harm. To conduct the study, patient photographs were e-mailed to a central location in the United States, where the randomization was performed. This study used a two-tiered system of prayer—the first group of intercessors prayed for a successful pregnancy for the patients to whom they were assigned, whereas a second group prayed for the success of the first group's prayers, as "prayer amplifiers."

The results of this study were striking—the group receiving the prayer intervention had a significantly higher pregnancy rate compared to the controls (50% vs 26%, $p = 0.0013$). The implantation rate of embryos was also significantly higher in the patients receiving prayer (16.3% vs 8%, $p = 0.0005$). The authors had no other explanations to account for their findings and suggested a repeat study to validate their results.

FUTURE DIRECTIONS IN HEALING PRAYER STUDIES

Although the application of prayer for healing purposes is an ancient cultural practice in traditions throughout the world, the scientific literature addressing this area can only be regarded as immature. There is no definitive weight of evidence that could support changes in practice standards or guidelines in cardiology or any other medical discipline. With any newly evolving area of medical research, one of the first points of concentration in planning future clinical trials is the development of well-defined, common nomenclature for key descriptors, methodologic variables, and end-point measures.

In addition to standardizing terminology, it is imperative that qualitative descriptors and, wherever possible, objective measures of patient characteristics, prayer methods, and outcomes be gathered as meticulously and as comprehensively as possible. In the absence of mechanistic knowledge, randomized controlled outcomes studies have the potential to support models to help elucidate mechanistic clues based on outcome observations. Such models may help to develop more mechanistically oriented hypotheses in the future (e.g., whether there is a dose–response relationship to the timing, duration, content, or number of intercessors providing healing prayer).

Issues regarding blinding patients and providers are also important. Trials must be conducted to exclude any possible placebo effect, because if a patient is merely participating in a trial or anticipates "receiving" prayer, he or she may influence outcome. However, as we will see below, this notion is also one that is debated, because it is possible that part or all of the success of a prayer intervention might stem from the knowledge or connection between the one who prays and the recipient. By definition, blinding would remove this connection.

As noted previously, the concept of "dosing" prayer, if it is to be treated as any other therapy with risks and benefits, is one that must be considered. Appropriate end-points must be measured in these trials, which may or may not include the "traditional" cardiovascular end-points of major adverse cardiac events of death and myocardial infarction (MI). For example, whether death is a negative outcome in a trial of prayer therapy is debatable, and quality-of-life outcomes may become more important. Safety issues must also be considered, with the implication that if prayer therapy has the potential to be beneficial, it also has the potential be harmful.

An important component of the quality and credibility of future research will depend on funding and funding sources. Perhaps most important among these are federal funding sources. In 2001, the National Center for Complementary and Alternative Medicine (NCCAM) at the National Institutes of Health (NIH) issued a request for applications for "frontier medicine" therapies, defined as "widely practiced medical therapeutics for which there is no plausible explanation," including healing prayer. The participation of the NIH will undoubtedly encourage research protocols to develop strong scientific rationales and statistical analysis plans.

Another important and evolving step for future research in healing prayer is the involvement of professional societies. As noted earlier, the American College of Cardiology has formally commissioned a consensus paper on complementary therapies, including spirituality and prayer.

This paper most likely addresses issues like the ethics and recommended approaches to issues, such as the need for informed consent from patients participating in study protocols using prayer therapies.

The involvement of federal agencies and professional societies may also help future research to stay focused on the health care agenda that is central to this area of systematic study. Issues, such as how God responds to prayer, whether there is proof that God exists, or which ethnic type of prayer is best, may make for interesting topics of philosophical debates but have little to do with safety and efficacy assessments of prayer as a novel adjunctive therapy for patients with CVD or other diseases. Similarly, whether prayer may affect human beings only at some ineffable level must be considered an issue outside of what is relevant to health care. Healing prayer of scientific and therapeutic significance can, in part, be defined by the requirement that at least some somatic manifestation of the healing effect is measurable.

Recently, a paper was published by Chibnall et al. arguing against the validity of applying scientific methods with statistical analysis to the constructs of prayer and spirituality *(19)*. They argue that the use of the null hypothesis is inappropriate in prayer and spirituality studies (in other words, "Assuming that God cannot heal at the bequest of human intercessors, what is the probabililty of getting these results?" *(19)*. They also argue that blinding healers or intercessors to patients is inappropriate, especially when the human connection of the intercessors might be part of what makes the intervention successful. Their article provides a thorough list of possible questions and concerns regarding prayer research, including the amount of prayer; the type, form, duration, frequency, level of fervency, and number of prayers; team vs individual prayer; specific faith involved; and the entity to whom the prayer is directed. The authors challenge the application of a deterministic model and the concept of causality to study prayer. The paper raises several interesting concerns regarding future research, although these critiques cannot simply be said to support the conclusion that research in this area is intrinsically meaningless.

CURRENT PERSPECTIVES ON CLINICAL APPLICATION OF HEALING PRAYER

With no insight into the mechanism and immature scientific literature to date, the weight of evidence does not support changing recommendations or developing specific guidelines for the systematic incorporation of healing prayer into health care delivery in general. Participation in investigational protocols of intercessory prayer that combine reasonable scientific study design with ethical compliance to standards for the protection of human subjects should be considered, like any patient participation in trials of novel therapeutics. However, any recommendations for physicians to prescribe prayer systematically apart from such protocols is premature.

With no safety issues identified to date and recognizing the ancient and global cultural belief systems in the role of prayer in health and illness, spiritual support services can and should continue to be offered to patients charitably. They should also be evaluated as a component of health care systems and as part of an ongoing quality improvement in health care. If a patient or family wants to pray, the presence of an on-site chapel or a chaplain who can be of assistance is both reasonable and important.

CONCLUSIONS

Intercessory prayer trials have shown varied results. In cardiovascular medicine, two of three trials were interpreted as "positive" for intercessory prayer in CCU patients; however, the clinical relevance of the composite scores used is unclear. The third trial shows no benefit. Similarly, intercessory prayer trials conducted with other diseases use different methods and end points and have differing results. Further research should be conducted to ensure standardization of methods and terms, as well as the safety and efficacy of spirituality as an intervention. Questions exist regarding the validity of applying scientific methods to the study of a field that, by its nature, transcends science as we currently understand it. Regardless of the ability of the scientific and medical communities to provide data on prayer and clinical outcomes, many patients, their families, and their friends will undoubtedly continue to pray for themselves and their sick loved ones, with the goal of affecting outcomes, as well as providing spiritual support.

REFERENCES

1. King DE, Bushwick B. Beliefs and attitudes of hospital inpatients about faith healing and prayer. J Fam Pract 1994;39:349–352.
2. Maugans TA, Wadland, WC. Religion and family medicine: a survey of physicians and patients. J Fam Pract 1991;32:210–213.
3. Eisenberg DM, Davis RB, Ettner SL, et al. Trends in alternative medicine use in the United States, 1990–1997: results of a follow-up national survey. JAMA 1998:280:1569–1575.
4. Princeton Religion Research Center. Religion in America. The Gallop Poll, Princeton, NJ, 1996.
5. Koenig HG, McCullough ME, Larson DB. Handbook of Religion and Health. Oxford University Press, London, 2001.

6. Halperin, EC. Should academic medical centers conduct clinical trials of the efficacy of intercessory prayer? Acad Med 2001;76:791–797.

7. Astin, JA, Harkness E, Ernst E. The efficacy of "distant healing": a systematic review of randomized trials. Ann Intern Med 2000;132:903–910.

8. Dossey L. Healing Words—The Power of Prayer and the Practice of Medicine. Harper, San Francisco, 1993.

9. Benor DJ. Spiritual Healing: Scientific Validation of a Healing Revolution. Vision Publications, 2001.

10. Byrd, RC. Positive therapeutic effects of intercessory prayer in a coronary care unit population. Southern Med J 1988;81:826–829.

11. Harris WS, Gowda M, Kolb JW, et al. A randomized, controlled trial of the effects of remote, intercessory prayer on outcomes in patients admitted to the coronary care unit. Arch Intern Med 1999;159:2273–2278.

12. Aviles JM, Whelan E, Hernke DA, et al. Intercessory prayer and cardiovascular disease progression in a coronary care unit population: a randomized controlled trial. Mayo Clin Proc 2001;76:1192–1198.

13. Krucoff MW, Crater SW, Green CL, et al. Integrative noetic therapies as adjuncts to percutaneous intervention during unstable coronary syndromes: Monitoring and Actualization of Noetic Training (MANTRA) feasibility pilot. Am Heart J 2001;142:760–767.

14. American College of Cardiology Clinical Expert Consensus Document on Alternative Medicine, September 2001.

15. Mueller PS, Plevak DJ, Rummans TA. Religious involvement, spirituality, and medicine: implications for clinical practice. Mayo Clin Proc 2001;76:1225–1235.

16. Matthews, DA, Marlowe, SM, MacNutt, FS. Effects of intercessory prayer on patients with rheumatoid arthritis. Southern Med J 2000;93:1177–1186.

17. Sicher F, Targ E, Moore D, Smith H. A randomized double-blind study of the effect of distant healing in a population with advanced AIDS. Western J Med 1998;169:356–363.

18. Kwang YC, Wirth DP, Lobo RA. Does prayer influence the success of in vitro fertilization-embryo transfer? Report of a masked, randomized trial. J Reprod Med 2001;46781–787.

19. Chibnall JT, Jeral JM, Cerullo MA. Experiments on distant intercessory prayer. Arch Int Med 2001;161:2529–2536.

10 Massage Therapy and Cardiovascular Disease

Patricia Cadolino, LMT, CIMI

CONTENTS

INTRODUCTION

Manual therapy, such as massage therapy, is one of the oldest forms of treatment in the world, probably older than that of recorded time. Massage was referred to in ancient Greek and Roman texts and was also mentioned in the writing of Asclopiades and Herodicus. Dating back to at least 1800 BC. Hippocrates defined medicine as "the art of rubbing" and stated that "the physician must be experienced in many things...but assuredly in rubbing. For rubbing can bind a joint that is too loose, and loose a joint that is too tight" *(1)*.

From: *Contemporary Cardiology*
Complementary and Alternative Cardiovascular Medicine
Edited by: R. A. Stein and M. C. Oz © Humana Press Inc., Totowa, NJ

Massage therapy is widely used in the United States and abroad and noted in our earlier medical texts, where it was often listed as a component of primary healing, along with diet and exercise. Massage therapy was all but abandoned from the American medical scene in the 1940s during the pharmaceutical revolution but has become popular as part of the focus of interest on complementary and alternative medicine (CAM) therapies. This may relate, in part, to the observation that Americans are relatively touch deprived in comparison with other cultures *(2)*. As the historical trend toward integration between CAM modalities and mainstream health care evolves the medical community is increasingly seeking evidence that massage is effective and safe, despite its long and positive history.

Massage therapy has value regarding facilitating growth, reducing pain and stress, increasing alertness, lowering depression levels, and enhancing immune functions. Studies have indicated that touch can stimulate physiological changes that positively affect on cognitive, emotional, physical, and neurological development *(3,4)*. Our skin is the largest sensory organ. It is the first sense to be developed *in utero* and accommodates millions of touch receptors. When the skin is stimulated by massage, neuro impulses are sent via the spinal column to the brain, potentially triggering adaptive responses in all organ systems.

Every culture has an attitude on how to approach the body. Western medicine has traditionally separated the healing of the body from healing of the mind. Many patients and health care providers now view the two as inseparable. Body work (massage) addresses both mind and body in the context of physical and psychological healing. Massage is defined as the systematic manual or mechanical manipulations of the soft tissues of the body for therapeutic purposes, such as promoting blood circulation and lymph, muscle relaxation, pain relief, metabolic balance restoration, and other physical and mental benefits. Systematic manual or mechanical manipulations include such movement as rubbing, kneading, pressure, rolling, or tapping *(5)*.

CLINICAL RESEARCH

The Touch Research Institute, founded in 1992 under the direction of Dr. Tiffany Field, is one of the first centers to focus on the scientific study of touch and its effects on disease. The institute has demonstrated that the physiological consequences of massage are mediated, in part, by release of gastrointestinal (GI) hormones, increases in endorphins levels, reduction in stress hormones (cortisol, norepinephrine, and adrenaline) and increases in dopamine and serotonin levels *(6–9)*.

Dr. Saul Schanberg conducted research using rats to support the use of touch as therapy for enhancing growth. The effect of touch deprivation was assessed by comparing the outcomes in rat pups that were taken away from their mother with pups left with their mothers (controls). Schanberg noted a decrease in growth hormone (GH) (ornithinedecarboxylase) in all body organs, including the heart, liver, and brain (cerebrum, cerebellum, and brainstem) in the pups that were removed from their mothers (touch deprived). The values returned to the normal range when the pups were given stimulation techniques that replicated the mother's behavior. Researchers mimicked the stimulation by using a paintbrush dipped in water and briskly stroked all over, mimicking their mother's tongue. The data suggest that stimulation of pressure receptors is critical for facilitating growth, and the researchers postulated that an alteration in genetic expression, triggered by touch, led to protein synthesis. Shanberg stated, "Maternal touch is not just a nice thing for children to have; you damn well need it if you want them to grow!" *(10,11)*.

Mind–Body Connection

Tight contracted tissues are perceived by the massage therapist to result from emotional stress turned inward and from physical insults and trauma. Tissues are programmed to contract as a response to being irritated. One of the main goals of massage is not to allow accumulation of contracted or tight muscle tissue throughout the body. In theory, this reduces spasm and prevents scar-like tissue accumulation. Thus, a patient with episodes of pain over time, who treats the pain only with medication, will suffer increasingly muscular and soft tissue levels of dysfunction.

Spinal Alignment

Observation of the influence of postural mechanics on function and symptomatology have led to the hypothesis that posture moderates several physiologic functions, including breathing, hormone production, spinal pain, headache, mood, blood pressure, pulse, and lung capacity. The most significant noted influences of posture are on respiration, oxygenation, and sympathetic function. Massage therapy is, in part, based on the belief that homeostasis and autonomic regulation are intimately affected by posture *(12)*. Tension to the spine causing postural deviations is viewed as leading to degenerative changes. That may interfere with the normal function of the central nervous system (CNS) leading to maladaptive alteration in function and coordination of the systems in the body. Massage is believed to sustain muscles at their normal resting length, as opposed to a tight and constricted state. Additionally, increases local circulation, potentially enhancing oxygen delivery of nutrients that may help to normalize muscle anatomy and physiology *(13)*.

THE EFFECTS OF MASSAGE ON THE NERVOUS SYSTEM

Numerous studies have demonstrated the effects of massage on the nervous system; however, these effects are limited to the massage period. Four separate studies have demonstrated the effect of massage therapy on the amplitude of H-Reflex response. The H-Reflex is a measure of neuromuscular excitability measured by using skin electrodes. It is increased in spinal cord injury and in patients who are suffering from muscular cramps or spasms. Decreasing the H-Reflex response correlated with increased patient comfort and decreased cramps and spasms. The massage therapy related reduction in the H-Reflex amplitude (60–80%); however, lasts only during the massage. The importance of this observation is the implication that local massage therapy mediates changes in H-Reflex, which reflects a change in the excitability of motor nerves in the spinal cord *(14–18)*.

Massage either sedates or stimulate a person's nervous system, depending on its application. Most commonly, massage will sedate the nervous system. Massage can downregulate the sympathetic nervous system and enhance the parasympathetic nervous system activity. In contrast, in preevent sport massage, the body worker stimulates the sympathetic nervous system activity so that the athlete is "ready for action" *(19)*.

Massage may mediate an increase in parasympathetic activation to slow the heart rate and may decrease body temperature, enhance digestion and elimination, and reduce stress-related hormone levels, such as cortisol norepinephrine and adrenaline *(20)*.

Blood and Coagulation

Massage enhances functional red blood cell number and white blood cells and platelet counts *(21)*. Thrombosis from impaired venous return may be prevented by massage, as indicated in one study of burn patients. In this study, unilateral lower extremity massage decreased the incidence of deep vein thrombosis (DVT) in the massaged limb by 82%, in comparison with the untreated limb *(22)*. Arm massage also decreases DVT incidence *(23)*.

Blood Pressure

Massage mechanically assists venous blood flow return to the heart and stimulates tissue release of histamines and acetylcholine *(24)*. Massage increases systolic stroke volume via a decreased heart rate, thus increasing diastolic filling. The reduction in heart rate is effected by a decrease in stimulation of the sympathetic the increase in parasympathetic activity. One small study demonstrated a reduction in systolic and diastolic blood pressures after 30 min of massage on the back area. The systolic pressure was reduced from mean values of 142 to 133 mmHg. After massage, the patients scored significantly lower on anxiety, depression, and hostility scales and had a decrease from premessage levels in salivary and urinary cortisol hormone levels *(25)*. Another recent study of 52 people demonstrated a significant decrease in blood pressure after a 15-min chair massage *(26)*.

THE EFFECTS OF MASSAGE
ON THE CIRCULATORY SYSTEM

One of the most widely recognized physiologic effects of body work is an increase in peripheral and central blood flow. Studies dating back to the 1930s described increases in blood flow resulting from massage, with a dilation of superficial blood vessels and a consequent decrease in peripheral vascular resistance *(27)*.

Studies that have examined the increase in the number of open capillaries and the rate of blood flow before and after massage have noted an effect similar to exercise, with an enhanced amount of open capillaries. The peak open capillary count per mm^2 of muscle was 1400 after massage and 3500 after peak exercise. Resting capillary counts were a mean of 37. This effect was noted to last for approx 24 h and, as with exercise, the more frequent and intense the stimulus (massage) the longer the capillaries stayed open at rest. In addition, massage has been reported to increase lymph circulation *(28,29)*.

Pain Reduction

Massage therapy is often effective in reducing pain and can help to reduce muscle tension and muscle contraction, which is generally present in a pain-type condition. The author has found that often, when there is a complaint of pain, it is accompanied by contracted skin, fascia, and muscle. When moderate therapeutic pressure is applied directly on the skin, the tissue is softened and normalized and discomfort eased. This is important, because the underlying tissues must be kept healthy. It is believed that tight contracted tissues "squeeze" pain receptors, blood vessels, and nerves, resulting in pain, fatigue, and weakness. Massage decreases pain by releasing endorphins, enkephalins, and other pain-modulating neurochemicals. In addition, the general relaxation brought on by massage therapy has, in the author's experience, an admonishing effect on pain.

Massage may inhibit pain by interfering with inceptive information (the "gateway" concept), which enters the spinal cord through stimulation of cutaneous thermoreceptors and mechanoreceptors. Sensations that are produced by massage have the potential to suppress painful stimuli. Massage is believed to mechanically effect pain receptors (e.g., golgi tendon organs) and alter the neural signals. This is termed "neuromuscular reeducation" *(30)*.

THE EFFECTS OF MASSAGE
FOR THE RESPIRATORY SYSTEM

Massage slows down the rate of respiration via stimulation of the parasympathetic nervous system. The mechanical loosening and discharge of phlegm in the respiratory tract is increased with the rhythmic alternating pressures induced by massage. Tapotement (cupping) and vibration on the rib cage are often used to enhance this effect. Phlegm loosening and discharge are further enhanced when combined with certain postural body positions to promote drainage. By freeing tight respiratory muscles, massage can be used to increase vital capacity and pulmonary function *(31)*.

CARDIAC MEDICATIONS

Aspirin, Coumadin, and other antiplatelet drugs are often associated with easy bruising and bleeding. Manual methods, such as compression, friction, deep sustained pressure, or trigger-point work, should generally be avoided in patients on these medications. Light pressure massage may be valuable. Patients who are taking diuretics may complain of pain, muscle weakness, and cramping or spasms. These are common symptoms that are treated by massage and may be a sign of electrolyte imbalance. Calcium channel blockers and other vasodilators may cause swollen feet and ankles. Caution is advised, because some of these patients may be at an increased risk for developing DVT *(32)*.

THE EFFECTS OF MASSAGE
FOR THE URINARY SYSTEM

Massage, especially abdominal work, increases urine output possibly by activating dormant capillary beds and recovering lymphatic fluids for filtration and enhancing parasympathetic activity. Massage increases the excretion of nitrogen, inorganic phosphorus, and sodium chloride. The levels of these metabolic wastes are elevated in urine after massage *(33)*.

SPECIAL CONSIDERATIONS FOR MASSAGE

There are several situations where massage is relatively contraindicated, depending on the extent of the condition. The general rule is that massage should maintain a patient's internal stability and avoid promoting the spread of any disease, infection, or blood clot. Generally, relative contraindications will apply to an area being treated and not to the entire body. However, appropriate caution is always advised (*see* Table 1).

MANUAL HEALING TECHNIQUES:
A BRIEF DESCRIPTIVE GLOSSARY

The following list provides a brief description of various manual and "touch" therapies that your patient may encounter.

Alexander technique: Gentle touch motions and manual therapy are aimed at achieving a more balanced and poised state. The outcome is relief of physical tension through reeducation of the "kinesthetic sense." A practitioner will aim to make a series of adjustments to the body to improve posture.

Aromatherapy: The use of essential oils is an age-old technique. Various scents added to massage oil therapy could selectively influence the massage to be relaxing and stimulate healing.

Craniosacral: This is a type of myofascial release addressing tensions in the craniosacral system. It is a light-touch procedure aimed at remedying distortions in the structure and function of the craniosacral mechanism. It is believed to help alleviate neck and low back pain and stress-related problems.

Feldenkrais: A system of physical reeducation. The practitioner provides gentle manipulation in helping patients to avoid bad posture and movements that reflect disruptions in the nervous system. Strives to improve posture to free a person to become more flexible.

Myofascial release: This is used to loosen contractile connective tissues, muscles, and fascia. Gentle traction, pressure, and positioning are used to coax muscles in spasm to relax and to break adhesions in the fascia.

Neuromuscular therapy: This is soft-tissue manipulation that is aimed at balancing the CNS with the musculoskeletal system. Moderate to deep pressure is applied to break stress–tension–pain cycles. The aim is to relax muscles, especially those that are compressing nerves to increase circulation.

On-site massage: A 15- to 20-min chair massage fully clothed with concentration on the shoulders, neck, back, head, and arms.

Polarity: This is a blend of Western therapies, traditional Chinese medicine, and ayurveda. Practitioners aim to rebalance the energy flow

Table 1
Special Considerations for Massage

Acute infection	Massage is relatively contraindicated for areas of acute infection. This could include infections of the bone, (osteomyelitis), joints (septic arthritis), skin (dermatitis), muscle (myositis), or subcutaneous (cellulites). Avoid affected areas if inflammation is localized. Do not apply massage if a fever is present.
Acute rheumatoid arthritis	Avoid affected joints.
Aplastic anemia	Massage is systemically contraindicated. Physician verification is needed.
Hemolytic anemia	Massage is systemically contraindicated. Physician approval necessary.
Aneurysm	Massage is systemically contraindicated for patients with known aneurysms. Physician must verify that the patient can handle the increase in circulation and pressure. With abdominal aneurysm, local massage is absolutely contraindicated.
Angina pectoris	Massage systemically contraindicated during acute episodes of angina but can continue after symptoms are relieved.
Arteriosclerosis	Massage can help to reduce stress and anxiety levels and may promote general relaxation.
Cancer	There is no research indicating that body work causes cancer to spread. Research has shown that informed, caring touch can have a positive effect on the immune system. Avoid deep pressure. Cancer massage is effective in the management and treatment of cancer in these following areas: reducing cancer pain—managing nausea, treating lymphedema, reducing anxiety, and enhancing relaxation *(34–44)*.
Cardiomyopathy	Massage can be used with physician verification that patient can tolerate treatment.
Congestive heart failure (CHF).	Massage should be light and of short duration. Patients with CHF may be candidates for massage; however, the treatment is not a general kneading massage. Care must be given to ensure that the patient's chest is elevated and that the

(continued)

Table 1 (Continued)

	massage does not mobilize sufficient extracellular fluids to produce symptoms of congestion. Avoid deep work, excessive elevation, and large range of motion movements, because this could activate sympathetic nervous system response. It is important not to lay the patient in a prone position. The goal of the massage is to reduce stress using relaxing and soothing techniques. Designing a treatment plan with limb work first helps to reduce peripheral resistance.
Postcardiac surgery	During the early recovery phase from coronary bypass surgery, massage is contraindicated. Saphenous vein resection sites and chest incision sites should be healed. Foot massage to induce relaxation is recommended. Collaboration is essential between therapist and attending physician.
CVA	Massage is systemically contraindicated during early recovery but indicated during the later recovery phases.
Decubitus ulcers	Massage is a good preventive modality to increase general circulation. Massage at or near unhealed ulcers is contraindicated.
Diabetes mellitus	Massage may be appropriate with diabetes, under the right circumstances. Patient must have healthy responsive tissues with good blood supply, and medical clearance is appropriate. Caution should be used in patients with diabetic neuropathy because of their lack of sensation and propensity to develop skin ulcers.
Edema	When edema results from CHF or renal failure, massage therapy that may "mobilize fluids" is relatively contraindicated. Venous insufficiency-related edema is a reasonable setting for massage therapy. Pitting edema is contraindicated.
Heart murmur	Massage is beneficial for general relaxation.
Hypercholesterolemia	Massage is beneficial for general relaxation.
Hematomas	Massage should avoid any areas where foreign

(continued)

Table 1 (Continued)

	bodies may exist or potentially cause damage. In addition, massage should avoid areas of hematomas in the first few days after injury so blood clots are not disrupted.
Hemophilia	Massage is systemically contraindicated.
Hypertension	In patients with borderline hypertension not requiring medications, conservative massage can help to lower blood pressure and reduce stress levels. Massage is beneficial for general relaxation. A good general guideline is that the patient's blood pressure on treatment should be less then 160/90. When the blood pressure is higher than that, deep abdominal work is contraindicated. When the blood pressure at rest is over 190/100, massage is contraindicated. Observing signs that massage could be overchallenging the body, such as clamminess, bogginess, and possible edema, in the days after the treatment is important. Patients who are on medication for hypertension or who are known to have atherosclerosis should consult a doctor before receiving a massage.
Insomnia	Massage therapy can offer a good night's sleep, brought about by restoration of balance between parasympathetic and sympathetic nervous system.
Joint inflammation	Massage is indicated after the acute phase. Massage should be applied using strokes to promote draining, which pushes edema fluid toward the heart and increase, lymphatic circulation.
Myocardial infarction	After the acute phase, patients can benefit from massage for relaxation. It is suggested that this therapy be offered in collaboration with the attending physician.
Phlebitis, thrombosis, or other diseases blood vessels	If the patient is taking any type of medication or for these conditions he or she should get of medical clearance before receiving massage. In moderate to severe cases, massage is contraindicated both locally and distally.

(continued)

Table 1 (Continued)

Raynaud's syndrome	As long as any dangerous underlying causes for the vasoconstriction have been ruled out, patients with Raynaud's syndrome are candidates for massage. Massage may work with the parasympathetic nervous system to stimulate reflexive vasodilatation and help to restore normal circulation.
Renal failure	Massage is systemically contraindicated for both acute and chronic failure.
Skin conditions	Avoid areas that are contagious.
Transient ischemic (TIA)	Massage is contraindicated during acute attack episode but beneficial to patients after the early recovery phase.
Varicosities	Local massage is contraindicated in the areas where the veins are elevated from the skin and are visibly distorted. If the vein is not elevated, local massage may be appropriate; however, the pressure applied should be light. For spider veins, local massage is usually safe.
Vascular disorders	Any condition involving damaged blood vessels requires extreme caution for massage. Massage changes the internal environment d diles some blood vessels and constricts others.
Viruses	Massage should be given with caution for patients with active viral infections. For example, formononucleosis, the area at or near liver or spleen avoided.

by touch, nutritional advice, exercise, and counseling. Energy blocks can, in this theoretical framework, be released by body work, diet, exercise, and self awareness. The aim is to "balance the energy in the body."

Reflexology: Based on the theory that the body has "reflex areas" on the hands and feet that correspond to glands, organs, and different parts of the body. Manipulating those certain areas has a direct effect on corresponding organs and body parts.

Reiki: This is a form of nonmovement Japanese spiritual healing and a gentle hands-on technique to reduce stress, relieve pain, and facilitate healing. This does not involve manipulation of the muscles or other soft tissue. A practitioner holds his hands on or over the body in 12 basic

positions for approx 5 min each while channeling Ki or life energy. This
is believed to balance the body's energy.

Rolfing: A form of deep-tissue pressure massage that promotes well-
being and soft-tissue manipulation through deep manipulation. This
technique aims to balance the whole body into vertical alignment and
increase range of motion.

Shiatsu: Based in traditional Chinese medicine, this system is based on
the body's energy meridians, somewhat related to acupuncture. This
procedure is achieved by applying pressure on various points throughout the body to influence and stimulate energy flow.

Swedish massage: This is primarily designed to relax muscles. The
strokes and manipulations of Swedish massage are each conceived as
having specific therapeutic benefits. One of the primary goals of Swedish massage is to speed venous return from the extremities. Swedish
massage is believed to shorten recovery time from muscular strain by
enhanced local blood flow increasing the clearance, from the muscles,
of lactic acid, uric acid, and other metabolites. Because it can help to
reduce emotional and physical stress, it is often recommended as part
of a regular program for stress management.

Trager: A gentle therapy that employs light rocking, stretching, and
swinging-type movements to achieve deep relaxation and a sense of
well-being.

SUMMARY

Massage therapy can have a significant effect on the health and functioning of the body and potentially has beneficial effects on multiple
organ systems. Of course, it is not the preeminent answer for most serious medical problems. A knowledge of the indications, contradictions,
and precautions is necessary to provide safe and effective massage. There
is no greater gift than that of nurturing touch to patients that is provided
by successfully integrating massage therapy, as an adjunct modality,
with mainstream medicine.

STATUS OF THE PROFESSION

Educational requirements vary tremendously from state to state and
from school to school. The national education requirements are 500 to
650 h of training. Today, it is more common that massage programs are
1000 h, with an associate degree-equivalent to a 2-yr program.

REFERENCES

1. Tarver M. A historical perspective of massage. In: Massage Therapy Principles and
   Practice. W B Saunders, Philadelphia, 1999, pp. 4–8.

2. Field,T. Touch therapy effects on development. Int J Behav Devel 1998;22:779–797.
3. Field T. Massage therapy. Contemp Pediatr 1999;16:77–94.
4. Field T. Massage therapy for infants/children. Develop Behav Pediatr 1995;16:105–111.
5. Beck MF. Theory and Practice of Therapeutic Massage. 1999, (3rd ed.). 3, 17–18.
6. Field T. Pregnant women benefit from massage therapy. J Psychosomat Obstet Gynecol 1999;18:31–38.
7. Field T. Burn injuries benefit from massage therapy. J Burn Care Rehab 1998;19:241–244.
8. Field T. Massage therapy effects on depression and somatic symptoms in chronic fatigue syndrome. 1997;3:43–51.
9. Field T. Touch therapy effects of development. Int J Behav Devel 1998;22:779–797.
10. Health and Discovery. Quote Dr. Saul Schanberg. Newsday November, 1998, p. B-29.
11. Field T, Schanberg S. Touch therapy effects on development. Int J Behav Devel 1998;22:779–797.
12. Lennon S, Cady M, Cox. Am J Pain Manage. Postural and respiratory modulation of autonomic function. Pain Health 1994;4:36.
13. Akio S. The reflex effects of spinal somatic nerve stimulation on visceral function. J Manip Physiol Ther 1992;15:57–61.
14. Goldberg J. The effect of two intensities of massage on H-reflex amplitude. Phys Ther 1992;72:449–457.
15. Goldberg J. The effects of therapeutic massage on H-reflex amplitude in persons with spinal cord injury. Phys Ther 1994;74:728–737.
16. Mason M. The treatment of lymphoedema by complex physical therapy. Austr Physiother 1993;39:41–45.
17. Morelli M. H-reflex modulation during manual muscle massage of human triceps surea. Arch Phys Med Rehab 1991;72:915–919.
18. Sullivan S, Williams L, Seaborne D, Morelli M. Effects on massage of alpha motoneuron excitability. Phys Ther 1991;71:555–560.
19. Burch S. Recognizing Health and Illness. Health Positive Publishing, Lawrence, Kansas, 1997, pp. 37–39.
20. Salvo S. Effects on the Nervous System. In: Massage Therapy. WB Saunders, Philadelphia, PA, 1999, p. 259.
21. Salvo S. Effects on Blood cell counts. In: Massage Therapy. WB Saunders, Philadelphia, PA, 1999, pp. 430–432.
22. Gotes GC. Massage the scientific basis of an ancient art: part 2: physiologic and therapeutic effects. Br J Sports Med 1994;28:153–298.
23. Gotes GC. Massage the scientific basis of an ancient art: part 2: physiologic and therapeutic effects. Br J Sports Med 1994;28:153–156.
24. Salvo S. Effects on Cardiovascular. In: Massage Therapy Principles and Practice. WB Saunders, Philadelphia, PA 1999, p. 298.
25. Field T. High blood pressure reduced by massage therapy. J Body Work Movement Ther. 2000;4:31–38.
26. Barr J, Taslitz N. "Influence of back massage on autonomic functions. Phys Ther 1970;50:1679–1691.
27. Gotes GC. Massage the scientific basis of an ancient art. Physiologic and therapeutic effects. Br J Sports Med 1994;28:153–156.
28. Wine. Massage treatment for vascular dysfunction's. Massage Mag 64:122–123.
29. DeDomenico G. Mechanical, physiological, psychological, and therapeutic effects of massage. In: DeDomenico G, Woods E, eds. Beard's Massage (4th ed.) WB Saunders, 1997, pp. 56–57.

30. Anderson K. Massage physiology—nervous and endocrine systems. In: Salvo SG, ed. Massage Therapy Principles and Practice. WB Saunders, 1999, pp. 432–433.
31. Massage for respiratory conditions. In: De Domenico G, Wood E, eds. Beard's Massage (4th ed.) WB Saunders, Philadelphia, 1997, pp. 149–155.
32. Persad R. Massage Therapy & Medication. Curties-Overzet Publications Inc., 2001, pp. 12–13.
33. Effects on the Urinary System. In: Salvo SG, ed. Massage Therapy. WB Saunders, 1999, p. 344.
34. Barbour LA, McGuire DB, Kirchhoff KT. Nonanalgesic method of pain controls used by cancer out patients. Oncol Nurs Forum 1986;13:56–60.
35. Dalton J. Pain relief for cancer patients. Cancer Nurs 1998;11:332–328.
36. Daut RL, Cleeland CS. The prevalence and severity of pain in cancer. Cancer 1982;50:1913–1918.
37. Dibble S. Acupressure for nausea. Oncol Nurs Forum 2000;27:41–47.
38. Dorrepaal KL, Aaronson NK, van Dam FS. Pain experience and pain management among hospitalized cancer patients. A clinical study. Cancer 1989;63:593–598.
39. Ferrell BR, Schneider C. Experience and management of pain at home. Cancer Nurs 1988;11:84–90.
40. Ferrell-Torry A, Glick O. The use of therapeutic massage as a nursing intervention to modify anxiety and the perception of cancer pain. Cancer Nursing 1993;16:93–101.
41. Grealish L. Foot massage—a nursing intervention to modify the distressing symptoms of pain and nausea in patients hospitalized with cancer. Cancer Nurs 2000;23:237–243.
42. Bruce I. Post mastectomy lymphoedema treatment and measurement. Med J Austr 1994;161:125–128.
43. Hernandez-Reif M, Field MT, Ironson G, Weiss S, Katz G. Immunological responses of breast cancer patients to massage therapy. Touch Research Institute, 2001.
44. Weinrich SP, Weinrich MC. The effect of massage on pain in cancer patients. Appl Nurs Res 1990;3:140–145.

11 Acupuncture in Cardiovascular Disease

Soeren Ballegaard, MD

CONTENTS

HISTORICAL BACKGROUND

What is Acupuncture?

The word *acupuncture* comes from the Latin words *acu* (needle) and *punctura*. Therefore, acupuncture is the treatment of illness by sticking needles in the skin.

Acupuncture originated in China, and the first acupuncture needles, which were made of flint, date back to approx 800 yr BC. Acupuncture is believed to be based on the discovery of the existence of points on the body's surface through which symptoms of illness could be influenced. A systemization of these points was first described in the second century BC, in the book *Huang-di Nei-jing (1)*.

At that time, scholarship was flourishing in China. The educated were individuals who had personally acquired wisdom and who passed it on to their students through many years of training, following the master–apprentice model: a model that is still seen in the Far East today. In addition to observing nature, the educated formulated theories to explain

From: *Contemporary Cardiology*
Complementary and Alternative Cardiovascular Medicine
Edited by: R. A. Stein and M. C. Oz © Humana Press Inc., Totowa, NJ

what they observed. These theories put the many and various observations into systems, making it possible to pass on experience to students meaningfully. The theories were like glue that held the many independent observations together. The formulation of these theories was based on, simply, the world view that predominated at that time—Taoism. In Nei-jing, the historical and empirical discovery of sensitive points—and their effects on disease—has been chained together in a Taoistic model. Points with related functions are held together by binding them with lines called meridians. The book also describes how the body works and how illnesses arise and can be treated.

The individual masters developed their own personal variations on the common theoretical theme. That is why today there are many different ways of doing acupuncture not only different from country to country but also in China.

The role of the doctor in classical Chinese society was different from the modern Western role. The doctor was only paid if he kept his patients well. Once a year, at the end of the year, people gave the doctor his pay, based on how effectively he had helped them to look after their health in that year. In addition, he had to hang a red lamp outside his practice every time one of his patients was sick. This enabled travelers to gauge the quality of his work and to avoid the doctors who had many red lamps hanging outside their doors. Patients made it possible for their doctors to keep them in good health by seeing them regularly, when their complaints were minor and before their illnesses were so advanced that they couldn't work.

When these Chinese patients went to their doctors, the doctors thoroughly analyzed their total life situations. All symptoms from every part of the body were considered and viewed as a significant part of the total problem. The patient's psychological and social situation was also evaluated. The doctor had many different ways to guide and help the patient. Acupuncture was just one of these. Chinese society had formulated various fixed rules of life, which its citizens were advised to follow to maintain good health. These included dance; massage; Taoist psychological techniques; breathing exercises, such as Qigong *(2)*, and special gymnastic exercises, such as Thai Qi. The patient was to do such exercises every day to maintain control over his or her body and to maintain good health. This is also a fundamental element in the Eastern fighting disciplines, such as karate and judo/jujitsu, both of which are derived from Thai Qi. Regarding purely medical options, in addition to acupuncture, the doctor could offer a range of herbal medicines. The various treatment options were often combined, so that the patient received acupuncture and dietary instructions and was required to do gymnastic and breathing exercises and take various herbs.

To understand how acupuncture can be used to treat an illness in its early stages, we must assume that the Chinese diagnostic system is sensitive and picks up signals early in the illness progression. Therefore, the body must emit signals at an early stage. The signals that the Chinese discovered were sore points, which developed on the skin in connection with certain illnesses.

We also have to assume that the body has a healing system—a system that, when stimulated, can lead to healing the patient's illness and that sticking a needle in the skin's sore points, the acupuncture points, activates and stimulates such a healing process.

Classical Chinese Medical Theory

When you begin to talk about classical Chinese medical theory, you run into words such as Tao, yin, yang, and the five elements: wood, fire, earth, metal, and water. It is important to understand that these concepts belong to a philosophical model, which the Chinese constructed to explain the natural phenomena they saw around them. The Chinese worldview is characterized by a holistic understanding in which all phenomena in the universe are a part of the same ultimate reality—Tao. Tao can never become demonstrable knowledge or be described adequately with words, because it lies in that region between the senses and the intellect *(3)*.

Tao, which is unity, reality, and harmony in the universe, is divided into two opposing forces, yin and yang. The relationship between them is described as "the law of the unity of opposites." They shape, consume, support, and transform into one another.

The idea that they shape one another shows that they don't exist in isolation but only in their interaction with their opposite part. Yin and yang respectively symbolize minus and plus, cold and warm, woman and man, inward and outward, downward and upward, darkness and light, passive and active, and earth and heaven.

Something that is yin in one situation can be yang in another, because they are relative concepts. For example, the skin on the back is yin (back) relative to the skin on the chest, which is yang (front). At the same time, the skin on the back is yang (outward) relative to the inner organs, which are yin (inward).

Because of their relationship of mutual opposition, the weakening or loss of one will automatically influence the other. Therefore, weakening of yin leads to the relative strengthening of yang, and a strengthening of yin will lead to a relative weakening of yang and vice-versa. The balance between them is not static but always dynamic. Under normal conditions they will be in relative balance, but under conditions of strain, one of them can dominate too much and the other become too weak and then illness occurs. The goal of treatment is to reestablish the relative balance.

The five elements—wood, fire, earth, metal, and water—are considered to be the basic components of the material world. A relationship of mutual interdependence and control exists among the elements, which is used to classify natural phenomena, body tissues and organs, and human feelings *(4,5)*. In practice, the theories of yin and yang and the five elements are tied together so that the individual elements are divided into yin and yang parts. For example, the liver and the gallbladder belong to the wood element, where the gallbladder is the yang and the liver is the yin.

The theories of yin and yang and the five elements are not seen as stiff theoretical systems but rather as poetic models, which can be applied as needed. In Chinese medicine, they are used to describe the body's functions and illness development. They also assist in diagnosing and treating in daily clinical work. Man is seen as a miniature universe, a microcosm with an indwelling life force, "qi," which balances between the two opposing forces, yin and yang. Man is not viewed as an isolated phenomenon but, on the contrary, as tightly connected to the whole, the universe. The goal of human life is to live in harmony with this.

The Body's Composition

According to traditional Chinese medicine, the following components are the basic elements in the human body *(6)*: (1) the inner organs, (2) meridians and communication channels, (3) Qi ("life energy," pronounced "chee" as in "cheese"), and (4) blood and body fluids.

An important assumption in traditional Chinese medicine (TCM) is that the inner organs are connected to the body's surface through a complicated network of channels (meridians), whose main purpose is to supply all the parts of the body with life energy, "qi." These meridians generally lie deep beneath the skin and touch the body's surface only at particular points, the so-called acupuncture points. There are 12 meridians that are connected to the body's various organs. Energy flows through the organs in a fixed order and then starts again at the end of each cycle. A full cycle is believed to take 24 h. The individual organs are believed to be most active when their energy level is at its peak.

TCM has a view of man that differs from the Western view in two key ways. Man is viewed as an integrated part of the total universe, and the human biological processes are viewed as being controlled by the circulation of qi. The concept of qi does not exist in Western medicine; even the description of the body differs from the Western model. Although the same words are used from time to time, they mean different things. For example, the spleen is not the same in classical Chinese medicine as it is in the West, because it also looks after the functions that, in Western medicine, belong to the pancreas. The pancreas does not exist in Chinese medicine, nor do the hormone-producing glands or the nervous system, including the brain.

Although organs are well-defined structures in Western medicine, in Chinese medicine they are not viewed as solid components whose existence can be proven. Instead, they are defined by their functions and their mutual relationships. Therefore, Chinese medicine describes organs that don't exist in the Western sense. The *Sanjiao* organ does not exist as an anatomical structure but as a functional relationship between the organs, which influence the body's water metabolism. Feelings are also attached to the organs; for example, anger and a hot temper are linked to the liver, whereas happiness is linked to the heart.

The ancient Chinese masters were not particularly interested in proofs—that these things (qi, meridians, and organs) didn't exist in the physical sense doesn't matter. The important thing is that in the context of the culture, the system works and, therefore, the descriptions should be understood as a poetic expression of the things we can observe.

Can poetry be proved? It can be used, and we can decide whether it is worth listening to.

How Acupuncture Works According to Chinese Theory

Acupuncture generally works by harmonizing the body's energy balance. In parts of the body where there is too much energy, the needles help to remove the excess and bring the body back into balance. Acupuncture in the foot to treat a headache works by taking the surplus energy away from the head. Another type of headache is best treated using needles in the hand, but from a Chinese perspective, the mechanism is still the same—the removal of an energy surplus in an acupuncture meridian. This time it is just a different meridian which is out of balance.

It is important to understand that headaches can be treated in many different ways in Chinese medicine, depending on the nature of the headache and the patient's general state. The Chinese doctor will construct a complete picture of the patient's situation and then work out his or her treatment based on this.

If the Chinese doctor decides that there is an energy deficiency somewhere in the body, the goal of the acupuncture treatment will be to supply the person with energy and to harmonize the energy that already exists in the body. This is the theory behind moxibustion, where a special herb is burned on the needle to heat it, and this heat is transferred to the patient's body.

As one of the cornerstones in the process of working out an acupuncture treatment, the Chinese doctor will examine the patient and identify sore points (trigger points). The existence of these points assists the doctor in diagnosing, because the doctor's testimony can be weighed against the patient's account of his or her symptoms. Such trigger points always constitute an important element in treating the patient and are usually combined with other acupuncture points, which don't necessarily have to be sore. Of the approx 400 Chinese acupuncture points, only some can be used for diagnosis, whereby soreness has implications for the patient's treatment. Many of the acupuncture points are not sore, even when the patient is sick, just as certain acupuncture points can be sore without the patient necessarily being sick.

The traditional Chinese doctor, when talking to the patient, can home in on the location of the problem. By examining the patient's body, the doctor may find sore points, which can confirm the diagnosis. The doctor can then treat the patient with acupuncture, and, if the patient's problem has been helped, the same points will be less sore or free from soreness. The patient can be trained to be familiar with his or her own acupuncture points and apply acupressure when they flare up, starting treatment early. The acupressure may even be used for preventive measures.

Another cornerstone of acupuncture is understanding the courses of the meridians. Although the existence of these meridians is speculative, there have been times when a patient's ailment could not be fully explained using Western medical knowledge and when only a knowledge of the meridians' flows helped to understand and treat the problem.

Lisa P.'s illness is one such example. Four years ago, she had to have a tissue sample taken from her lung. A surgical cut was made in the skin over her breastbone, perpendicular to the bone. The scar healed, but some time later it began to hurt. The discomfort increased gradually until she had constant pain in her scar for the last few months. The pain had also spread to the skin around the scar. The skin in the whole region had become incredibly oversensitive, so that even the touch of clothing or the wind caused her discomfort. She couldn't get any explanation or any treatment that relieved the pain within the realm of conventional medicine. Two further operations had not even helped. From an acupuncture perspective, her discomfort could be explained by the surgical cut over her breastbone having been straight across a meridian, and, unfortunately, the "energy" could no longer find its way. The treatment was simple. Because the author knew which way the "energy" had to run in the meridian, he put a needle through the scar in the direction of the energy flow. The patient immediately described a feeling of "pins and needles" on the other side of the scar. After waiting some time, a needle was placed in the scar in the opposite direction.

The patient then said that the "pins and needles" stopped—she felt a calmness and a normal, comfortable feeling. At the end of the treatment, the scar and the surrounding area were hot. On her next visit, she told the author that the discomfort had been gone for 2 d. The treatment was repeated, and after a few visits, the patient's discomfort was alleviated.

If we imagine energy streaming along the meridians like water in a river, it's not difficult to see how a scar across the direction of flow could cause a blockage, like a dam in a river. We can also understand how pricking a hole in the blockage could allow the energy to flow again.

If we compare how acupuncture works with how common medical and surgical treatments work, there is a significant difference. While both medicine and surgery can be viewed as treatments of the symptom or the disease through an active intervention that tries to block biological processes, acupuncture works by stimulating the body's own healing resources, so that the body heals itself. I have asked patients who were undergoing angina pectoris treatment using acupuncture what were the effects they experienced. Although their comments can't be taken as proof that these things are true, they are certainly thought provoking. The needles make them relax, so that when they face situations that normally make them stressed and irritable and lead to angina, they instead find they are much more relaxed. They also discover, to their surprise, that they don't get heart pain. They describe it as a contrast to treatment with medicine, which indeed prevents their heart pain but doesn't change their feeling of stress. In addition, as with conventional treatment, they experience an improved physical performance.

CONTEMPORARY USE OF ACUPUNCTURE

Global and Local Variation

The practice and the teaching of acupuncture vary considerably throughout the world, from a close adherence to the rules of the TCM to a western "prescription" use of acupuncture. This implies a variety in the use of diagnostic procedures, treatment approach, dosage, choice of acupuncture points, use of electrical stimulation, and treatment frequency. Most practitioners adopt a personal style, which is developed from a mix of inspiration from various sources, combined with their own clinical experience, and this variety shows up in clinical and scientific studies, as illustrated later in this chapter. Only a few attempts at systematic development and improvement of the technique, such as the Swedish studies on skin flap survival, have been conducted (*see* Ischemic Skin Flaps section). This is in contrast to the industry-supported development of transcutaneous electrical nerve stimulation (TENS) and spinal cord stimulation (SCS).

The use of acupuncture, acupressure combined with numerous other remedies, all supporting the same aim—to help the body to heal itself and the person to live in balance with nature—has produced encouraging results in the treatment for angina pectoris. The results of one such treatment complex, called integrated rehabilitation, are presented later in this chapter (*see* Evidence Level B Observational Studies section).

Safety

In an English study of 34,000 acupuncture treatments, no serious side effects were encountered. Accordingly, it was concluded that when compared with medical treatment, acupuncture must be seen as a relatively gentle treatment *(7)*. However, in treating heart disease, the locations of the acupoints are close to vital organs, and the risk of serious complications, such as cardiac tamponade or pneumothorax, does exist *(8–10)* although such incidences are extremely rare.

CLINICAL AND SCIENTIFIC STUDIES AND EVIDENCE REGARDING USE OF ACUPUNCTURE

Methodological Considerations

INTRODUCTION

The double-blind randomized trial is the hallmark of the Western scientific world when assessing the effects of a new treatment. The purpose of the randomization is to ensure a balanced distribution of baseline variables between the treatment groups. The double-blinding eliminates patient and investigator biases. However, in acupuncture trials, it is not possible that *the treatments being compared are identical to the patient and the practitioner*. The consequences of this are discussed below and more comprehensively elsewhere *(11)*.

PATIENT BIAS

Genuine acupuncture entails the penetration of the skin at specific sites related to the condition of the patient, repeated physical contact between the hands of the acupuncturist and patient's skin, and a unique physical sensation when the needle affects the acupuncture point. This sensation is described as a soreness, an aching, or a burning and is different from the sensation related to penetration of the skin. Consequently, a truly nonactive control treatment, which feels like genuine acupuncture is not possible, and therefore patient bias cannot be eliminated.

Acupuncturist Bias

When compared with surgery and pharmacological treatment, the risk of inducing bias is far greater in acupuncture treatment because of the extensive and prolonged contact between patient and doctor: 10–12 consultations of 45 min, for a 3-wk period, in patients with angina pectoris. Accordingly, it is important to address the possible bias from the "Rosenthal Effect" induced by the acupuncturist. This effect is present in a range of experimental settings, for example, reaction time, animal learning, human learning, and ability testing *(12)*. Furthermore, the size of this effect is substantial, with 95% confidence limits ranging from 0.62–1.22 standard deviations *(13)*. The importance of this in cardiovascular disease (CVD) is underlined by observations of the lethal, healing, and conditioning power of words *(14)*, as well as the following examples of the physiological effects of human touch, a distinctive feature of acupuncture. Rats receiving a high-cholesterol diet and a one-to-one relationship with the investigator, including touch three times daily, showed a 60% reduction in diet-induced arteriosclerosis when compared with an untouched control group *(15)*. When touched daily, premature infants in incubators increased their weight faster than infants in the same condition who were not touched *(16)*. In patients with unconscious arrhythmias, manual pulse taking had a normalizing effect on the heart rhythm *(17,18)*. In conclusion, acupuncture trials require an adjustment concerning the Rosenthal effect.

Comments Concerning the "Grading" of Clinical and Scientific Studies According to Evidence Level

The Agency for Health Care Policy and Research (AHCPR) of the US Public Health Service has suggested that studies be "graded" according to the following criteria:

1. Well-designed, well-conducted, controlled trials
2. Observational studies and small clinical studies
3. Expert opinion/panel consensus

As indicated in the previous section, this "grading" requires an adjustment in acupuncture trials. Accordingly, for the present evidence analysis, the "grading" has been adjusted as follows:

1. Well-designed, well-conducted, controlled trials that demonstrate an effect of acupuncture at a 1% significance level. Alternatively, well-designed, well-conducted trials that have eliminated patient and acupuncturist bias and demonstrate an effect of acupuncture at a 5% significance level.

2. Observational studies and randomized studies, which demonstrate an effect at a 1% and 5% significance level, respectively.
3. Consensus reports.

Clinical Trials Evaluating the Clinical Effect of Acupuncture in Cardiovascular Disease

The effects of acupuncture and acupressure are described side-by-side with other treatments, which stimulate the nerves of the skin. These related treatment methods involve electrical stimulation of the nerves, either through the skin (TENS) or through an electrode implanted in the spinal cord (SCS). Even though these are different kinds of treatments, they employ the same basic mechanism—stimulating sensory nerves of the skin.

ANGINA PECTORIS

Level A Randomized Clinical Trials. For nearly two decades, a Swedish research group has carried out well-conducted studies on the effects of TENS and SCS. In an early study, 21 patients with severe angina pectoris were randomly allocated to 10 wk of TENS or no treatment (control) after a 3-wk run-in period. Compared to the control group, the TENS group experienced increased exercise tolerance and decreased ST depression and recovery time (all $p < 0.001$) *(19,20)*. TENS was prescribed 3 times 1 h daily, plus during angina attacks. To elucidate the underlying mechanism, the group conducted a series of invasive studies *(19–22)*, in which the effect of pacing with and without TENS was compared, using intracoronary measurements of hemodynamics. Although the treatments were not allocated randomly, they are mentioned in this chapter, because the results underline the clinical findings and randomization was used, for example, when the effect of naloxone was compared to the effect of a saline injection *(22)*. Naloxone produced no significant difference when compared to a saline injection. The main results of the studies were a decrease in lactate production and in afterload during pacing with TENS.

Other Level A Clinical Trials. To eliminate the potential bias from patient and acupuncturist expectancy, a triple-design was used for a study of 49 patients with stable exercise-induced angina pectoris: three individual tests on the same patients were performed by three separate research teams, each of which was unaware of the outcome of the other tests *(11,23–25)*. The patients were initially given a psychosocial test, which included the patients' treatment outcome expectations for angina pectoris.

Second, the patients were randomized to genuine or sham acupuncture for their angina pectoris, using clinical data, exercise tolerance, and electrocardiogram (ECG) data as effect variables. Sham acupuncture was performed outside the Chinese acupoints but in the same spinal segment. This design permitted blinding of the observers. By correlating the results of this trial with the psychosocial testing, detecting whether such factors influenced the outcome of the acupuncture for the treatment of angina pectoris was possible.

Third, all patients received traditional acupuncture from a different acupuncturist; the changes in skin temperature, pain threshold, and pain tolerance threshold were recorded on the index finger (close to the acupuncture site) and on the hallux (distant to the acupuncture site). Correlating results from the two acupuncture trials resulted in "the Rosenthal effect" from acupuncturist bias being eliminated.

When the results from the first and second parts were correlated, no significant influence from patient expectation and psychosocial factors on the antianginal effect of acupuncture was observed. No significant difference was noted between the effects of the genuine and sham acupuncture on angina pectoris, both demonstrating a significant effect on anginal attack rate and nitroglycerin consumption ($p < 0.005$). Patients who received genuine acupuncture increased exercise tolerance ($p < 0.005$), increased pressure-rate-product ($p < 0.05$), and had a delayed onset of pain ($p < 0.05$), when compared to pretreatment values but not when compared to sham acupuncture. Because a significant effect of acupuncture and sham acupuncture was observed, these data do not address the role of placebo effect.

When the results from the second and third parts of the study were correlated, a significant correlation was observed between antianginal and neurophysiological variables: the change in anginal attack rate, nitroglycerin consumption, exercise tolerance, and pressure-rate-product correlated significantly to the change in local skin temperature. This correlation was absent regarding change in remote skin temperature and change in pain thresholds locally as well as remotely (all $p > 0.1$). This finding suggests a mutual mechanism underlying the antianginal effect and change in skin temperature, although the same is not valid for change in pain thresholds. Furthermore, a Rosenthal effect induced by acupuncturist bias can be excluded, because this effect would have produced a similar correlation in local and remote change in skin temperature. This interpretation is underlined by the change in exercise tolerance being significantly correlated to the change in pressure-rate-product, indicating that the improvement in exercise tolerance after acupuncture results from positive hemodynamic alterations. The correlation between the antianginal effect and change in skin temperature on the index finger was significant for both sham and genuine acupuncture, suggesting either a strong placebo effect or that segmental nerve stimulation is important rather than exact choice of Chinese acupuncture points. The combined study suggests a mutual mechanism underlying the acupuncture-induced improvement in pressure-rate-product during exercise and an increase in local skin temperature; a decrease in sympathetic tone, induced by segmental nerve stimulation is a possible explanation.

Level A Scientific Studies. Several experiments on animals support the clinical findings in patients with angina pectoris.

In one study, experimental myocardial ischemia was produced in 30 rabbits by ligation of the ventricular branch of the left coronary artery. The rabbits were randomly allocated to electroacupuncture at Per. 5 (acupoint Jianshi) (60 Hz for 10 min) or no treatment. Using ST depression as a measurement of myocardial ischemia, the acupuncture group showed a decrease in ST depression after release of the ligation, when compared to the control group ($p < 0.05$), and a normal ST amplitude was obtained after 50 min in the acupuncture group only *(26)*. In another study with the same design, 48 rabbits were randomly allocated to (1) control, (2) acupuncture, (3) electrolytic destruction of the hypothalamus without acupuncture, and (4) electrolytic destruction of the hypothalamus with acupuncture. Again, when compared to the control group, the acupuncture group showed improved recovery after release of the ligation, measured as ST depression ($p < 0.05$). Although lesion of the hypothalamus did not affect the recovery, the effect of acupuncture in the group with a destroyed hypothalamus was no longer significant when compared to the control group *(27)*.

A Chinese American group of scientists have conducted a series of impressive experiments on anesthetized cats, elucidating the effects of acupuncture on bradykinin stimulated, reflex-induced myocardial ischemia *(28–30)*. To produce a controlled reduction in regional coronary blood flow (CBF), the left anterior ascending artery was totally (5 cats) or partially occluded (7 cats). Regional wall movement measured by Doppler was used to assess myocardial function in response to the induced ischemia. Electroacupuncture at the median nerve (corresponding to acupoint Per. 6: Neiguan) significantly improved wall function when compared to controls ($p < 0.05$). The improvement in regional function with stimulation of the median nerve was accompanied by a diminished pressor response, as indicated by significantly reduced increments in blood pressure and pressure-rate-product ($p < 0.05$). The inhibitory effect of acupuncture on the reflex-induced myocardial ischemia was blocked by naloxone, administered either intravenously or directly into the cardiovascular reflux center of the medulla spinalis, suggesting that the decrease in myocardial oxygen demand was mediated by stimulation of opioid receptors in the medulla spinalis exercising an inhibitory effect on cardiovascular sympathetic reflexes *(29)*.

Evidence Level B Observational Studies. In studies where acupuncture is used as part of a comprehensive management program (termed integrated rehabilitation), the studied effects should include prospective long-term cost-benefit analysis and quality-of-life measurements, along with clinical outcomes. Our ongoing observational study of a cohort of patients with stable, severe angina pectoris *(31–33)* includes 103 consecutive patients who were candidates for invasive treatment. During an average of 3-yr observation, noted that 82% of the cohort no longer had required invasive therapy and that in-hospital days were reduced by 96% and the use of medication by 78%, and the 3-yr death rate was 2.0% (compared to 6.4% in the general Danish population matched for age and sex). The health care expenses were reduced by $12,000 per patient per year *(33)*.

In integrated rehabilitation, the patients receive 12 consultations for a 4-wk period and training in self-care. The acupuncture is performed with the patient in the supine position and in agreement with traditional Chinese practice *(6)*. Principal points are used: Shanzhong (C.V. 17), Jueyinshu and Xinshu (U.B. 14 and 15), Neiguan (Per. 6), and Zuzanli (St. 36). A book containing a comprehensive presentation of the program, as well as the long-term results, has been submitted for publication in the United States *(35)*.

Level B Randomized Clinical Trials. More than 50 yr ago, substantial indications of an antianginal effect of cutaneous stimulation occurred when application of local anesthetics in trigger areas of the precordial muscles produced complete relief of anginal pain in all 31 patients with angina pectoris and in several cases led to monthlong relief *(36)*.

More recently, 21 patients with stable angina pectoris were randomized to acupuncture and a placebo pill in a crossover design for two 4-wk periods. A clinical effect was observed in the treatment period when compared to the placebo period ($p < 0.01$) *(37)*. In contrast, in a study of 26 patients with angina pectoris who were resistant to medical treatment, genuine acupuncture was compared to sham acupuncture, and a significant difference could not be demonstrated regarding the clinical effect variables although it was found concerning tolerance ($p < 0.001$) *(38)*.

The effect of TENS was studied in 34 patients with myocardial ischemia and no coronary artery stenosis, in 15 patients with coronary artery stenosis, and in 16 heart transplant patients. Measurement of coronary resting blood flow were obtained by Doppler. TENS was associated with a significant increase for the first two groups ($p < 0.001$) but not for the third group. There was no change in coronary arterial diameter as a result of the neurostimulation. There was a significant decrease in epinephrine levels for the first two groups ($p = 0.01$) but not for group 3

(39). This study suggested that neural mechanisms are involved in the coronary artery hemodynamic response to acupuncture.

Several studies have been conducted concerning the effect of SCS on angina pectoris, with results similar to those obtained by TENS: an increase in exercise tolerance and a decrease in ST depression *(40,41)*. In contrast, a nonrandomized study using positron emission tomography (PET) showed no change in CBF in response to SCS *(42)*. In one study, in which 104 patients were randomly allocated to bypass surgery or SCS, no effect from SCS on exercise test variables could be found, although the patients experienced a pronounced effect in anginal attack rate and nitroglycerin consumption when compared to pretreatment values $(p < 0.0001)$ *(43)*.

ISCHEMIC SKIN FLAPS

Evidence Level A Randomized Clinical Trials. A series of studies performed in Sweden on skin flap survival provide an excellent example of scientific exploration of acupuncture. Different treatment parameters were tested against each other using sets of 10 rats in each group *(44–46)*.

Regarding 6-d survival, manual acupuncture (two needles inserted at the base of the flap to a depth of 0.5 cm and rotated backward and forward through 180° every 5 min for 10 s during a 1-h period) was superior to superficial acupuncture (two needles inserted at the base of the flap to a depth of 0.1 cm and retained for 1 h) $(p < 0.002)$. Electroacupuncture was superior to manual acupuncture $(p < 0.02)$, high-intensity electroacupuncture superior to low-intensity acupuncture $(p < 0.05)$, whereas no difference was found between high-frequency (80 Hz) and low-frequency acupuncture (2 Hz). Repeated treatment was superior to a single treatment $(p < 0.02)$ and postoperative treatment superior to preoperative treatment $(p < 0.05)$ *(44)*. In a different study, similar results were found concerning TENS *(45)*. A third study, using laser Doppler measurement of skin blood flow, demonstrated that acupuncture increased skin blood flow when compared to controls $(p < 0.001)$ *(46)*.

Level B Randomized Clinical Trials. Blood flow was measured by laser Doppler flowmetry in ischemic skin flaps of 20 patients undergoing reconstructive surgery and who received TENS and placebo-TENS in randomized order. Active treatment increased blood flow significantly $(p < 0.001)$, whereas placebo treatment did not. No between-group comparison was made, and no long-term follow-up was done *(47,48)*.

HYPERTENSION

Evidence Level A Scientific Studies. The effect of electric sciatic nerve stimulation (3 Hz for 30 min) was studied in rats. When compared to five normotensive rats, an hour-long depressor response was observed in 16 spontaneous hypertensive rats ($p < 0.001$). The magnitude of the depressor response correlated significantly to the initial blood pressure ($r = 0.75; p < 0.001$). The response was reversed by iv naloxone, as well as by chloralose-urethane anesthesia. No significant change in blood pressure was observed in the normotensive group *(49)*. However, the depressor response could not be reproduced in a different group of hypertensive rats, in which the hypertension was not associated with sympathetic hyperactivity *(50)*.

Level B Randomized Trials. In 50 patients with essential hypertension, the effect of acupuncture was compared to the effect of rest in a crossover design with a 30-min observation period. A significant decrease was demonstrated for both treatments, and the one for acupuncture was associated with a decrease in plasma rennin activity. No between-group comparison was made, and there was no random allocation between the treatments *(51)*.

APOPLEXY

Evidence Level A Randomized Clinical Trials. A review based on nine randomized trials, with a total sample size of 538 patients concluded that there is not sufficient evidence to indicate that acupuncture is effective in stroke rehabilitation *(52)*.

CARDIOVASCULAR EFFECTS IN HEALTHY HUMANS

Evidence Level A Scientific Studies. In a randomized crossover design, the effect of electroacupuncture on acupoint LI4 (Hegu) and LI10 (Shousanli) (2 Hz for 20 min) was compared to that of a placebo pill, with respect to myocardial work capacity (expressed as pressure-rate-product) and skin blood flow in 23 healthy subjects. The study demonstrated that acupuncture increased initial low values of maximum pressure-rate-product and decreased initial high values, whereas intermediate values were not affected ($r = 0.70, p < 0.0002$) *(53,54)*.

Clinical Trials Evaluating the Clinical Effect of Acupuncture in Noncardiovascular Disease

NAUSEA

Evidence Level A Randomized Trials. Although not directly related to an evaluation of the cardiovascular effects of acupuncture, three studies of the antiemetic effect of acupuncture and acupressure deserve attention, because the acupuncture points used are commonly used in acupuncture and acupressure treatment of ischemic heart disease. These studies demonstrate an effect of stimulation of sensory nerves of the skin and symptoms related to the inner organs, in this case nausea *(55–58)*.

LEVEL B RANDOMIZED CLINICAL TRIALS EVALUATING THE CLINICAL EFFECT OF ACUPUNCTURE IN OTHER CVDS

Heart Failure. The effect of genuine vs dummy acupuncture on left ventricular ejection fraction (LVEF) was examined in 22 subjects with angiographically proven coronary artery disease (CAD) and 22 normal subjects in a nonrandomized crossover design. Genuine acupuncture increased LVEF significantly ($p < 0.05$) in the heart patients, whereas dummy acupuncture did not. No changes were observed in the normal subjects (59).

Peripheral Arterial Insufficiency. In a nonrandomized study of 34 candidates for limb amputation, only 38% of the patients who received SCS underwent amputation during a 16-mo follow-up period, compared to 90% in a comparable group of unstimulated patients (60).

Placental Ischemia. The effect of TENS in 33 patients with placental ischemia was compared to bed rest in 22 control subjects in a nonrandomized study. A significant increase in blood flow was observed in the umbilical artery and fetal aorta of the TENS group ($p < 0.05$), whereas no change was observed in the control group (61).

EVIDENCE LEVEL B SCIENTIFIC STUDIES ON THE EFFECT OF ACUPUNCTURE IN CVD

More than 50 yr ago, indications of circulatory effects on the inner organs from cutaneous stimulation were observed. In decerebrated cats, application of moderate localized warming or vacuum cups produced vasodilatation in the cutaneous stimulation area and in the corresponding segmental area of the gastrointestinal (GI) tract. However, in animals that had been subjected to bilateral section of the splanchnic nerves and extirpation of the lumbar trunk of the sympathetic trunk, no such changes were observed (62). In 22 cats, the cardiac effects of painting the skin of the chest with a skin irritant solution were studied, using painting at the skin of the gluteal region in seven cats as a control. ECG recordings revealed that when compared to the control group, stimulation of the chest influenced heart activity. Histological examinations showed that stimulation caused vasodilatation, hyperemia, inflammation, and, in some cases, myocytes necrosis (63).

EVIDENCE LEVEL C CONSENSUS REPORTS

The National Institutes of Health (NIH) in the United States has held a consensus conference on acupuncture. Acupuncture was considered to be effective in treating postoperative and chemotherapy-induced nausea and vomiting and dental pain. There are other situations, such as addiction, stroke rehabilitation, headache, menstrual cramps, tennis elbow, fibromyalgia, myofascial pain, osteoarthritis, low back pain, carpal tunnel syndrome, and asthma, in which acupuncture may be useful as an adjunct treatment or an acceptable alternative or be included in a comprehensive management program *(64)*. The British Medical Association (BMA) has approved acupuncture as an effective treatment in the management of back and dental pain, nausea and vomiting, and migraine *(65)*. An evaluation of acupuncture in CVD (not characterized as effective) is included in the NIH and BMA reports. However, the latter of the studies presented in this analysis were not available at the time of their evaluation.

EVIDENCE-BASED SUMMARY

Introduction

An editorial in *JAMA* suggests that when the effect is large and the risk associated with the treatment is small, prospective observational studies suffice to support clinical recommendations *(66)*.This is an important consideration when discussing the level of evidence needed to support the clinical use of acupuncture alone or in combination with comprehensive management programs, such as integrated rehabilitation, for angina pectoris. Furthermore, although invasive treatments and medication are based on level A evidence when compared to placebo *(67,68)*, the evidence level is C when compared to several natural remedies *(31–33,69–80)*.

Conclusions

1. Level A evidence exists concerning a clinical effect of acupuncture in angina pectoris and ischemic skin flaps.
2. Level A evidence exists concerning some of the possible physiological mechanisms underlying the observed clinical effect of acupuncture in angina pectoris.
3. Level B evidence exists concerning a clinical long-term effect of acupuncture, when performed in its classical Chinese context as part of a comprehensive treatment complex for angina pectoris.
4. Level B evidence exists concerning the use of acupuncture in essential hypertension.
5. Level B indications of an effect on heart failure, peripheral arterial insufficiency, and placental ischemia exist.

Request

Clinicians who wish to explore the potential of integrated rehabilitation on their heart patients are urged to contact the author of this chapter to include your data into a mutual clinical database.

REFERENCES

1. Klassisk kinesisk Medicin Veith I. The Yellow Emperor's Classic of Internal Medicine (2nd ed.). University of California Press, Los Angeles, CA, 1972.
2. Cohen KS. Qigong. The Art and Science of Chinese Energy Healing. Ballentine Books, New York, 1997.
3. Tse I. Tao te King, Visdommens bog. Sphinx, København, 1982.
4. Porkert M. The Theoretical Foundations of Chinese Medicine. MIT Press, Cambridge, MA, 1974.
5. Kaptchuk TJ. Chinese Medicine. The Web That has No Weaver. Rider, Great Britain, 1983.
6. Beijing College of Traditional Chinese Medicine: Essentials of Chinese Acupuncture. Beijing, Foreign Languages Press, 1980.
7. MacPherson H, Thomas K, Walters S, Fitter M. The York acupuncture safety study: a prospective survey of 34,000 treatments by traditional acupuncturists. Br Med J 2001;323:486–487.
8. Halvorsoen TB, Anda SS, Naess AB, Levang OW. Fatal cardiac tamponade after acupuncture through congenital sternal foramen. Lancet 1995;345:1175.
9. Kataoka H. Cardiac tamponade caused by penetration of an acupuncture needle into the right ventricle. J Thoracic Cardiovasc Surg 1997;114:674–676.
10. Valenta IJ, Hengesh JW. Pneumothorax caused by acupuncture. Lancet 1981;2:322.
11. Ballegaard S. Acupuncture and the cardiovascular system. A scientific challenge. Med Acupunc 1998;10;5–11.
12. Rosenthal R. Interpersonal expectations: effects of the experimenters hypothesis. In: Rosenthal R, Rosnow RL, eds. Artifact in Behavorial Research. Academic, New York, 1969, pp. 182–279.
13. Rosenthal R. Experimenter Effects in Behavioral Research. Enlarged ed. Irvington Publishers, New York, 1976, pp. 441–479.
14. Lown B. Introduction. In: Norman Cousins. The Healing heart. Avon, New York, 1983, pp. 11–25.
15. Nerem RM, Levesque ML, Cornhill JT. Social environment as a factor in diet-induced atherosclerosis. Science 1980;208:1475–1476.
16. Helders PL, Cats BP, Van der Net J. The effect of tactile stimulation/range-finding program on the development of very low birth weight infants during initial hospitalization. Child Care Health Dev 1988;14:34–54.
17. Lynch JL, Thomas SA, Mills ME, Malinow K, Katcher AH. The effects of human contact on cardiac arrhythmia in coronary care patients. J New Ment Dis 1974;158:88–99.
18. Lynch JL, Flaherty L, Emrich C, Mills ME, Katcher A. Effects of human contact on the heart activity of curarized patients in a shock trauma unit. Am Heart J 1974;88:160–169.
19. Mannheimer C, Carlsson CA, Vedin A, Wilhelmsson C. Transcutaneous Electrical Nerve Stimulation (TENS) in angina pectoris. Pain 1986;26:291–300.
20. Mannheimer C, Carlsson CA, Emanuelsson H, et al. The effects of Transcutaneous Electrical Nerve Stimulation in patients with severe angina pectoris. Circulation 1985;71:308–316.
21. Emanuelsson H, Mannheimer C, Waagstein F, et al. Catecholamine during pacing-induced angina pectoris and the effect of transcutaneous electrical nerve stimulation. Am Heart J 1987;114:1360–1366.

22. Mannheimer C, Emanuelsson H, Wagstein F, Wilhemsson C. Influence of naloxone on the effect of high frequency transcutaneous electrical nerve stimulation in angina pectoris during pacing. Br Heart J 1989;62:36–42.
23. Ballegaard S, Pedersen F, Pietersen A, Nissen VH, Olsen NV. Effects of acupuncture in moderate stable Angina pectoris. J Intern Med 1990;227:25–30.
24. Ballegaard S, Meyer CN, Trojaborg W. Acupuncture in angina pectoris: does acupuncture have a specific effect? J Intern Med 1991;229:357–362.
25. Ballegaard S, Karpatschof B, Holck JA, Meyer CN, Trojaborg W. Acupuncture in angina pectoris. Do psycho-social and neurophysiological factors relate to the effect? Acupunt Electrother Res Int J 1995;20:101–116.
26. Cao Q, Wang S, Liu J. Effect of acupuncture on acute myocardial ischemic injury in rabbits. J Trad Chin Med 1981;1:83–86.
27. Liu J, Cao Q, Zhuang D. Role of hypothalamus in the recovery of acute ischemic myocardial injury promoted by electro acupuncture in rabbits. J Trad Chin Med 1984;4:119–126.
28. Li P, Pitsillides KF, Rendig SV, Pan HL, Longhurst JC. Reversal of reflex-induced myocardial ischemia by median nerve stimulation. Circulation 1998;97:1186–1194.
29. Li P, Tjen-A-Looi S, Longhurst JC. Rostral ventrolateral medullary opioid receptor subtypes in the inhibitory effect of electroacupuncture on reflex autonomic response in cats. Autonomic Neuroscience 2001;89:38–47.
30. Chao DM, Shen LL, Tjen-A-Looi S, Pitsillides KF, Li P, Longhurst JC. Naloxone reverses inhibitory effect of electroacupuncture on sympathetic cardiovascular reflex responses. Am J Physiol 1999;276(6 Pt 2):H2127–H2134.
31. Ballegaard S, Nørrelund S, Smith DF. Cost-benefit of combined use of acupuncture, shiatsu and lifestyle adjustments for treatment of patients with severe angina pectoris. Acupunct Electro Therapeut Res Int J 1996;21:187–197.
32. Ballegaard S, Johannesen A, Karpatschof B, Nyeboe J. Addition of acupuncture and self-care education in the treatment of patients with severe angina pectoris may be cost beneficial: an open, prospective study. J Altern Complement Med 1999;5:405–413.
33. Ballegaard S, Borg E, Johannessen A, Karpatschof B, Nyboe J. Three-year follow-up on Integrated Cardiac Rehabilitation in patients with severe angina pectoris, in press.
34. Ornish D, Brown SB, Scherwitz LW. Can lifestyle change reverse coronary heart disease? Lancet 1990;336:129–133.
35. Ballegaard S. Heal Your Heart, in press.
36. Rinzler SH, Travell J. Therapy directed at the somatic component of cardiac pain. Am Heart J 1948;35:248–268.
37. Richter A, Herlitz J, Hjalmarson AA. Effect of acupuncture in patients with angina pectoris. Eur Heart J 1991;12:175–178.
38. Ballegaard S, Jensen G, Pedersen F, Nissen VH. Acupuncture in severe, stable angina pectoris: a randomized trial. Acta Med Scand 1986;220:307–313.
39. Chauhan A, Mullins PA, Thuraisingham SI, Taylor G, Petch MC, Schofield PM. Effect of transcutaneous electrical nerve stimulation on coronary blood flow. Circulation 1994;89:694–702.
40. Sanderson JE, Brooksby P, Waterhouse D, Palmer RBG, Neubauer K. Epidural spinal electrical stimulation for severe angina: a study of its effects on symptoms, exercise tolerance and degree of ischaemia. Eur Heart J 1992;13:628–633
41. De Jongste MJL, Haaksma J, Hautvast RWM, et al. Effect of spinal cord stimulation on myocardial ischemia during daily life n patients with severe coronary artery disease. Br Heart J 1994;71:413–418.
42. Landsherre CD, Mannheimer C, Habets A, et al. Effect of spinal cord stimulation on regional myocardial perfusion assessed by positron emission tomography. Am J Cardiol 1992;69:1143–1149.

43. Mannheimer C, Eliason T, Augustinsson LE, et al. Electrical stimulation versus coronary artery bypass surgery in severe angina pectoris. Circulation 1998;97:1157–1163

44. Jansen G, Lundeberg T, Samuelson UE, Thomas M. Increased survival of ischemic musculocutaneous flaps in rats after acupuncture. Acta Physiol Scand 1989;135:555–558.

45. Kjartansson J, Lundeberg T, Samuelson UE, Dalsgaard CJ, Heden P. Calcitonin-gene-related-peptide (CGRP) and transcutaneous electrical nerve stimulation (TENS) increase cutaneous blood flow in a musculocutaneous flap in the rat. Acta Physiol Scand 1988;134:89–94.

46. Jansen G, Lundeberg T, Kjartansson J, Samuelson UE. Acupuncture and sensory neuropeptides increase cutaneous blood flow in rats. Neurosci Lett 1989;97:305–309.

47. Lundeberg T, Kjartansson J, Samuelson UE. Effect of electrical nerve stimulation on healing of ischaemic skin flaps. Lancet 1988;24:712–714.

48. Kjartansson J, Lundeberg T. Effects of electrical nerve stimulation (ENS) in ischemic tissue. Scand J Plast Reconstr Hand Surg 1990;24:129–134.

49. Yao T, Andersson S, Thorén P. Long-lasting cardiovascular depression induced by acupuncture-like stimulation of the sciatic nerve in unanesthetized spontaneously hypertensive rats. Brain Res 1982;240:77–85.

50. Hoffmann P, Thoren P. Long-lasting cardiovascular depression induced by acupuncture-like stimulation of the sciatic nerve in unanaesthetized rats. Effects of arousal and type of hypertension. Acta Physiol Scand 1986;127:119–126.

51. Chiu YJ, Reid IA. Cardiovascular and endocrine effects of acupuncture in hypertensive patients. Clin Exper Hypert 1997;19:1047–1063.

52. Park J, Hopwood V, White AR, Ernst E. Effectiveness of acupuncture for stroke: A systematic review. J Neurol 2001;248:558–563.

53. Ballegaard S, Muteki T, Harada H, Ueda N, Tsuda H, Tayama F, Ohishi K. Modulatory effect of acupunture on the cardiovascular system: A cross-over study. Acupunct Electrother Res 1993;18:103–115.

54. Karpatschof B, Nyboe J, Ballegaard S, Trojaborg W. Two-level regression for the test of a stabilizing effect of acupuncture. in press.

55. Dundee JW, Chesmutt WN, Ghaly RG, Lynas AGA. Traditional Chinese acupuncture: a potentially useful anniemetie. Br Med J 1986;293:583–584.

56. Dundee JW, Bell PF, Sourial FBR, Ghaly RG. P6 acupressure reduces morning sickness. J Royal Soc Med 1998;81:456–457.

57. Dundee JW, Ghaly RG, Fitzpatrick KTJ, Lynch GA, Abram WP. Acupuncture to prevent cisplatin-associated sickness. J Royal Soc Med 1989;82:268–271.

58. Dundee JW, Gordy RG, Fitzpatrick KTJ, Lynch GA. Abram WP. Acupuncture to prevent cisplatin-associated vomiting. Lancet 1987;1:1083.

59. Ho FM, Huang PJ, Lo MH, Lee FK, Chern TH, Chiu TW, Liau CS. Effect of acupuncture at nei-kuan on left ventricular function in patients with coronary artery disease. Am J Chin Med 1999;27:149–156.

60. Augustinsson LE, Carlson CA, Holm J, Jivegaard L. Epidural electrical stimulation in severe limb ischemia: Pain relief, increased blod flow and possible limb-saving effect. Ann Surg 1985;202:104–110.

61. Enzelsberger H, Skodler WD, Kubista E. Zur Verbesserung der Doppler-Sonographiebefunde nach transkutaner Elektrostimulation bei Frauen mit Plazentainsuffizienz. Z Geburtsh u Perinat 1991;195:172–175.

62. Kuntz A, Haselwood LA. Circulatory reactions in the gastrointestinal tract elicited by localized cutaneous stimulation. Am Heart J 1940;20:743–749.

63. Pastinszky I, Kenedi I, Faber V. Experimental studies of the dermato-cardiac reflex effect. Acta Physiol Acad Sci Hung 1964;25:89–95.

64. NIH Concensus Development Panel on Acupuncture. JAMA 1998;280:1518–1524.
65. Silvert M. Acupuncture wins BMA approval. Br Med J 2000;321:11.
66. Radford MJ, Foody JM. How do observational studies expand the evidence base for therapy? JAMA 2001;286:1228–1229.
67. Eagle KA, Guyton RA, Davidoff R, et al. ACC/AHA guidelines for coronary artery bypass graft surgery: Executive summaries and recommendat ions. A report of he American College of Cardiology/American Heart Association task force on practise guidelines. Circulation 1999;100:1464–1480.
68. Gibbons RJ, Chattererjee K, Daley J, et al. ACC/AHA/ACP-ASIM guidelines for the management of patients with chronic stable angina pectoris. A Report of the American College of Cardiology/ American Heart Association task force on prac-tise guidelines. J Am Coll Cardiol 1999;33:2093–2190.
69. Hasdai D, Garratt KN, Grill DE, et al. Effect of smoking status on the long-term outcome after successful percutaneous coronary revascularization. N Engl J Med 1997;336:755–761.
70. Calle EE, Thun MJ, Petrelli JM, Rodriguez C, Heath CW, Jr. Body-mass index and mortality in a prospective cohort of U.S. adults. N Engl J Med 1999;341:1097–1105.
71. Leon AS, Connett J, Jacobs D, et al. Leisure-time physical activity levels and risk of coronary heart disease and death. JAMA 1987;258:2388–2395.
72. Hakim AA, Petrovitch H, Burchfiel CM, et al. Effects of walking on mortality among non-smoking retired men. N Engl J Med 1998;338:94–99.
73. de Lorgeril M, Salen P, Martin J-L, et al. Mediterranean Diet, Traditional Risk Factors, and the Rate of Cardiovascular Complications After Myocardial Infarction. Final Report of the Lyon Diet Heart Study. Circulation 1999;6:779–785.
74. Fraser GE, Sabate J, Beeson WL, Strahan TM. A possible protective effect of nut consumption on risk of coronary heart disease. The Adventist Health Study. Arch Intern Med 1992;52:1416–1424.
75. Hu FB, Stampfer MJ, Manson JE, Rimm EB, Colditz GA, Rosner BA, Speizer FE, Hennekens CH, Willett WC. Frequent nut consumption and risk of coronary heart disease in women: prospective cohort study. Br Med J 1998;317:1341–1345.
76. Thun MJ, Peto R, Lopez AD, Monaco JH, Henley SJ, Heath CW Jr, Doll R. Alcohol consumption and mortality among middle-aged and elderly U.S. adults. N Engl J Med 1997; 337:1705–1714.
77. Nerem RM, Levesque MJ, Cornhill JF. Social environment as a factor in diet-induced atherosclerosis. Science 1980;208:1475–1476.
78. Ornish D, Brown SE, Scherwitz LW, et al. Can lifestyle changes reverse coronary heart disease? The Lifestyle Heart Trial. Lancet 1990;336:129–133.
79. Ornish D, Scherwitz LW, Billings JH, et al. Intensive lifestyle changes for reversal of coronary heart disease. JAMA 1998;280:2001–2007.
80. Schnyder G, Roffi M, Pin R, et al. Decreased rate of coronary restenosis after lowering of plasma homocystein levels. N Engl J Med 2001;345:1593–1600.

12 Chelation Therapy for Cardiovascular Disease

Steven C. Halbert, MD

CONTENTS

INTRODUCTION
EDTA PHARMACOLOGY
CLINICAL STUDIES
MECHANISMS OF ACTION
CLINICAL APPLICATIONS
CONCLUSIONS
REFERENCES

INTRODUCTION

The primary Food and Drug Administration (FDA)-approved indication for chelation therapy with ethylene diamine tetraacetic acid (EDTA) is the treatment of lead intoxication. However, for more than three decades, EDTA chelation therapy has been widely used by alternative medicine practitioners as a controversial treatment for atherosclerotic disease and other degenerative conditions. In 1993, it was estimated that 500,000 people per year in the United States are treated with off-label use of chelation therapy (1). A recent Canadian study revealed that 8% of patients who had undergone cardiac catheterization and responded to a survey used chelation therapy (2). This conservative estimate translates to approx 100,000 patients, at a cost of $400 million annually. Clearly, the magnitude of the use of EDTA chelation therapy as an alternative therapy has become a public health issue. Despite decades of use, EDTA chelation therapy studies on athersclerosis have been

From: *Contemporary Cardiology*
Complementary and Alternative Cardiovascular Medicine
Edited by: R. A. Stein and M. C. Oz © Humana Press Inc., Totowa, NJ
189

extremely few, small in size, and poorly designed, offering few conclusions concerning its effectiveness. If chelation therapy is proved safe and effective in treating ischemic heart disease or peripheral vascular disease, it would represent a new therapeutic modality and would gain widespread application. However, if chelation therapy is ineffective for coronary artery disease (CAD), these data will provide important information to the public and allow for informed decision making.

This chapter attempts to put chelation therapy in perspective for the clinician. It is important for physicians to ask patients who are using or intending to use chelation therapy to determine their concerns, expectations, misconceptions, and to discuss treatment options before patients undergo chelation therapy.

Topics addressed in this chapter include:

1. EDTA pharmacology
2. An evidence-based review of EDTA as a therapy for atherosclerotic disease
3. Mechanisms of action
4. Clinical applications

EDTA PHARMACOLOGY

EDTA is an amino acid that was first synthesized in 1930. It is currently approved by the FDA for removal of toxic metal cations, such as lead. The term *chelation* derives from the Greek *chele*, which refers to the claws of a crab or a lobster. Chelation is the chemical reaction in which a molecule surrounds and bonds with a metal cation to form a heterocyclic structure. The compound resulting from a chelating agent and a metal is described as a metal chelate. Metal chelates are widely represented in biologic systems. For example, hemoglobin, chlorophyll, and vitamin B_{12} are metal chelates of iron, magnesium, and cobalt, respectively. EDTA is a tetrabasic acid with four replaceable hydrogen ions. It is poorly soluble in water, but it is soluble in alkaline hydroxides. In the United States, the commercially available salts are the disodium and the calcium disodium salts of EDTA. In these formulations, EDTA is widely used as an in vitro anticoagulant for blood collection and as an antioxidant synergist, stabilizer, and preservative for pharmaceutical preparations. Calcium EDTA is used for lead toxicity, whereas disodium EDTA is used to treat atherosclerosis.

EDTA binds with divalent and trivalent metal cations, such as iron, copper, calcium, magnesium, zinc, mercury, aluminum, and lead, with differing affinities. EDTA is poorly absorbed from the gastrointestinal (GI) tract. After iv administration, EDTA is found primarily in plasma.

It is distributed in the extracellular fluid, and it does not penetrate cells. Only approx 5% of the plasma concentration is found in spinal fluid. The half-life is 20–60 min. It is excreted mainly by the kidney, with approx 50% excretion in 1 h and more than 95% within 24 h. Almost none of the compound is metabolized.

CLINICAL STUDIES

Initial Reports

In 1955, Norman Clarke suggested that atherosclerosis could be treated with EDTA. He observed that patients who were treated for lead toxicity and had concomitant atherosclerosis experienced improvements in their vascular disease (3). Clarke later reported on the successful use of EDTA in the management of angina pectoris and occlusive vascular disease (4,5). Meltzer and Kitchell initially confirmed Clarke's work, and then in 1963, after further investigation, concluded that chelation therapy was no more beneficial than existing therapies for coronary artery disease (CAD) (6–8). This placebo-controlled, double-blind, crossover study of nine patients with coronary heart disease (CHD) assessed treadmill performance as a primary end point. In the group treated with EDTA, two of four patients showed benefit at 12 wk. However, only two patients enrolled in the second phase, and neither showed improvement. No statistical analysis was reported. Until this year, this report was the only controlled trial assessing chelation therapy for ischemic heart disease.

Observational Studies and Small Clinical Studies

The majority of the clinical literature describing the benefits of chelation therapy in patients with CAD or peripheral arterial, noncarotid disease is in case reports and case series. Cranton reported that by 1993, there were more than 4600 published case reports and case series supporting the potential benefits of chelation therapy (9). A large, retrospective analysis of 2870 patients with vascular and other degenerative diseases was reported by Olszewer, which suggested a beneficial effect of chelation therapy (10). Chappell and Stahl conducted a meta-analysis covering 19 studies and a total of 22,765 patients with vascular disease treated with EDTA chelation. This analysis revealed a measurable improvement in approx 87% of patients (11). However, two large uncontrolled retrospective studies dwarfed the other 17 studies in the analysis. It also involved a mixture of patients with CAD, peripheral vascular disease, and cerebrovascular disease, which make the results difficult to interpret for any one condition.

EDTA chelation has also been used in patients with cerebrovascular disease. The claims of efficacy with EDTA therapy in this population are based on subjective clinical improvement and, in some studies, improved cerebral perfusion or reduction in degree of carotid stenosis, as assessed by noninvasive testing *(6,10,12–18)*. However, the patient populations were generally small. Most importantly, the studies were without appropriate controls, and, in some, there was criticism of methodology. Particularly in the older data, the observations were subjective and descriptive. Thus, there are no well-designed randomized trials of EDTA in the treatment of cerebrovascular disease.

Randomized Controlled Trials

There have been three interpretable, randomized trials of EDTA chelation for patients with atherosclerotic vascular disease. A fourth trial, the Pilot Trial to Assess Chelation Therapy (PACT), is currently ongoing.

Two prospective trials conducted by vascular surgeons in Denmark and New Zealand have evaluated the use of EDTA in peripheral vascular disease. In 1992, the Danish trial randomized 153 patients with stable intermittent claudication to receive either 3.0 g EDTA or placebo *(20,21)*. The treatment regimen consisted of 20 infusions administered over 5 to 9 wk. The primary end-points were walking distance and ankle/brachial indices. The changes observed in the pain-free and maximal walking distances, measured on a treadmill, were similar in the two groups. During the 3-mo ($n = 149$) and 6-mo ($n = 123$) follow-up period, no long-term therapeutic effect of EDTA could be demonstrated. This trial was criticized for the high dropout rate at 6 mo. Additionally, the blinding protocol was violated, and the Danish Committee on Scientific Dishonesty criticized various methodological study aspects *(22)*.

In 1994, the New Zealand group randomized 32 patients and compared EDTA with placebo in the treatment of stable intermittent claudication *(23)*. There were 32 patients recruited who had peripheral vascular disease confirmed by angiography. Patients with diabeties were excluded, and patients were required to stop smoking. The active infusion consisted of 3.0 g of EDTA, 0.76 g magnesium chloride, and 0.84 g sodium bicarbonate in normal saline. The placebo infusion was normal saline. There were no significant differences reported in pain-free walking distance or total walking distance when the EDTA-treated group was compared to the placebo group. However, at 3 mo after treatment, resting ankle-brachial indices showed some improvement in the chelation group in both legs, with a significant between-groups effect favoring chelation. An extensive analysis of quality of life also was performed in the research subjects, with mixed results. Although there were no differences in scales relating to general health and effect of poor circulation on life activities, chelation patients scored better on two scales that rated the level of physical activity ($p < 0.05$ for between-groups differences) 3 mo after therapy. Despite the quality of this study, the small number of patients enrolled precludes any definitive conclusion concerning the efficacy of chelation therapy in peripheral vascular disease.

The Program to Assess Alternative Treatment Strategies to Achieve Cardiac Health (PATCH) was a 6-mo randomized trial that measured exercise capacity in 84 stable patients with angina randomized to receive either EDTA treatment or placebo (24). Patients were eligible to participate in the trial if they were over the age of 21 had proved CAD, and stable angina pectoris, and ≥ 1 mm ST-segment depression within 2–14 min on a gradually ramping treadmill test. A total of 39 patients were ultimately randomized to the treatment groups, receiving iv solutions of EDTA 40 mg/kg, up to a maximum of 3.0 g, or placebo (0.9% sodium chloride). Patients received treatment 2 times/wk for 15 wk, then once per month for 3 mo, for a total of 33 treatments. Importantly, both groups received iv magnesium (750 mg) and ascorbic acid (5 g) in the infusate. All patients were given oral multivitamins. There were no significant differences in clinical outcomes or quality-of-life scores between the treatment groups. There were no deaths and no myocardial infarctions (MIs), and there were nine hospitalizations for worsening angina (six in the chelation group and three in the placebo group). Both groups increased their exercise times approx 1 min, an improvement that the investigators attributed to placebo or "training" effect. Unfortunately, in this trial, the "placebo" contained vitamin C (antioxidant effect) and magnesium (vasodilator and antiarrhythmic effects), and the study was underpowered to assess clinical event rates.

MECHANISMS OF ACTION

The original hypothesis underlying the use of chelation therapy was that EDTA would remove calcium from atheromatous plaques producing favorable effects (25,26). Unfortunately, there are little data to support the decalcifying hypothesis. Other postulated mechanisms of EDTA action include (1) inhibition of platelet aggregation, (2) parathormone (PTH) release stimulation that, in turn, mobilizes calcium from plaques and reduces progressive calcification; (3) an antioxidant effect by complexing with transitional metals thus interfering with free radical production and lipid peroxidation; (4) effects on serum iron, and (5) transient lowering of serum cholesterol (27–30). Some of these hypotheses may be valid, but there are no confirmatory mechanistic studies.

Endothelial cell dysfunction contributes to the pathogenesis of cardiovascular disease (CVD) and is modified by risk-reduction therapies. A more current understanding of the mechanisms underlying atherogenesis would suggest that chelation therapy may act by reducing oxidative stress in the vascular wall, leading to improved vascular function, reduced inflammation, and reduced risk for CVD events.

Chelation therapy may improve vascular function by several mechanisms. One possibility is direct removal of calcium from the vascular wall. Studies in animal models suggest a relationship between endothelial function and arterial calcification *(31)*. As mentioned, removal of calcium from lesions and the vessel wall by EDTA chelation therapy has been questioned. However, if operative, such an effect would likely result in an improved response to both endothelium-dependent and independent vasodilators.

Another potential mechanism is chelation of redox active transition metals, such as iron and copper. Transition metals ions are a well-recognized source of oxidative stress in the vasculature *(32)*. Iron is a catalyst for the formation of the highly reactive hydroxyl radical via the Fenton reaction, and similar chemistry exists for copper *(32)*. Free copper and iron also induce lipid and protein oxidation *(33,34)*. On the basis of these observations, investigators have proposed that transition metals may contribute to atherogenesis by stimulating low-density lipoprotein (LDL) oxidation. In support of this proposal is the observation that human atherosclerotic lesions contain redox active iron and copper *(35,36)*, whereas normal tissue does not *(32)*.

In addition to impairing endothelial function by stimulating LDL oxidation and forming reactive oxygen species (ROS), metal ions may also have direct effects that may contribute to atherogenesis and vascular dysfunction. For example, there is evidence that iron contributes to NFκB activation *(37)* and the expression of vascular cell adhesion molecule-1 (VCAM-1) in endothelial cells *(38)*. The interactions with iron and nitric oxide (NO) may also be relevant. NO reversibly binds to heme iron and activates guanyl cyclase, which results in vasodilation. However, nonprotein-bound iron may directly inactivate endothelium-derived NO *(39)*. Recently, iron chelation with iv deferoxamine improved NO-dependent vasodilation in the coronary arteries of patients with diabetes mellitus *(40)*. A similar effect has been demonstrated in patients with angiographically proven CAD *(41)*. However, EDTA is a less effective chelator of iron and copper than deferoxamine and other more specific agents. Furthermore, there is data to suggest that iron, but not copper, may remain in a redox active state when bound to EDTA *(42)*. Importantly, this effect does not occur when there is a molar excess of EDTA, as is the case in plasma after high-dose EDTA infusion *(43)*.

One study has examined the effect of EDTA chelation therapy on endothelial function *(44)*. In an unblinded study of eight patients with CAD, endothelium-dependent forearm blood flow responses to acetyl-choline were examined at baseline, after 10 sessions of chelation therapy with EDTA alone, and after 10 additional sessions with EDTA plus magnesium, thiamine, riboflavin, pyridoxine, and vitamin B_{12}. Interestingly, there was a trend toward improved endothelium-dependent vasodilation after EDTA alone and significantly improved flow responses after the additional course of treatment with EDTA plus B vitamins.

Another somewhat larger mechanistic trial of EDTA in CAD is currently in progress. The PACT is a double-blind trial evaluating 40 patients with established CAD, randomized to receive 15 infusions of either EDTA chelation solution or placebo. PACT will test the hypothesis that chelation therapy reverses endothelial dysfunction in patients with CAD by reducing oxidative stress. End-points include measurement of endothelium-dependent forearm blood flow, plasma concentrations of soluble intercellular adhesion molecule (ICAM)-1, endothelin, C-reactive protein, 8-epi-PGF$_{2\alpha}$ (a specific marker of arachidonic acid oxidation), and ascorbic acid at baseline and after the completion of the infusions.

CLINICAL APPLICATIONS

Up to 40% of the US population uses some form of alternative therapy. However, the majority of these individuals are not forthcoming about such treatment with their primary care physicians *(45)*. Awareness of this dichotomy has prompted physicians to inquire directly about their patient's use of alternative healing modalities. Increasingly, it is likely that physicians will encounter questions from their patients regarding EDTA chelation therapy for atherosclerosis. Therefore, this section is intended to provide the clinician with an understanding of the clinical applications of EDTA chelation therapy as promulgated by the American College for Advancement in Medicine (ACAM).

Coronary Artery Disease

Clinical observations and case studies suggest that if EDTA chelation was clinically efficacious, it would require 3–6 mo of weekly iv infusions to produce clinical benefit. Therefore it would not have a role in patients with acute coronary syndromes who should be so counseled. Patients who have spontaneous or provocable ischemia, in the face of reasonable medical therapy, are candidates for angiography and possibly coronary revascularization, not chelation therapy.

Patients with chronic stable angina, which has been well controlled on medical therapy, with no evidence of left ventricular dysfunction would, if EDTA chelation therapy was found to be effective, be considered a target population. In contrast, those individuals who have high-risk coronary disease suggested by significant left main coronary disease, three-vessel disease with left ventricular dysfunction, and two-vessel disease with proximal LAD involvement are clearly candidates for surgical revascularization. These patients often have had coronary angiography because of medical therapy failure or high-risk predicted by clinical findings or stress testing. Patients who refuse angiography for these indications may inquire about chelation therapy as a therapeutic alternative. It is best to counsel patients against chelation therapy in this setting, because these patients are at high risk for sudden cardiac death.

Patients with stable angina and significant left ventricular dysfunction should avoid chelation therapy. The additional sodium and fluid load imposed by chelation can cause left ventricular decompensation. Additionally, a subset of these patients may benefit from revascularization.

The 1999 American Heart Association/American College of Cardiology Guidelines for the Management of Chronic Ischemic Heart Disease lists EDTA chelation therapy under Class III treatments, which signifies that the authors and reviewers found only an intermediate level of scientific evidence to support its effectiveness and where in some cases the treatment may be harmful *(46)*.

Peripheral Vascular Disease

Patients with acute limb ischemia should not be managed with chelation therapy. This subgroup requires prompt angiography and definitive endovascular or surgical intervention. In chronic peripheral arterial occlusive disease, patients may inquire about chelation therapy as a nonsurgical option. Symptoms range from stable intermittent claudication to more severe symptoms of disabling claudication and rest pain. Presently, other than smoking cessation and exercise conditioning, there is little evidence that medical interventions improve outcomes or relieve symptoms in peripheral vascular disease. A retrospective analysis of more than 2800 patients receiving chelation therapy reported marked improvement in 91% of patients with peripheral vascular disease, as opposed to 77% of those with CAD, and only 24% with cerebral vascular disease *(10)*. Therefore, given the limited therapeutic choices, in a patient who refuses revascularization or is a nonsurgical candidate, one might consider chelation therapy as a treatment option.

Toxicity and Contraindications

When used by physicians properly trained in its use, EDTA chelation therapy has a low morbidity rate. Renal toxicity is directly related to the rate and dose of EDTA infused. Adherence to dosing protocols based on lean body mass, creatinine clearance, and infusion rate minimizes toxicity *(47)*. Liberal fluid intake is encouraged to reduce the risk of renal injury. Nephrotoxicity is reversible and responds promptly to EDTA treatment cessation. A conservative approach would be to advise patients with a serum creatinine above 2.5 mg/dL to avoid chelation therapy.

Patients with congestive heart failure (CHF) are at risk for clinical decompensation that could occur secondary to fluid and sodium (sodium ascorbate in the infusion) overload or from the negative inotropic effect of transient hypocalcemia induced by EDTA. Patients with mild compensated CHF can be managed successfully, with attention to restricting iv fluid volume and additional diuretic therapy, if necessary. However, with moderate to severe left ventricular dysfunction, it is best to avoid EDTA chelation therapy.

Patients who are receiving anticoagulation therapy with warfarin can safely receive chelation therapy. Pregnancy, known allergy to EDTA, and active liver disease represent contraindications. A summary of contraindications to EDTA chelation therapy is shown in Table 1.

The toxicity of EDTA chelation therapy, apart from the potential for nephrotoxicity, is minimal. Relatively common symptoms during a course of treatment include fatigue and muscle cramping. Correcting mineral deficiencies usually alleviates these symptoms. Mild hypocalcemia is particularly common. Hypoglycemia may occur during treatment, particularly in patients who are calorically deprived before receiving an infusion. Transient hypocalcemia induced by chelation has the potential to induce arrhythmias; however, clinically this is exceedingly uncommon.

Treatment Protocol

A treatment course of chelation therapy usually consists of a series of 30–40 iv infusions of disodium magnesium EDTA, adjusted for appropriate osmolality and buffered with sodium bicarbonate. The most common solution contains 3 g (or 50 mg/kg) of EDTA in 500 mL of sterile water, which is infused for 3 h and administered weekly. Typically, 2 g of magnesium chloride, 7 g of ascorbic acid, and the B vitamins thiamine, pantothenic acid, and pyridoxine are added.

CONCLUSIONS

For 40 yr, EDTA chelation therapy for vascular disease has remained controversial and of unproven clinical benefit. Hundreds of thousands of Americans expose themselves to treatment with EDTA chelation therapy. If this therapy proves helpful, then additional as-yet-untreated

Table 1
Contraindications to EDTA Chelation Therapy

1. Acute coronary syndromes
2. Acute limb ischemia
3. Severe left ventricular dysfunction, with left ventricular ejection fraction < 30%
4. Angiographic indications for coronary revascularization (left main, two-vessel with proximal LAD, and three-vessel with left ventricular dysfunction)
5. Serum creatinine > 2.5 mg/dL
6. Pregnancy
7. Active hepatic disease
8. Allergy to ethylene diamine tetraacetic acid

patients may benefit from it. Conversely, if EDTA chelation were without clinical merit, then physicians, administrators, and regulatory authorities would be able to reject it on solid scientific evidence. The few double-blind, prospective trials that have been performed were either underpowered or methodologically flawed. The general acceptance of EDTA chelation therapy in treating CVDs will need more rigorously designed clinical studies to establish its efficacy and safety. Fortunately, a large multicenter trial Trial to Assess Chelation Therapy (TACT) has been initiated by the National Institutes of Health to assess the effects of EDTA chelation on quality of life, clinical outcomes, cost-effectiveness, and plasma markers of oxidative stress and endothelial dysfunction. Until such a trial is completed, physicians can intelligently counsel patients inquiring about EDTA chelation therapy by adhering to the guidelines presented.

REFERENCES

1. Grier MT, Meyers DG. So much writing, so little science: a review of 37 years of literature on edetate sodium chelation therapy. Ann Pharmacotherapy 1993;27:1504–1509.
2. Quan H, Ghali WA, Verhoef MJ, Norris CM, Galbraith PD, Knudtson ML. Use of chelation therapy after coronary angiography. Am J Med 2000;111:686–691.
3. Clarke NE, Sr., Clarke NE, Jr., Mosher RE. The "in vivo" dissolution of metastatic calcium. An approach to atherosclerosis. Am J Med Sci 1955;229:142–149.
4. Clarke NE. Treatment of angina pectoris with disodium EDTA. Am J Med Sci 1956;232:654–666.
5. Clarke NE, Atherosclerosis, occlusive vascular disease and EDTA. Am J Cardiol 1960;6:233.
6. Kitchell JR, Meltzer LE, Seven MJ. Potential uses of chelation methods in the treatment of cardiovascular diseases. Prog Cardiol Dis 1961;3:338–349.

7. Meltzer LE, Kitchell JR, Palmon F, Jr. The long term use, side effects and toxicity of disodium ethylenediamine tetraacetic acid (EDTA). Am J Med Sci 1961;242:51–57.
8. Kitchell JR, Palmon F, Aytan N, Meltzer L. The treatment of coronary artery disease with disodium EDTA: a reappraisal. Am J Cardiol 1963;11:501–506.
9. Cranton EM, Frackelton JP. Current status of EDTA chelation therapy in occlusive arterial disease. J Holistic Med 1982;1:24.
10. Olzsewer E, Carter JP. EDTA chelation therapy: a retrospective study of 2,870 patients. J Adv Med 1989;2:137–139.
11. Chappell LT, Stahl JP. The correlation between EDTA chelation therapy and improvement in cardiovascular function: a meta-analysis. J Adv Med 1993;6:139–160.
12. Clarke NE, Sr., Clarke NE, Jr., Mosher RE. Treatment of occlusive vascular disease with disodium ethylene diamine tetraacetic acid. Am J Med Sci 1960;239:732–744.
13. Nikitina EK, Abramova MA. Treatment of atherosclerosis with Trilon B (EDTA) Kardiologiia 1972;12:137–139
14. Lamar CP. Chelation therapy for occlusive arteriosclerosis in diabetic patients. Angiology 1964;15:379–395.
15. Brucknerova O, Tulacek J. Chelates in the treatment of occlusive atherosclerosis. Vnitrni Lek 1972;18:729–735.
16. McDonagh EW, Rudolph CJ, Cheraskin E. An oculocerebrovasculometric analysis of the improvement in arterial stenosis following EDTA chelation therapy. J Holistic Med 1982;4:21–23.
17. Rudolph CJ, McDonagh EW. Effect of EDTA chelation and supportive multivitamin trace mineral supplementation on carotid circulation: case report. J Adv Med 1990;3:5–11.
19. Rudolph CJ, McDonagh EW, Barber RK. A non-surgical approach to obstructive carotid stenosis using EDTA chelation. J Adv Med 1991;4:157–166.
20. Sloth-Nielson J, Guldager B, Mouritzen C, et al. Arteriographic findings in EDTA chelation therapy on peripheral arteriosclerosis. Am J Surg 1991;4:122–125.
21. Guldager B, Jelnes R, Jorgensen SJ, et al. EDTA treatment of intermittent claudication—a double-blind, placebo controlled study. J Int Med 1992;231:231–267.
22. Udvalget Vedrorenmde Videnskabelig Uredelighed (UVVU). The Committee on Scientific Dishonesty. Conclusions concerning complaints in connection with trial of EDTA versus placebo in the treatment of atherosclerosis. January 1994.
23. Van Rij AM, Solomon C, Packer SGK, Hopkins WG. Chelation therapy for intermittent claudication: a double-blind, randomized, controlled trial. Circulation 1994;90:1194–1199.
24. Knudtson ML,Wyse, GD, Galbraith PD, et al. Chelation therapy for ischemic heart disease: A randomized controlled trial. JAMA 2002;287:481–486.
25. Bolick LE, Blankenhorn DH. A quantitative study of coronary arterial calcification. Am J Path 1961;39:511.
26. Wilder L, DeJode L, Milstein SR. Mobilization of atherosclerotic plaque calcium with EDTA utilizing the isolation-perfusion principle. Surgery 1962;52:793.
27. Kindness G, Frackelton JP. Effect of ethylene diamine tetraacetic acid (EDTA) on platelet aggregation in human blood. J Adv Med 1989;2:519–530.
28. Rudolph CJ, McDonagh EW, Barber RK. Effect of EDTA chelation on serum iron. J Adv Med 1991;4:39–45.
29. Schroeder H. A practical method for the reduction of plasma cholesterol in man. J Chron Dis 1956;4:461.
30. Olwin J, Koppel J. Reduction of elevated plasma lipid levels in atherosclerosis following EDTA therapy. Proc Soc Exp Biol Med 1968;128:1137.

31. Niederhoffer N, Lartaud-Idjouadiene I, Giummelly P, Duvivier C, Peslin R, Atkinson J. Calcification of medial elastic fibers and aortic elasticity. Hypertension 1997;29:999–1006.
32. Heinecke JW. Sources of vascular oxidative stress. In: Keaney JF, Jr., ed. Oxidative stress and vascular disease. Kluwer Academic Publishers, Boston, 2000, pp. 9–25.
33. Esterbauer H, Striegl H, Puhl H, Rotheneder M. Continuous monitoring of in vitro oxidation of human low density lipoprotein. Free Radic Res Commun 1989;6:67–75.
34. Huggins TG, Wells-Knecht MC, Detorie NA, Baynes JW, Thorpe SR. Formation of o-tyrosine and dityrosine in proteins during radiolytic and metal-catalyzed oxidation. J Biol Chem 1993;268:12,341–12,347.
35. Swain J, Gutteridge JM. Prooxidant iron and copper, with ferroxidase and xanthine oxidase activities in human atherosclerotic material. FEBS Lett 1995;368:513–515.
36. Smith C, Mitchinson MJ, Aruoma OI, Halliwell B. Stimulation of lipid peroxidation and hydroxyl-radical generation by the contents of human atherosclerotic lesions. Biochem J 1992;286:901–905.
37. Lin M, Rippe RA, Niemela O, Brittenham G, Tsukamoto H. Role of iron in NF-kappa B activation and cytokine gene expression by rat hepatic macrophages. Am J Physiol 1997;272:G1355–G1364.
38. Olbrych MT, Khan BV, Alexander RW, Medford RM. Metal dependent and independent regulation of redox-sensitive VCAM-1 gene expression in human vascular endothelial cells [abstract]. Circulation 1995;92:I–229.
39. Cooper CE. Nitric oxide and iron proteins. Biochim Biophys Acta 1999;1411:290–309.
40. Nitenberg A, Paycha F, Ledoux S, Sachs R, Attali JR, Valensi P. Coronary artery responses to physiological stimuli are improved by deferoxamine but not by L-arginine in non-insulin-dependent diabetic patients with angiographically normal coronary arteries and no other risk factors. Circulation 1998;97:736–743.
41. Duffy SJ, Biegelsen ES, Holbrook M, et al. Iron chelation improves endothelial function in patients with coronary artery disease. Circulation 2001;103:2799–2804.
42. Galey J-P. Potential use of iron chelators against oxidative damage. In: Sies H, ed. Antioxidants in Disease: Mechanisms and Therapy. Academic, San Diego, 2001, pp. 167–203.
43. Heinecke JW, Baker L, Rosen H, Chait A. Superoxide mediated modification of low density lipoprotein by arterial smooth muscle cells in culture. J Clin Invest 1986;77:757–761.
44. Green DJ, O'Driscoll JG, Maiorana A, Scrimgeour NB, Weerasooriya R, Taylor RR. Effects of chelation with EDTA and vitamin B therapy on nitric oxide-related endothelial vasodilator function. Clin Exp Pharmacol Physiol 1999;26:853–856.
45. Astin JA. Why patients use alternative medicine: results of a national study. JAMA 1998;279:1548–1553.
46. ACC/AHA guideline for the Management of Stable Angina. J Am Coll Cardiol 1999;33:2092–2197.
47. Rosema T. The protocol for safe and effective administration of EDTA and other chelation agents for vascular disease, degenerative disease and metal toxicity. J Adv Med 1997;10:5–100.

13 Energy Medicine, Energy Therapies, and Cardiovascular Disease

Glen Rein, PhD
and Maria Syldona, PhD

Contents

INTRODUCTION

Energy medicine is an emerging field that is based on the principle that energy is related to, interacts with, and underlies all biomolecular processes to promote and maintain good health. The treatment modalities' mechanisms of action that comprise energy medicine involve modulation and regulation of the intrinsic energy fields in the body. The energy to which we refer in energy medicine therapies includes energy that is either externally applied (extrinsic) or internally generated (intrinsic). Extrinsic energy therapies can be either man-made (electromagnetic/

From: *Contemporary Cardiology*
Complementary and Alternative Cardiovascular Medicine
Edited by: R. A. Stein and M. C. Oz © Humana Press Inc., Totowa, NJ

acoustic/light therapy, acupuncture, or homeopathy) or of human origin (laying-on of hands healing and external Qigong). Some of the intrinsic energy modalities are also categorized as mind–body medicine. Intrinsic energy modalities include meditation, imagery, biofeedback, stress management (relaxation training), internal Qigong, Tai chi, and Hatha Yoga. For an extensive and relatively scientific treatment of energy medicine, see the recent reviews by Gerber *(1)* and Oschman *(2)*.

Several double-blind randomized clinical trials in orthopedics have demonstrated the efficacy of electromagnetic (EM) fields to increase the rate of bone healing. Currently the Food and Drug Administration (FDA) has approved the use of these devices only for bone healing, soft tissue wound healing, pain, and electroacupuncture. Although there are also several scientific studies suggesting the efficacy of extrinsic energy therapies in the treatment of cardiovascular disease (CVD), most of these devices are not FDA approved and can only be used as investigational devices for research purposes. Nonetheless, some manufacturers of energy therapy devices are in the process of obtaining FDA approval. Some extrinsic energy therapies, notably auditory acoustic energy and magnets, are not regulated by the FDA. More evidence-based research using contemporary scientific methodologies is clearly required to evaluate which, if any, of the energy medicine therapies are effective in the treatment and/or prevention of heart disease.

THE INTRINSIC ENERGY SYSTEM ACCORDING TO EASTERN SCIENCES

The ancient Eastern sciences and traditions for millennia have included energy therapies as an integral part of their medical sciences. The existence of a global, intrinsic energy system within the body has been thoroughly described in the Eastern Sciences of Life, such as the Vedic, Yogic, Taoist, and Buddhist traditions. The Eastern sciences describe a subtle energy body that underlies and interpenetrates the physical body. Because all matter is energy at the subatomic level, the physical body is, in fact, also an energy body. The subtle energy body in this context can be viewed as matter. It would be of a finer or higher vibration than the vibration of the visible, physical body. Both bodies exist in the same place at the same time. This phenomenon is akin to that of radio waves occupying the same place as the physical body when a person is in their path. The radio waves and the physical body coexist in the same space and time, even though the radio waves are not detectable without a radio.

Within the subtle body is a circulatory system that in oriental medicine is called the meridian (acupuncture) system and in Ayurvedic medicine is called the nadi system. The energy that flows through this system is called chi in the meridian system and prana in the nadi system. The subtle body is also the realm of the mind, if not synonymous with the mind and, thus, the primary mechanism by which mental and emotional processes affect the body. This is why meditation and imagery are considered energy medicine modalities. All of these techniques were incorporated in ancient Eastern psychologies.

THE INTRINSIC ENERGY SYSTEM ACCORDING TO WESTERN SCIENCE

The subtle body was originally described in the Eastern traditions as "light". The intrinsic energy system of the body has been studied by Western scientists using optical techniques. These studies have been pioneered by Popp, who first demonstrated that biological systems emit ultraweak and highly coherent light (visible and ultraviolet [UV]) (3). Popp concludes that the body contains a quantum coherent energy field, which acts nonlocally to regulate all physiological processes.

However, most Western scientists studying bioelectricity have characterized the electrical system of the body by measuring surface electrodermal potentials. Indeed, electroencaphalogram (EEG) and electrocardiogram (ECG) measures have provided useful diagnostic information. Such EEG and ECG potentials are believed to arise from underlying alternating currents generated by ion movement. In turn, these ionic currents induce endogenous electric and magnetic fields, typically believed to accompany membrane depolarization in excitable tissues. According to traditional neurophysiology, these endogenous EM fields are, therefore, considered a byproduct of underlying electrochemical processes.

From the energy medicine perspective, the exact opposite is true—the intrinsic energy system is postulated to underlie and regulate biochemical processes. Furthermore, traditional electrophysiologists consider endogenous electric fields as locally acting within specific regions of the nervous system and the cardiovascular system. In energy medicine, the body's endogenous energy system is considered to be global. If we consider the brain and the heart as separate electrical oscillators, under certain conditions (associated with meditation) the two oscillators couple to and synchronize with one another (4). Under these conditions (referred to as psychophysiological coherence), other oscillating systems in the body (e.g., the respiratory system) can also resonate harmoniously with the two main coupled oscillators (5). These results offer experimental support for the existence of a global intrinsic energy field.

Additional support for such a global field was presented by Burr, who first measured DC electrodermal potentials. Burr concluded that "all living systems possess an Electro-dynamic field... of the whole organism" (6). More recently, Becker established a role for DC potentials in wound healing (7), and he noted their role in the acupuncture meridian system by studying DC potentials on and off acupoints (8). Slydona has studied the fluctuations in DC potentials on acupoints as subjects practiced mental healing and meditation techniques (9,10). An intrinsic energy field of the body, also referred to as the "biofield," is believed to be the source of intrinsic energy therapies and the target for extrinsic energies.

PART I: EXTRINSIC ENERGY THERAPIES

Extrinsic energy therapies fall into two categories—energies generated by man and those generated by machine. These studies suggest that man-made devices, which generate EM, acoustic, and optical energy, have a variety of biological effects at the cellular and systemic levels. The scientific data regarding their use in cardiology are discussed in the next two sections. Despite limited use in the United States (due, in part, to FDA regulations), European, Japanese, and Russian physicians and practitioners use these devices in clinical settings. Some commercially available devices have FDA approval, whereas others are designed for home use only. A relevant example that demonstrates these points is the popular use of magnets. Several scientific studies reviewed below demonstrate that weak DC magnetic fields may, in fact, have beneficial effects. Parameters like the strength and polarity of the magnets, the duration of treatment, exposure conditions (continuous vs interrupted exposure), and the method of application (placement on/off acupuncture points) have been selected from clincial experience. In some cases, there is a scientific rationale for the choice of the parameters, although they were determined by trial and error. For many of the studies described, appropriate clinical usage parameters have not yet been defined.

Bioelectromagnetics

The bioelectromagnetics community is actively involved with scientific and clinical research (and publication of a peer-reviewed journal) of the biological effects of EM fields. During the last 40 yr, research has focused on both beneficial and detrimental biological effects of EM fields. Generally, strong EM fields produce thermal biological effects, which are often detrimental, whereas weak fields produce nonthermal effects that in select cases have been clinically beneficial. Government funding has been available for studying the detrimental effects of computer terminals, power lines, and, more recently, cell phones.

Under certain conditions, residential and occupational exposure to power lines and other types of man-made EM fields can produce detrimental effects. Potential detrimental effects on the cardiovascular system have also been evaluated. Several reviews of radiowave/microwave EM fields concluded that in order to see changes in heart rate and blood pressure, relatively high field strengths (kW/cm^2) are required (11). A recent review of cardiovascular effects of low-frequency EM fields concludes that ECG, heart rate, and blood pressure effects require field strengths of several Tesla (12). An extensive study was unable to reveal any cardiovascular effects using low-intensity (100 mT) fields over a wide range of low frequencies (13). These studies concluded that weak 60Hz EM fields do not have a detrimental effect on the measured cardiovascular parameters (11).

Beneficial Effects of Electromagnetic Fields on Cardiovascular Disease

Because they can be easily generated using commercial flat magnets with north/south (N/S) poles on opposite faces, clinical studies using DC magnetic fields have been conducted. Studies of animals using DC or static magnetic fields have noted improved blood flow after topical application of various strength magnets for relatively short time periods. For example, a recent study in mice measured the ability of weak (1 mT) magnetic fields to increase capillary blood flow velocity in tibialis anterior muscles (14). The effect required only 10 min of exposure and lasted for an extended period after removal of the magnets. Another recent animal study noted effects on microvascular dynamics after only 1 min of exposure, although somewhat stronger magnets (10 mT) were required (15). Long-term exposure for several weeks resulted in vasodilation of arterioles in a rabbit model (16). In a rabbit hypertension model, whole-body exposure to magnets (approx 10 mT) increased capillary blood flow, and, in some cases, concomitant changes in blood pressure were recorded. (17).

It was discovered in the late 1980s that, in addition to stimulating heart muscle with electrical currents, high-frequency (11 MHz and 29 GHz) EM fields of relatively low amplitude (5 mW/cm^2) increased the tension of heart muscles made to contract by standard electrical stimulation (18). This study pioneered the use of EM fields in cardiology. More recently, an EM cardiac pacemaker was developed, which generates a weak magnetic field (160 uT), with frequencies similar to those in the power spectrum of the ECG (19).

Clinically, application of force fields using noninvasive technology may be more advantageous than applying current. This possibility has opened the market to a flood of EM field-generating devices, with a wide variety of healing claims. Many are unsubstantiated claims, but some of the devices were tested using contemporary scientific methods, and the results published in mainstream, peer-reviewed journals. This section reviews studies in the latter category to determine which EM generators emit fields with beneficial effects on the cardiovascular system, whether tested with human subjects or animals, in vitro or in vivo. Therefore, in some cases, healthy benefits in humans can only be inferred.

Contemporary researchers have used specific waveforms generating unique frequencies and harmonics, which are designed to specifically interact with transmembrane ionic conductances, notably calcium ions *(20)*. A commercially available device, the Diapulse, reduces calcium efflux from central nervous system (CNS) tissues *(21)*. This device is FDA approved for postoperative treatment of edema and pain associated with soft-tissue wounds. A similar low-frequency device was used to prevent the calcium accumulation that follows spinal cord injury *(22)*. It is possible that selected EM field therapies that alter calcium ion flux will have a beneficial effect on ischemia, arrhythmias, and hypertension.

Several studies have demonstrated the beneficial effects of EM fields on ischemic tissue damage. An early study demonstrated that pulsed electrical stimulation (35 mA at 128 Hz for 30 min) improved the survival and reduced the necrosis of ischemia-induced tissue injury in pig skin flaps *(23)*. In animal studies, EM fields have been efficacious in the treatment of acute ischemic injury to both the brain and the heart. Using a rabbit model, an Italian group demonstrated the beneficial effects of a weak (3 mT) EM field (75 Hz repetition rate) on transient focal ischemia *(24)*. After occlusion of the carotid artery and 4 h of reperfusion in the presence of the EM field, ischemic injury was assessed using magnetic resonance imaging (MRI) and histology. EM field treatment reduced ischemic injury by 65–69%. The authors suggest that EM field therapy may be potentially valuable in the clinical treatment of ischemic stroke.

A second animal study by the Italian group used a rat model for acute experimental myocardial infarctions (MIs) *(25)*. Ligation of the left anterior descending artery for 1 h was used to induce acute ischemic injury to the heart. Myocardial tissue damage was evaluated using histochemical staining. EM treatment for 18 h postsurgery resulted in a significant reduction in the size of the necrotic area and an increase in the survival of the most peripheral areas of the infarct. Chronic effects were also monitored after continuous EM treatment during the next 6 d. Increased vascular invasion of the necrotic area was noted, with no changes in actual necrosis. A study of short-term exposure of unorganized bovine aortic endothelial cells to weak, low-frequency EM fields resulted in their reorganization into complex three-dimensional structural vessels *(26)*. Low-frequency EM fields have been noted, as discussed previously, in selected animal studies to induce angiogenesis both in vitro and in vivo, suggesting that EM fields may be useful in reducing ischemia-induced myocardial damage.

Effects of Acoustic Energy on Cardiovascular Disease

Soundmyography has been used to detect and measure sound emissions from the body *(27)*, suggesting that extrinsic acoustic energy therapies may have direct biological effects. Acoustic energy can be delivered in the form of mechanical vibrations, which generate sound waves, and is primarily characterized in terms of its frequency relative to the auditory range (20 Hz to 100 kHz). Ultrasound uses frequencies higher than this range, and infrasound uses frequencies lower than this range. Sound therapy uses auditory range acoustic energy, which is not FDA regulated.

A growing body of in vitro and animal research has addressed the scientific basis for the therapeutic application of low-intensity acoustic energy. This research area, bioacoustics, is now the subject of scientific inquiry *(28)* and the focus of a professional society: The Acoustic Society of America. Selected bone-healing experiments have indicated that acoustic energy produced effects similar to those observed with EM fields and that mechanical vibrations, generated from a noise generator, produced protective effects against subsequent hypoxic stress, as has been noted with EM fields *(29)*.

THERAPEUTIC ULTRASOUND AND INFRASOUND

Selected animal studies have indicated that ultrasound energy may stimulate angiogenesis as has been noted with EM fields. One study using a wound-healing model in rats demonstrated that that after 5 d of ultrasound (100 mW/cm^2, 750 kHz) treatment there was a significant increase in new blood vessel formation *(30)*. A recent report noted the efficacy of low-intensity ultrasound for 2 wk to promote the healing of pressure ulcers in patients *(31)*.

One study in rats directly applied ultrasound to cardiovascular tissue and evaluated changes in cardiac function. Rat hearts were subjected to ultrasound (2 W/cm^2, 1000 kHz) for 15 min and ventricular pressure and pressure time intervals were measured. There was no noted effect of ultrasound to improve healthy isolated heart hemodynamic performance *(32)*. In contrast, studies in Russia using long-term treatments with 8 Hz infrasound have produced preliminary evidence for increased myocar-

dial functional activity *(33)*. A recent review of the applications of therapeutic ultrasound to cardiology foresees a possible future role for acoustic energy in treating CVD *(34)*.

AUDITORY ACOUSTIC ENERGY

In addition to these studies using ultrasound, an unpublished but intriguing clinical study regarding the effect of auditory acoustic energy on the
cardiovascular system is worth mentioning. Acoustic resonance therapy,
developed at the Neuroacoustic Research Institute, was a new method
aimed at modulating the activities of the sympathetic and parasympathetic nervous systems. Real-time heart rate variability was calculated
and monitored as the subject was exposed to a sweep of auditory frequencies from 50 to 220 Hz. The primary frequency, which produced the
best balance of sympathetic and parasympathetic acitivity, was then fed
back to the subject in a chord using three octaves. Preliminary data
suggest a lowering of blood pressure when the sounds are played to
subjects with CVD *(35)*. It will be interesting to see if further studies
confirm this finding.

Other studies using auditory acoustic energy have been done with
new-age music and specially designed music. Biological effects beyond
the expected generalized relaxation and stress reduction response have
been noted, including altered mental and emotional balance *(36)*, brain
synchronization *(37)*, and immune system enhancement *(38)*. Meaning-
ful clinical studies that address the effect of sound therapies on the cardiovascular system would, if positive, present intriguing therapeutic
opportunities.

Effects of Lasers on Cadiovascular Disease

As mentioned in the introduction, cells emit and are sensitive to
ultraweak visible and UV light, suggesting their utilization of biophoton
energy in intercellular communication.

Several biological effects at the cellular level have been reported in
the literature for both incoherent *(39)* and coherent (laser) light *(40)*.
Different types of lasers use different physical mechanisms (YAG, CO_2,
etc.) to generate light of varied wavelengths in the visible and infrared
portion of the EM spectrum. In contrast to low-intensity laser therapy,
the use of strong lasers to burn holes in tissues is not considered part of
energy medicine.

Several different types of low-intensity lasers have been used for
wound healing *(41)*. For example, one study, used low-intensity lasers
to promote the healing of skin ulcers induced by ionizing radiation *(42)*.
Another study used an animal model (rats) for ischemic injury to the

heart and MI. A reduction in infarct size and a reduced ventricular dilation were observed with low-intensity laser treatment *(43)*. In both studies, laser-induced effects were mediated by an increase in the number of blood vessels.

Extrinsic Energy Therapies of Human Origin

All the extrinsic energy therapies described so far used man-made EM, acoustic, and optical energies. As mentioned in the introduction, a second category of extrinsic energy therapies can be considered using energy generated and projected from the human body.

Some long-established schools and organizations provide instruction in such "healing arts." These include the Rosalyn Bruyere School, the Reiki Alliance, the Barbara Brennan School, and Therapeutic Touch, which is taught to nurses and used in some hospitals. In addition to healing, external Qigong can be considered an extrinsic energy therapy, because these practitioners are taught to project their Qi to heal others. The National Qigong Association offers trainings and lists of practitioners throughout the country. Although some studies have suggested that these healing techniques produced physiological responses, to date there is no significant evidence of direct effects on the cardiovascular system.

PART II: INTRINSIC ENERGY THERAPIES

Although much research is still necessary concerning intrinsic energy therapies, there exists some consensus among practitioners and researchers regarding their application in heart disease. The general consensus is that intrinsic energy therapies, such as meditation, cognitive restructuring, and relaxation training/stress management, are most effective as preventive measures for heart disease and hypertension. The extensive clinical experience of Udupa suggests that Hatha Yoga postures, such as Shavasana, in selected situations can be an effective treatment modality *(44)*.

The most effective ways for a patient to learn intrinsic energy techniques is to work with a certified practitioner or go to a mind-body medicine clinic. Several such clinics, such as the ones at the University of Massachusetts and Beth Israel Hospital, are affiliated with university hospitals. Schools of yoga, such as Iyengar Yoga, are producing well-trained and qualified instructors of Hatha Yoga. Therapists and instructors of imagery, stress management, and cognitive behavioral therapy can be found in the fields of health psychology and behavioral medicine. Biofeedback and hypnosis are allied fields. Meditation techniques are offered by organizations, such as Transcendental Meditation, Self-Realization Fellowship, SYDA Foundation and the Vedanta Society. The most important factors to consider for a patient who uses intrinsic energy therapies is his or her interest level and finding a certified practitioner with whom he or she can work.

Effect of Intrinsic Energy Therapies on Cardiovascular Disease

Because of the relative youth of energy medicine in the West, few scientific studies have been conducted. Rigorous scientific studies in cardiology are lacking; however, a few clinical studies have yielded promising results. Meditation (invoking the relaxation response) and cognitive behavioral interventions are the best studied intrinsic energy therapies, because they overlap with mind–body medicine, which has been receiving more research attention to date.

One of the earliest clinical studies involving intrinsic energy therapies was done by Udupa (44). In this noncontrolled study, 25 patients with hypertension (five with previous drug treatment) were selected at random from a hypertension clinic and matched with 25 normotensive subjects. All 50 subjects were observed for 6 to 8 wk, without any therapy for blood pressure stabilization. All 50 were then given the Shavasana (relaxation) yoga posture to perform for 30 min/d for 3 mo. Both systolic and diastolic blood pressures decreased significantly in the no-drug group who performed Shavasana posture. Blood pressure decreased even more significantly in the five patients who received Shavasana and drug therapy, indicating that the yoga posture treatment could be combined with drug therapy to achieve a significant result in a shorter time.

The relaxation response, which is evoked through meditation, visualization, and related techniques, and cognitive restructuring have been used successfully in treating cardiovascular disorders, including hypertension and heart disease (45), particularly when they are stress related. The relaxation response, combined with cognitive restructuring, lowers hostility in heart attack survivors (46). In the studies performed by Dr. Dean Ornish, CVD has been effectively treated with a comprehensive lifestyle and diet intervention involving relaxation techniques (47).

Relaxation techniques are also effective against stress, and studies have demonstrated that mental stress and negative emotional states have a detrimental effect on the cardiovascular system (48). It is also worth noting that positive emotions have a beneficial effect on the immune system (49).

The Institute of HeartMath has developed several techniques based on mental and emotional management. One of the fundamental techniques involves focusing the attention on the heart while recalling a prior positive emotional experience. The Institute has also been initiating clinical research to evaluate the beneficial effects of its techniques on the cardiovascular system. Specifically, it has demonstrated a balancing of heart rate variability *(50)*.

Several recent studies *(51–53)* indicate that Transcendental Meditation is effective in reducing hypertension, has a beneficial impact on cardiovascular functioning in adolescents who are at risk for hypertension, and is associated with a reduced carotid atherosclerosis measurement, compared with a health-education control group in African Americans with hypertension.

Numerous studies on the effect of internal Qigong practice on CVD have been conducted in China. Their methodological details are unclear, resulting from, in part, language translation difficulties. However, Qigong practice is used as a treatment modality in the Shanghai Research Institute for Hypertension, where it is generally acknowledged as a cure for many patients with hypertension *(54)*. In *101 Miracles of Natural Healing*, Chan *(55)* interviewed 101 patients at "The World's Largest Medicineless Hospital" who, through Chi-Lel (a specific form of Qigong), were cured of several diseases, including heart disease.

In one such uncontrolled study performed in China, Lee *(56)* studied the physiological effects of Korean traditional internal Qigong training on changes in blood pressure, heart, and respiratory rates before, during, and after Qigong. For 12 normal healthy trainees, heart rate, systolic blood pressure, and rate-pressure product were significantly decreased after practicing this technique. In a study by Kuang *(57)* TCM was used to treat coronary heart disease (CHD) and Qigong was used to treat hypertension. It was reported that the frequency and severity of angina pectoris in CHD and the blood pressure in essential hypertension were significantly decreased. A recent review published in the *Journal of Alternative and Complementary Medicine* evaluated 30 studies selected from peer-reviewed scientific publications, the database from the Qigong Institute of San Francisco, and books and newsletters from Qigong institutes in China. The authors concluded, with one dissenting author: "in hypertensive patients, the practice of Qigong positively affects blood pressure, other blood flow measures, cardiovascular outcome measures and other aspects of health" *(58)*.

EDITORS' ADDENDUM

Safety and Efficacy of Energy Therapies in Humans

When limited to commercial flat magnets, auditory range acoustic energy and extrinsic healing arts (e.g., Rikki, Qigong, and Therapeutic Touch) and intrinsic meditation practices (e.g., yoga, Transcendental

Meditation, and the relaxation response) extrinsic energy therapies for CVD do not represent conceptual or reported issues of patient safety. Small clinical trials of mediation, yoga, and the relaxation response have noted small but significant reductions in systolic and diastolic blood pressures in subjects with hypertension, suggesting a role for their use in appropriate subjects.

Animal studies and select small noncontrolled studies in humans indicate a possible future role for EM, sound, and laser energy therapies for CVD. Selected studies, as noted previously, are intriguing but do not yet form the basis for contemporary clinical use of these therapies in humans.

REFERENCES

1. Gerber R. Vibrational Medicine. Bear & Co., Santa Fe, NM, 1988.
2. Oschman JL. Energy Medicine: Scientific Basis of Bioenergy Therapies. Churchill Livingstone, London, 2000.
3. Popp FA, Gu Q, Li K. Biophoton emission: experimental background and theoretical approaches. Mod Phys Lett 1994;B8:1269–1296.
4. Strogatz SH, Stewart I. Coupled oscillators and biological synchronization. Sci Am 1993;269:102–109.
5. Tiller W, McCraty R, Atkinson M. Cardiac coherence: a new non-invasive measure of autonomic nervous system order. Alt Ther Health Med 1996;2:52–65.
6. Burr HS, Northrop FSC. The electro-dynamic theory of life. Q Rev Biol 1935;10:322–333.
7. Becker RO. The basic biological data transmission and control system influences by electric forces. Ann NY Acad Sci 1974;238:236–248.
8. Becker RO, Reichmanis M, Marino AA, Spadaro JA. Electrophysiological correlates of acupuncture points and meridians. Psychoenergetic Sys 1976;1:105–112.
9. Syldona M. Electrophysiological and Psychological Assessment of Mental Healing Practitioners. Doctoral dissertation. American Commonwealth University, San Diego, 1987.
10. Syldona M, Rein G. The use of DC electrodermal potential measurements and healer's felt sense to assess the energetic nature of Qi. J Alt Comp Med 1999;5:329–347.
11. Jauchem JR, Merritt JH. The epidemiology of exposure to electromagnetic fields: an overview of the recent literature. J Clin Epidemiol 1991;44:895–906.
12. Jauchem JR Exposure of low frequency electromagnetic fields: cardiovascular effects in humans. Int Arch Occup Environ Health 1997;70:9–21.
13. Silny J. Influence of low frequency magnetic fields on the organism. Proc 4th Symp Electromagnetic Compatability, Zurich, March 10, 1981, pp. 175–180.
14. Xu S, Okano H, Ohkubo C. Acute effects of whole-body exposure to static magnetic fields on microcirculation in anesthetized mice. Bioelectrochemistry 2001;53:127–35.
15. Ohkubo C, Okano H, Xu S, Gmitrov J. Modulator effects of static magnetic field exposure on microcirculation and systemic circulation in animals. Proc 24th Bioelectromagnet Soc Quebec City, June 23, 2002, pp. 72–73.
16. Xu S, Okano H, Ohkubo C. Subchronic effects of static magnetic fields on cutaneous microcirculation in rabbits. In Vivo 1998;12:383–389.

17. Okano H, Ohkubo C. Anti-pressor effects of whole body exposure to static magnetic field on pharmaclogically induced hypertension in conscious rabbits. Bioelectromagnetics, 2003;24:139–147.

18. Pozela J, Narusevicius E, Pauza A, et al. Contraction of frog myocardium in nonuniform electromagnetic fields. Gen Physiol Biophys 1987;6:321–326.

19. Van Bise WL, Rauscher EA. Magnetic field impulse cardiovascular stimulation for normalizing arrhythmias and/or heart blocks. Proc Bioelectromagnet Soc Meeting, St. Paul, MN, June 10, 2001.

20. Hernandez-Hernandez R, Velasco M, Armas-Hernandez MJ, et al. Update on the use of calcium antagonists on hypertension. J Human Hypertens 2002;16(Suppl 1):S114–S117.

21. Lieb RJ, Regelson W, West B, et al. Effect of pulsed high frequency electromagnetic radiation on embryonic mouse palate in vitro. J Dent Res 1980;59:1649–1652.

22. Young W. Pulsed electromagnetic fields alter calcium in spinal injury. Central Nerv Syst Trauma 1984;1:89–95.

23. Im MJ, Lee WPA, Hoopes JE. Effect of electrical stimulation on survival of skin flaps in pigs. Phys Ther 1990;70:37–40.

24. Grant G, Cadossi R, Steinberg G. Protection against focal cerebral ischemia following exposure to a pulsed electromagnetic field. Bioelectromagnetics 1994;15:205–216.

25. Albertini A, Zucchini P, Noera G, et al. Protective effect of low frequency low energy pulsing electromagnetic fields on acute experimental myocardial infarcts in rats. Bioelectromagnetics 1999;20:372–377.

26. Yen-Patton GP, Patton W, Beer D, et al. Endothelial cell response to pulsed electromagnetic fields: stimulation of growth rate and angiogenesis in vitro. J Cell Physiol 1988;134:37–46.

27. Yoshitake Y, Moritani T. The muscle sound properties of different muscle fiber types during electrically induced contractions. J Electromyogr Kinesiol 1999;9:209–217.

28. Au WW. Some hot topics in bioacoustics. J Acoust Soc Am 1997;101:2433–2441.

29. Di Carlo AL, White NC, Litovitz TA. Mechanical and electromagnetic induction of protection against oxidative stress. Bioelectrochemistry 2000;53:87–95.

30. Young SR, Dyson M. The effect of therapeutic ultrasound on angiogenesis. Ultrasound Med Biol 1990;16:261–269.

31. Selkowitz DM, Cameron MH, Mainzer A. Efficacy of pulsed low-intensity ultrasound in wound healing. Ostomy Wound Manage 2002;48:40–44.

32. Greenberg S, Finkelstein A, Raisman E, et al. Direct ultrasound application had no effect on cardiac hemodynamic performance in a baseline isolated rat heart model. Ultrasound Med Biol 2000;26:315–319.

33. Nekhoroshev AS, Glinchikov VV. Morpho-functional changes in the myocardium after exposure to infrasound. Gig Sanit 1991;12:56–58.

34. Nesser HJ, Karia DH, Tkalec W, et al. Therapeutic ultrasound in cardiology. Herz 2002;27:269–278.

35. Thompson J. Balancing the autonomic nervous system with physical resonance. Available at: http://www.neuroacoustic.com.

36. McCraty R, Atkinson M., Rein G, et al. Music enhances the effect of positive emotional states on salivary IgA. Stress Med 1996;12:167–175.

37. Bhattacharya J, Petsche H, Pereda E. Long-range synchrony in the gamma band: role in music perception. J Neurosci 2001;21:6329–6337.

38. Kuhn D. The effects of active and passive participation in musical activity on the immune system as measured by salivary immunoglobulin A. J Music Ther 2002;39:30–39.
39. Kubasova T, Horvath M, Kocsis K, et al. Effect of visible light on some cellular and immune parameters. Immunol Cell Bio 1995;73:239–244.
40. Karu T. Photobiology of low-power laser effects. Health Phys 1989;56:691–704.
41. Al-Watban FA, Zhang XY. Comparison of wound healing process using Argon and Krypton lasers. J Clin Laser Med Surg 1997;15:209–215.
42. Schindl A, Schindl M, Pernerstorfer-Schon H, et al. Diabetic neuropathic foot ulcer: successful treatment by low-intensity laser therapy. Dermatology 1999;198:314–316.
43. Yaakobi T, Shoshany Y, Levkovitz S, et al. Long-term effect of low energy laser irradiation on infarction injury in the rat heart. J Appl Physiol 2001;90:2411–2419.
44. Udupa KN, Singh RH, Settiwar RM. A comparative study on the effect of some individual yogic practices in normal persons. Indian J Med Res 1975;63:1066–1071.
45. Stuart EM, Caudill M, Leserman J, et al. Nonpharmacological treatment of hypertension: a multiple-risk-factor approach. J Cardiovasc Nurs 1987;4:1–14.
46. Williams R, Williams V. Anger Kills. Random House, NY. 1993.
47. Ornish D, Scherwitz LW, Billings JH, et al. Intensive lifestyle changes for reversal of coronary heart disease. JAMA 1998;280:2001–2007.
48. Ader R. (ed.). Psychoneuroimmunology. Academic Press, New York, 1981.
49. Rein G, Atkinson M, McCraty R. Effects of positive and negative emotions on salivary IgA. J Adv Med 1995;8:87–105.
50. McCraty R, Atkinson M, Tiller W, Rein G, Watkins AD. The effect of emotions on power spectrum analysis of heart rate variability. Am J Cardiol 1995;76:1089–1093.
51. Kondwani KA, Lollis, CM. Is there a role for stress management in reducing hypertension in African Americans? Eth Dis 2001;11:788–792.
52. Barnes VA, Treiber FA, Davis H. Impact of transcendental meditation on cardiovascular function at rest and during acute stress. J Psychosom Res 2001;51:597–605.
53. Castillo-Richmond A, Schneider RH, Alexander CN, et al. Effects of stress reduction on carotid atherosclerosis in hypertensive African Americans. Stroke 2000;31:568–573.
54. Xing ZH, Li W, Pi DR. Effect of qigong on blood pressure and life quality of essential hypertension patients. Zhongguo Zhong Xi Yi Jie He Za Zhi 1993;13:413–414.
55. Chan L. 101 Miracles of Natural Healing, Benefactor Press, Cincinnati, OH, 1997.
56. Lee MS, Kim BG, Huh HJ, et al. Effect of Qi-training on blood pressure, heart rate and respiration rate. Clin Physiol 2000;20:173–176.
57. Kuang AK, Chen JL, Lu YR. Changes in the sex hormones in female diabetics, coronary heart disease and essential hypertension and its relations with cardiovascular complications and the efficacy of traditional chinese medicine or qigong treatment. Zhong Xi Yi Jie He Za Zhi 1989;9:331–334.
58. Mayer M. QiGong and hypertension: a critique of research. J Alt Compl Med 1999;5:371–382.

14 Homeopathy and Cardiovascular Disease

Woodson C. Merrell, MD
and Amy Rothenberg, ND, DHANP

EDITORS' INTRODUCTION

Homeopathic medicine represents a unique challenge to traditional medicine, because the cognitive framework does not withstand Western medicine's scientific analysis. However, the homeopathic pharmacy is free of adverse effects, because its dilution is extraordinary by Western medicine standards and there are substantial allegorical reports of clinical success. To provide the readers with an understanding of how a homeopathic doctor approaches the patient and determines the selection of a homeopathic pharmaceutical (the experience your patient will have) and to provide a review and critique of the evidence for the clinical efficacy of homeopathy, this chapter is divided into two parts.

Dr. Amy Rothenberg, a practicing homeopathic physician, describes the rational and the thought process that is inherent in the selection of

From: *Contemporary Cardiology*
Complementary and Alternative Cardiovascular Medicine
Edited by: R. A. Stein and M. C. Oz © Humana Press Inc., Totowa, NJ

homeopathic pharmaceutical, with an emphasis of cardiovascular diseases (CVDs), and Dr. Woodson Merrell presents a critical analysis of the evidence, including relatively recent controlled clinical trials, regarding homeopathy. The editors are pleased with the "combination product" that they believe represents an insightful presentation of homeopathic medicine,

PART I. AN EVIDENCE-BASED REVIEW OF HOMEOPATHY AND CARDIOVASCULAR DISEASE

by Woodson C. Merrell, MD

Introduction

Complementary and alternative medicine (CAM) is fast entering American mainstream medical practice. Modalities that were once considered questionable or outright quackery are increasingly achieving an evidence basis and becoming recognized as having value in a more comprehensive approach to patient care. This approach is now more appropriately referred to as integrative medicine (1).

Acupuncture, mind–body practice (hypnosis, imagery, biofeedback, etc.), chiropractic practice, botanical medicines, diet, and nutraceutical therapies are now practiced by an increasing number of physicians, demanded by their patients (2), and taught in medical schools. One modality that is still believed to be outside the mainstream is homeopathy, despite that worldwide, homeopathy is one of the most used therapeutic approaches (3), and has recent studies to demonstrate its safety and efficacy against placebo and in some specific conditions (4).

Analysis of homeopathy's role in our health care system requires: knowledge of its historical background, philosophical and scientific tenets, mode of practice, training and education, and research findings.

Historical Background

Homeopathy was developed by the German physician Samuel Christian Hahnemann in the late 18th century. His work was based on case studies he performed using substances that in full potency would cause symptoms found in certain disease states. Serendipitously he found that when these substances were diluted, they stimulated the body to react against these symptoms. He discovered this initially on research with cinchona bark (containing quinine)—which, in full strength, causes symptoms similar to malaria, but when diluted can reduce a patient's symptoms, such as fever and toxicity, common to malaria and other illnesses. Hahnemann formulated the two guiding principles of homeopathy in his publication in 1796 in "Essay on the new Curative Principal" *(5)*. The first principle of homeopathy is called the Principle of Similars, in which a substance that is given in full strength can cause symptoms in a healthy person and can also stimulate self-healing in the same person with the illness. The second principle, the Principle of Dilutions, came from Hahnemann's discovery that as he diluted (and shook up—or successed) the substances, the more dilute they became and usually the more potent their effects.

Interestingly, Hahnemann's work was done at the same time that Edward Jenner was showing that diluted cowpox conferred immunity to humans for smallpox—a technique using diluted biologically active agents that took a more immediately successful path. However, by 1900, there were 22 homeopathic schools in the United States, including Boston University School of Medicine; Hahnemann Medical College (Philadelphia), and New York Medical College. After Harvard's Flexner Report and other changes in medical care in the United States, the number dwindled to four in 1922, and the last formal training program (part of Hahnemann Medical College) closed in 1949 *(6)*.

Use, Training, and Regulation

PUBLIC USE AND ACCEPTANCE

There is no doubt that homeopathy is enjoying a renaissance in the United States. After nearly a half century of dormancy, homeopathy's use and acceptance by patients has grown considerably in the last 20 yr. In one 7-yr study in the 1990s, the use of homeopathy grew approx 500% sales of homeopathic preparations have grown 20–30% per year in the 1980s and 1990s *(7)*.

PROFESSIONAL TRAINING

After the decline in homeopathy in the United States, Europe and India continued to recognize its ability. This recognition culminated in the 1990s in several formal reports on the usage of homeopathy in medical practice in Europe. In 1996, a Commission of the European Parliament (Homeopathy Medicine Research group) published a report that recommended homeopathy to be a part of medical practice *(8)*. In England in 1997, the Prince of Wales' Commission also recommended homeopathy's inclusion in the mainstream health care delivery system *(9)*. It was already part of the system, with one hospital—Glasgow Homeopathic Hospital—having been a part of the National Health Service for more than a decade. In 1998, the French equivalent of the American Medical Association (Conseil National de l'Ordre des Medicines) recommended that homeopathy be a part of undergraduate and postgraduate medical training *(10)*.

Formal training programs exist in Europe for physicians in homeopathy affiliated with conventional medical curricula, but they do not yet exist in the United States. Currently, there are also no CME courses and only cursory mention of homeopathy at most medical schools that offer instruction in integrative medicine in the United States. Some of the current independent training centers, such as the National Center for Homeopathy, continue to play a leadership role in quality courses, but currently there is no recognized formal medical certification. However, homeopathy is part of the formal curricula at most accredited American colleges of naturopathy, conferring a professional degree (ND) that is currently licensed in 13 states for primary patient care.

Homeopathy is a recognized practice with certification for professionals by three states: Arizona, Nevada, and Connecticut. The lay practice of homeopathy varies from state to state and remains unregulated, except in Minnesota, where unregulated practices by lay practitioners are allowed by the state under specific conditions.

SUBSTANCE REGULATION

Although homeopathy is not generally an accepted practice, homeopathic remedies have always been a part of the US pharmacopeia, officially recognized and regulated (with regular updates to the Homeopathic Pharmacopeia) as over-the-counter drugs. They were included in this federal compendium when the US Food and Drug Administration (FDA) was first established in 1938, under the Food Drug and Cosmetic Act (FDCA), 21 USC, paragraphs 321 (g-1A), and 351b, e.g., and still remain.

Many homeopathic substances are derived from common toxins, although they have been diluted to infinitesimal amounts. Quality control is certainly essential. The largest US homeopathic companies have pharmaceutical-standard manufacturing. As with all supplements (and unfortunately occasionally some pharmaceuticals), there is a potential for substandard manufacture. The FDA and Federal Trade Commission (FTC) are spread too thin to effectively monitor all companies' products. Having experienced providers who know the quality of the products they recommend is of utmost importance with all health care products, including homeopathy.

Practice

The heart and soul of homeopathic practice is based on the history. Few patients have ever had a conventional history taken that approaches the detail of that provided in a session with a homeopath. Classical homeopathy, done for the greatest impact for health transformation, is comprehensive in nature, with the totality of one's influences considered. There are some "cookbook" remedies that can be applied for specific use, such as arnica for bruises, but even this is not simple. The key is that for homeopathy to be maximally effective, it must be individualized.

Many homeopaths use an approach involving finding a patient's constitutional type. Woven into this essential makeup are the specific symptoms that are causing disease. Often all of this fits a polychrest—a confluence of information that suggests a specific remedy. If the remedy is not apparent, the practitioner will consult a *Repertory (11)*, which is a compendium of all known symptoms and corresponding provings from the homeopathic materia medica. This repertorization of homeopathic toxicology then leads to a remedy. Homeopathy is thus a comprehensive analysis of a patient's underlying makeup, with the presenting complaints leading to a particular remedy. Remedies are generally taken as sublingual pellets, with the homeopathic remedy on a small ball of lactose (an insignificant amount of lactose for those with lactose intolerance). Occasionally, sublingual liquids or topical preparations are used. Strengths or potencies are based on the amount of the dilution—remedies that have been diluted and shaken (succussed) in a series of dilutions of either: 10 times (X or D); 100 times (C); or 1000 times (M). For example, these dilutions are designated: for a thrice 10-fold dilution $(10^{-1 \times 3}) = 3X$; for a 10 times 100-fold dilution $(10^{-2 \times 10}) = 10C$.

Philosophical Tenets

As yet, homeopathy has no proven mechanism of action. Although not normally spoken of in this sense, homeopathy can be seen as a form of energy medicine. Many proponents explain its effects as changing the energy of the individual to a state that will promote change to a greater state of wellness. The principles of homeopathy are based on a vitalistic theory. This proposes that in disease states, there is an imbalance of one's *vital force*, which is similar to the traditional Chinese medical perspective of Qi, or Ayurveda's prana. This vitalistic theory is central to the practice of most all indigenous practices. It sees no division between mind and body and is comfortable that the changes coming from its practices are currently not explainable by conventional bioscience. (Western allopathic medicine is one of the earth's only health care approaches that does not recognize a principle of "energy" at its core.)

Because there is no explanation at present of homeopathy's core "energetic" mechanism of action, an examination of what scientific research there is for its mechanisms and current research on clinical outcomes are important to help to assess homeopathy's relative credibility.

Scientific Principles

Homeopathy was developed by Hahnemann by the use of careful clinical observation of patients. Hahnemann was first and foremost a scientist, embarking on some of the first controlled studies. He would take a substance (usually one with toxic properties at baseline concentration), record its effects at full potency, then see how each individual's response changed as the remedy was successively diluted (in sterile water) and successed (shaken). Hahnemann believed that the shaking of each successive dilution was critical for transferring the active substance/energy to the next dilution. The specific symptomatic response to the different strengths was called the *proving*. What became clear to Hahnemann after a series of provings on different individuals with different remedies at different strengths was that, perhaps at first counter intuitively, in many instances, the more dilute the remedy, the more powerful its effect in producing an improvement in the individual's problems. This was the original evidence basis for selecting the remedies for homeopathic practice developed by Hahnemann *(13)*.

One of the most elegant recent attempts to explain homeopathy's mechanisms is in a paper by Eskinazi. He examines mechanisms in homeopathy that are greeted with much skepticism by bioscientists but have much in common with current biomedical observations and practice *(7)*.

These focus on the following two great principals of homeopathy:

1. PRINCIPLE OF SIMILARS

This first principle states that a substance given in normal strength can produce symptoms in a healthy person can also ameliorate those symptoms when diluted and given to a person who is out of balance or ill *(13)*.

There are numerous of examples in conventional medicine where the same medicinal can either reduce or worsen a symptom based on the strength:

1. Immunization: This is the most well-known use of similars to induce a favorable biologic response against the substance given to the patient when it is diluted *(14)*.
2. Drugs, such as aspirin, reduce fevers at normal doses but can induce life-threatening fevers at higher doses *(15)*.
3. Cardiac medications that reduce angina (nitroglycerin), arrhythmias (digoxin), and vasoconstriction (epinephrine) can aggravate those symptoms at higher doses *(15)*.

2. PRINCIPLE OF DILUTIONS

As mentioned above, it is the dilution and succession of a substance from full strength that allows it to be active homeopathically. The potency of substances up to Avogadro's number (6.02×10^{23}) is well documented in conventional scientific literature. Common human physiologic substances are active when diluted 10^{-13} to 10^{-14} (somatostatin, tumor necrosis factor [TNF], and VAP), 10^{-16} to 10^{-18} (Substance P, VAP, and beta-endorphin), and 10^{-19} to 10^{-20} (leukotrienes and interleukin [IL]-1). From 15–150 molecules of pregnenolone improve memory in mice, and 1 molecule of pheromone increases neural firing *(7)*.

The real controversy in homeopathy comes when substances are diluted beyond Avogadro's number—beyond the dilution when you would expect nothing to exist of the original organic substance. Yet it is often exactly in this realm that homeopathy claims some of its most potent effects occur. There is currently no bioscientific explanation for these phenomena. Homeopaths' best explanation for this currently is more in the world of "energy" medicine, where there is some energetic effect ("vital force") transported to the water molecules that have been diluted and succussed. However, every explanation at this level is purely speculative.

The validation of homeopathy rests more in the clinical outcomes, but does it work?

Research

There is a rich tradition in conventional medicine of using medicinal substances that work before the mechanism of action is elucidated. Aspirin and the beta-blockers are two such examples. Of course, increasingly there is a burden for pharmaceutical companies to provide proof of both safety and efficacy and mechanisms of actions for new drugs. Although for many pharmaceuticals, such as psychotropics—drugs that alter some of our brain's most fundamental neurological transmissions, this is not possible.

As discussed above, remedies used in homeopathy have been selected on the basis of provings—by clinical examination of a particular ultra-diluted substance's ability to improve a pathologic state.

In the last 20 yr, studies have been undertaken on homeopathy using the current gold standard for research—randomized controlled trials. The following gives a synopsis of much of this literature to date.

PLACEBO STUDIES: META-ANALYSES

There have been six comprehensive systematic reviews of homeopathy in relationship to placebo *(16–21)*. Four of these show effects greater than placebo. Two show effects that cannot be distinguished from placebo. The largest studies *(16,17)* show significant differences in favor of homeopathy. Methodological flaws in many of the studies continue to be problems in the research into homeopathy, as expressed by the authors in all these analyses.

POSITIVE CLINICAL STUDIES

There have been several well-designed randomized studies of the safety and effectiveness of homeopathy for specific symptoms/illnesses.

Reilly et al. showed that homeopathic preparations (via both symptomatic and immunotherapy mechanisms) can reduce the severity and duration of *allergic asthma (22)*—individual study, with greater *p* value (increased from 0.003 to 0.0004) when results of 38 patients were combined with two other similar studies—*hay fever (23)*, and *allergic rhinitis (24)*. This last study found homeopathy's nasal effects to be similar to topical steroids.

Jacobs et al. published three clinical studies: two showed significant lessening of *diarrhea's* effects in children compared to placebo *(25,26)*. The other examined *acute otitis media*, and these results showed significant lessening in symptoms and (nonsignificant) lessening of treatment failures *(27)*.

A Harvard study in 1999 showed improvement in *mild traumatic brain injury (28)*.

A German study showed homeopathy's equivalence to beta-histine in treating vertigo *(29)*.

Vickers' meta-analysis of seven studies showed that the remedy oscillococcinum reduced the duration of influenza symptoms but not prevention *(30)*—although the overall quality of the studies was criticized.

NEGATIVE CLINICAL STUDIES

A common complaint of most authors of homeopathy meta-analyses is methodological flaws *(31)*. For example, the Cochrane review of asthma studies, which contradicts Reilly, concluded that design flaws precluded comment on efficacy *(32)*. Better design with larger studies unencumbered by belief systems are urgently needed *(33)*.

At this point, there are several well-designed studies that show no effect with homeopathy on specific conditions. These include:

> The use of arnica in surgery (meta-analysis of eight studies) *(34)* and postoperative hematomas *(35)*.
> Migraine headaches were not helped with homeopathy in three different studies *(36–38)*.
> Two meta-analyses of overall effects compared to placebo that conclude that the quality of the homeopathic studies cannot support its superiority over placebo *(20,21)*.

One issue that splits mainstream medicine and the homeopathic community alike is which remedies to use in homeopathic studies. Traditionally in homeopathy, each individual receives a remedy that is highly specific for his or her problem. At its core, homeopathy is not meant to fit the more reductionist Western bioscience model of one size fits (most) all. There are some general remedies that may work for most people, but this more often limits the effectiveness of the treatment according to homeopathic experience. Some published studies have used the same remedy for each study participant. Others individualized the treatments to each participant according to classical homeopathic principals— making the study more specifically about the homeopathic approach than a single remedy. An analogy of these different study designs would be asking, "Do antibiotics help cure infection?" and, perhaps, "If so, are there some that seem more reliably to do so?" rather than "Will erythromycin cure a particular type of bronchitis?" The issue of which research design is preferred for each study is still hotly contested and in need of clarification.

RESEARCH CONCLUSION

There are numerous quality studies in homeopathy to show its efficacy and safety for several conditions; however, methodological flaws still plague the field.

Use in Cardiology

The use of homeopathic remedies in CVDs is complex. There are no published controlled studies of homeopathy in cardiologic conditions. There are numerous anecdotal cases and guidelines presented in homeopathic journals *(39)* and reference books *(40)*. Guidelines for prescribing are based on the historical provings and their presentation in Kent's repertory (and more recent textual updates).

The use of homeopathic remedies in cardiology follows the general practice of homeopathy: take a careful detailed history and repertorize the symptoms and constitutional typing to determine a remedy that would help support a change in the patient's physical, mental, and emotional state.

The cardiology-related symptoms that are given prominence in Kent's repertory under "Chest" include *(11)* chest pain, congestion, constriction, fluttering, and palpitations, as well as sections of other associated symptoms, such as claudication, dizziness, dyspnea, and so on. Prescribing requires a trained practitioner with experience. Under chest pain alone, there are more than 1600 entries for general and specific symptoms and possible remedies. There are nearly 200 entries for palpitations and fluttering, with more than 110 possible remedy choices, depending on the constellation of personality, habits, environment, and symptoms unique to each person.

CVD management certainly does not lend itself to "cookbook" style treatments with one homeopathic remedy fitting all, which is common to allopathic medicine. The homeopathic experience and medical training of the homeopath becomes crucial in treating CVDs. This is a field in homeopathy needing controlled studies now.

Conclusion

Homeopathy is a two-century-old approach to health care that is still controversial. Use was based on provings and anecdotal experience until recently. In the last 20 yr, controlled studies have shown a trend to better the placebo effects and elucidated the use in some specific conditions.

However, in general, the quality of the research is not high. Larger and more carefully controlled studies are needed to better evaluate how to use homeopathy, who should use it, and in what form/strength. Most of Europe (and some of its most important regulatory bodies) has recognized that homeopathy has a place in the health care field. However, in the United States, although historically, a few methodologically sound studies and the controlled method of provings are important for guidance, more will be needed to convince health care leaders to include homeopathy as one of the basic approaches in integrative health care.

The jury is still out for specific treatments for specific conditions; however, homeopathy's benefits and safety clearly outweigh its risks, particularly for non-life-threatening, self-limited conditions. Health care providers, educators, and regulators should carefully evaluate and not be dismissive of the potential value of homeopathy: an inexpensive treatment approach with a track record of (some) proven efficacy and safety.

PART II. THE PRACTICE OF HOMEOPATHY FOR CARDIOVASCULAR DISEASE

by Amy Rothenberg, ND, DHANP

Homeopathy is a unique system of medicine that addresses the whole patient—physically, mentally, and emotionally. Symptoms are understood to occur, in large part, from the patient's straining to respond to both internal and external stressors. Symptoms are seen as the person's way of handling this dynamic. It is the gleaning and understanding of the details of and connections among these symptoms that lead the homeopath to prescribe a particular remedy (41).

Homeopathy was first conceived by Samuel Hahnemann (1755–1843), a German physician and chemist. Troubled by the harshness of medical protocols of his time as well as by personal family tragedies, he turned away from medical practice and devoted himself to the work of scientific translation. During his work on a translation of a popular book on botanical medicine, *Cullen's Materia Medica*, from the English into German, he became intrigued with the portion written on Cinchona bark, from which quinine was eventually derived, and the close relationship between its effectiveness and its toxicity. His curiosity was ignited.

He undertook what was essentially an early homeopathic drug study, known as a *proving*, giving healthy subjects samples of the substance in question and seeing what, if any, effect it had on them *(42)*. To his surprise, in the case of the Cinchona bark, several participants developed the symptoms that the herbal preparation was known to help.

From this observation was born *similia similibus curantur* from the Latin, "likes are cured by likes." This essential underpinning of homeopathic practice can be further defined as follows: any drug that is capable of producing morbid symptoms in a healthy individual will remove similar symptoms occurring as an expression of disease *(43)*.

In his lifetime, Hahnemann conducted provings on 106 substances. He worked diligently and wrote prolifically on topics of homeopathic philosophy, the treatment of chronic disease, and the *Materia Medica Pura*, one of the earliest homeopathic drug compendiums available.

Hahnemann also set out to determine what the optimal dosage of medication would be to achieve both the best clinical outcomes and the least side effects. His experimentations led to concepts of dilution and succussion, which are used in the potentization process of the homeopathic remedies.

Homeopathy is used to treat first aid problems, as well as acute and chronic diseases. First aid problems are addressed in rather "cookbook" fashion, for example, the homeopathic remedy *Arnica montana* for the treatment of trauma. Because traumatic events affect most people similarly, *Arnica* is one of only a handful of remedies to be considered. In other words, when the stress from the outside is severe, most individuals respond similarly. That response will point to one of only a few remedies.

For acute, self-limited problems, such as otitis media, cystitis, or diarrhea, patients present more individualized. For instance, one person with diarrhea might have copious flatulence, stomachache, and chills, whereas another might feel warm and simultaneously have a pounding headache. Although both have diarrhea, they would require and respond to two different homeopathic remedies. The homeopath addresses the whole person at any one time. With most acute illness, there are a limited number of remedies to choose from, because there are only so many ways an acute problem can manifest.

When patients present in the office with what appears to be an acute problem, it is interesting to understand if it is truly an acute problem or if it is rather a flare up of an underlying chronic condition. This would be true in illnesses for which flare-ups are common, such as multiple sclerosis, migraine headache, and premenstrual syndrome, but can also be found in those with upper respiratory tract infection, sinusitis, cystitis, or digestive complaints. Differentiating at this juncture informs treatment options and affects both the homeopathic remedy choice and the dosage.

For illnesses that are more chronic in nature, including most cardiovascular complaints, homeopathic practitioners prescribe constitutional remedies, which are based on the whole person, including his or her cardiac symptoms. There are many homeopathic remedies to be considered, although certain constitutional remedies are thought about more readily for patients with heart conditions. Homeopathic remedies are given for particular people, as opposed to particular diagnoses. One could have five patients with intermittent claudication, and they might receive five different remedies depending on how they experience the problem, i.e., how it actually feels, the type of pain or discomfort, what makes it better, what makes it worse, was there a clear initial etiology, does anything bring on each episode, are there any other simultaneous symptoms. The homeopath is interested in how the intermittent claudication fits into the rest of the person's physical health. In addition, it is central to perceive how those physical characteristics sit *vis-à-vis* the patient's mental and emotional health.

To the homeopath, all symptoms are context-dependent: one cannot see a symptom in isolation, rather the homeopath seeks to understand each symptom a patient reports as it relates to the whole person. The typical intake for a homeopathic physician is 1–2 h, allowing enough time to fully understand the patient and all aspects of his or her lifestyle and health.

This individualized approach would be used whether the presenting complaint was cardiovascular in nature, such as an arrhythmia, degenerative heart disease, valvular problem, peripheral vascular disease, or a condition relating to the gastrointestinal (GI) tract, urinary system, or the skin. For some patients, there are few outward symptoms related to their pathology (i.e., some patients with hypertension or those with poor cholesterol profiles), making it difficult for the homeopath to prescribe on such a chief complaint. However, the homeopath can prescribe based on presenting symptoms from all systems of the body and from general physical characteristics of the patient, as well as from his or her mental and emotional makeup. Homeopathic physicians give a remedy for the patient and expect his or her overall health to improve, including cardiac symptoms.

Many patients who present with heart symptoms are being simultaneously treated by cardiologists. For some of these patients, the problem is strictly functional and there is little to no tissue change and the results of diagnostic and laboratory tests are within normal limits. Homeopathy may be an excellent choice for these patients. It is believed that there are clear links between emotional and physical health. Some patients with mental and emotional concerns will somatosize issues into cardiovascular complaints. Helping address those underlying concerns with homeopathy proves effective in reducing or eliminating the outward signs of the problems. The functional cardiac disorder is fully treatable.

For those with more advanced disease, where tissue change is present, homeopathy can be used with allopathic medications and before and after cardiac surgery or other cardiac procedures to help promote healing and decrease pain. Homeopathy is gentle and nontoxic and does not interfere negatively with allopathic medicines; the remedies are low-cost and easy to administer.

The main risk involved in using homeopathy is the forfeiting of appropriate, timely, and effective allopathic treatment while seeking a "homeopathic cure." There are many patients who are wed to philosophical beliefs who put themselves at risk by not accepting effective treatment options available. Clearly, such patients are a liability to themselves, the prescribing homeopath, and the medical community at large. As the natural progression of certain cardiac conditions ensues, it is essential that each patient take full advantage of advances in the homeopathic, medical, and surgical approaches relevant to his or her case.

Like all practitioners of integrative medicine, the homeopath would ensure that the patient receive recommendation on the appropriate diet and exercise regimen, as well as on the appropriate therapeutic nutrition and botanical medicine supplements for his or her particular diagnoses, while taking into account his or her personal and family health history. For those homeopaths lacking such training, appropriate referral is expected.

As with many modalities in complementary medicine, it could be asked: Who goes to a homeopath? Most practitioners of homeopathy see a range of patients similar to what a family doctor would encounter. Perhaps nothing else is working for a particular patient. For some known or unknown reasons, there are patients who do not respond well to medications; some have paradoxical reactions to drugs, whereas some are allergic to pharmaceuticals or do not tolerate them well. Some patients merely want their medicine to be in accord with an overall health-oriented, "natural" lifestyle.

Some patients visit homeopaths because they have incurable conditions and are strictly seeking symptomatic relief. Some seek to enhance immune function, thereby reducing susceptibility to acute illness from which they suffer, along with chronic complaints. Others come to help address underlying mental or emotional concerns that accompany chronic physical complaints. The last group the homeopath may see are patients who do not feel well, yet there is nothing diagnostically wrong: the laboratory work, physical examination, and health history are unremarkable, yet their vitality is diminished, there are low-grade symptoms on various systems, and the mood is depressed. Some of these patients have clear and intense subjective symptoms, but they continue to pass all examinations. The goal of the homeopath is to offer that person increased energy and a feeling of well-being. One of the unique benefits of homeopathic care is that because homeopaths treat the patient, they do not have to wait until the patient presents with full-blown symptomotology. That there are no specific remedies for specific diagnoses may make some uncomfortable; it is contrary to the modern medical model where drug prescriptions are frequently diagnosis driven. However, if there is no clear pathologic diagnosis, it can difficult to choose correct medications or sometimes to provide any treatment at all.

What follows are general descriptions of several types of patients with cardiac complaints who present in the office. Although the chief complaint may be cardiac, the patient is seen in context of the whole patient. These are thumbnail sketches only, to give a sense of the type of symptomotology that may be present and the homeopathic remedies considered. There are fuller, more detailed descriptions of each of these remedies (*see* Resources section). Most assuredly, you will have many patients who do not fit these few descriptions regarding their physical complaints or their mental and emotional makeup. That means only that they would be prescribed a different homeopathic remedy than the ones addressed herein. Those new to homeopathy often ask: How is the correct remedy chosen? The case analysis portion of homeopathic practice is involved and will be discussed below.

The person who needs the constitutional remedy *Nux vomica* might present with palpitations that are worse when they are overworked, overexcited, or angry. The palpitations are exacerbated by any stimulants, including alcohol, spicy food, or caffeinated products. Their palpitations might also be aggravated while they eat or when they become chilly. They might also suffer from angina that is worse from the same, aforementioned situations.

Almost all patients, male or female, who need this remedy have a tendency for digestive tract problems, regardless of their chief complaint. GI disturbances include indigestion, constipation without urge, or history of peptic ulcer or irritable bowel syndrome. In many of these patients, there would be a tendency for hay fever or acute upper respiratory tract infections with frequent sneezing.

People who need this remedy have "Type A" personalities and are hard working, perhaps even aggressive and strong-willed. They are often in positions of power and take control easily. A patient who would respond favorably to this remedy would be irritable and impatient, be concerned with small details, and be conscientious about all manner of being: the way he or she dresses, the way he or she keeps home and office, and the quality of work he or she does. This tendency leads to competitiveness and exhaustive drive. They would expect the same high standards from others at home and work, hence the easy irritability and anger. They can have strong tempers and can be unapologetic. During acute illnesses, the emotional temperament of those who need *Nux vomica* is more extreme.

People needing *Nux vomica* suffer from insomnia, especially in the middle of the night when they find themselves awake, thinking about work, their responsibilities, and other tasks that need to be addressed. Patients requiring *Nux vomica* are chilly and feel worse in the cold weather. Sometimes if a patient has been this way for some time, he or she is in a state of exhaustion. Years of going at such a workaholic pace have taken their toll, and the physical symptoms have become stronger than he or she can ignore. Therefore, it is the physical symptoms that bring this patient to the doctor and that must be addressed, and the homeopath seeks to understand those symptoms in the context of the underlying issues.

When the symptoms match and this remedy is prescribed, the homeopath would expect all aspects of the *Nux vomica* patient to improve, from palpitations or angina to insomnia, constipation, and irritability. Lifestyle modification recommendations are made cautiously with a patient who needs *Nux vomica*, because he or she overdoes whatever suggestions are made.

Another constitutional remedy used in cardiac patients is *Glonoine* (nitroglycerine). Nitroglycerine was first used in medicine by the brilliant American homeopath, Constantine Hering (1800–1880), who used this substance some 30 yr before it was introduced into allopathic medical community. When prepared homeopathically, the nitroglycerine remedy is used for problems of *intense palpitation*, where there is visible throbbing of the carotids. The patient presents with severe pulsating headaches characterized by a sensation of congestion and fullness, which accompanies the heart symptoms. They are worse in warm temperatures and flush easily on the chest and face.

If the patient has angina, there would likewise be extreme redness to the face during episodes and the attendant headache. These attacks can be brought on by exposure to the sun or by becoming overheated. This temperature aggravation is exactly opposite to that of *Nux vomica*.

It is based on these types of individualizing symptoms that differentiate among the homeopathic medicines considered. Often these differences seem subtle—and indeed would be largely irrelevant to the allopathic doctor—but to a homeopath, that which is individually characteristic of the patient's complaint is paramount.

Patients who need the remedy *Glonoine* often suffer from fainting episodes. We can also think of this remedy for those patients with more advanced cardiomyopathy and for those whose cardiac symptoms alternate with headache symptoms. These people present with the tendency toward confusion that may worsen at night. They are better outside or in cool air. When the heart symptoms are aggravated, it may cause a hand tremor, making use of the hands difficult. This remedy is one of the ones considered when any symptom in the body is accompanied by throbbing and pulsation along with congestive headaches. *Glonoine* helps those patients in the acute phase of sunstroke, when the head is throbbing and bright red and they are worse from leaning forward and better with applying cold water to the face.

Those working with cardiac patients would not want to be without the remedy *Lachesis mutans*. There is a strong feeling of fullness in the chest in patients with heart arrhythmias. The feeling of fullness is so severe that the patient will describe it as a bursting sensation. They often are worse as they fall asleep and cannot tolerate sleeping on the left side. They prefer to sleep on the right side or in a sitting position. They are much worse in the heat and when they become overheated.

If the problem were angina, the *Lachesis* patient would describe a cramping pain in the chest, along with the sensation of fullness. It is not uncommon for those patients needing *Lachesis* to also have a concomitant cough during episodes of cardiac symptoms. Because the sense of fullness in the chest and the neck, these patients are unable to wear any clothing or jewelry that constricts those areas; in fact, they dislike any tight clothing, so they present with loose-fitting, collarless clothing. Because of their extreme warmth, the *Lachesis* patient commonly wears sandals year-round.

Patients with congestive heart failure (CHF) who require this remedy will have a tremendous feeling of suffocation. There will be a feeling of pressure on the chest that is difficult to escape; the patient is awakened by a feeling of choking and must sit up in bed to regain comfort. *Lachesis* can treat sleep apnea in patients with those general symptoms.

Many women will develop cardiac symptoms first during the perimenopausal years when they are markedly worse, physically and emotionally. It's as if without the monthly menstrual discharge, they suffer. Palpitations or angina may commence during these years. Menstruating women will be aggravated in all their symptoms the week before the menses and will be ameliorated when the flow begins. This will be true regarding heart symptoms and other physical complaints, as well as the mental and emotional sphere.

Those benefiting from *Lachesis* are worse in the heat. Many of their complaints are accompanied by bluish, purplish discoloration, whether in the face, skin lesion, or varicose veins. *Lachesis* patients are quite intense on physical, mental, and emotional levels. One can see a tendency for jealousy and even suspiciousness or paranoia. They can hold on interminably to past angers and insults and be difficult to reason with. These people are generally quite loquacious and full of ideas and thoughts and feelings, which must be shared with whomever is at hand. The doctor may feel overwhelmed by such patients.

For patients with peripheral vascular illness, homeopathy has much to offer. The remedy *Sepia* is used in the treatment of painful varicose veins, where there is a sensation of heaviness and drawing downward. This can be seen in men or women, although the remedy is used more frequently for women, especially after childbirth, where there remains an uncomfortable bearing down sensation in the pelvic area and the woman suffers from painful varicosities. These patients also tend to develop Raynaud's disease and phenomenon. In general, their circulation is poor, and they complain from cold weather. One finds constipation and an unusually sallow complexion. For these *Sepia* patients, chloasma is not uncommon and often persists long after parturition.

Someone who would respond well to *Sepia* presents with flat affect, feeling a degree of indifference to their loved ones and seeks solitude from children and family affairs. It is after the birth of several children that some women fall into this state, and taking the remedy can do much to restore health to the circulatory system, as well as to the spirit of the patient.

There are many many other homeopathic remedies employed when treating those with cardiovascular disorders. There are several philosophical approaches to case analysis. However, most agree that it is the individualizing nature of the physical symptoms, as well as the mental and emotional characteristics of the patient, that lead to finding the best homeopathic remedy for each patient.

Homeopaths study their medical art by focusing on several subjects. There is the ongoing study of *materia medica*: learning each remedy and how patients who need it would present regarding all physical symptoms (i.e., in a review of systems fashion). Homeopaths learn how each constitutional remedy type would present regarding the mental and emotional characteristics as well. The study of *materia medica* is a lifelong pursuit. Differential *materia medica*, in which remedies that are similar to each other are studied together, further helps the prescriber make the appropriate prescription. Authors are known based on their style of prose or on their practical experience.

The practice of homeopathy includes ongoing study of case-analysis techniques, with a focus on the long-term follow-up of patients. The goal is to treat a patient through his or her life, through the acute and chronic illnesses that may arise. Assessing efficacy and deciding the course of treatment requires a strong philosophical understanding of the homeopathic healing process and the nature of the person and his or her pathology. It is not uncommon to revisit the homeopathic philosophy books, particularly when faced with a complicated patient. The rich literature of this profession was recently highlighted in a book by Julian Winston entitled, *The Heritage of Homeopathic Literature: An Abbreviated Bibliography and Commentary (44)*.

To help facilitate recall of the approx 2000 remedies in use, many homeopaths study and then refer to repertories, which are books that list all the symptoms known and the homeopathic remedies that have helped to treat those specific symptoms. Repertories are organized by parts of the body. The mind section, so essential in our assessment, is followed by the head, eyes, ears, nose, face, mouth, teeth, throat, stomach, abdomen, rectum, stool, bladder, kidneys, prostate, urethra, urine, male genitalia, female genitalia, larynx and trachea, respiration, cough, chest (where we would find many of the cardiac symptoms), back, extremities, sleep, dreams, chill, fever, perspiration, skin, and generalities. These volumes are also available for use on a computer.

"Repertorization" of a patient's case can be done in a timely fashion after a full homeopathic interview, helping guide the homeopathic physician to a group of the most likely remedies to be considered for a particular patient. One still needs to perceive the correct symptomatology; to understand the patient in all aspects of his or her health, as even the best computer program would be of little use if the incorrect information is considered. Then, the prescribing homeopath must choose the correct remedy from a group of those suggested. Computers have made this analysis work less cumbersome and certainly less time-consuming. Additionally, computer technology allows the qualified homeopath to be flexible regarding various analysis techniques.

It should be added that homeopaths prescribe just as often by "pattern recognition." After one has treated 15 or 20 patients who responded well to the remedy *Nux vomica*, for instance, it is not difficult to recognize that pattern in the next patient who presents and needs the remedy. Therefore, even though a complete case is taken, by the end of the office visit the homeopath would ask questions that are geared at confirming a particular remedy and ruling out others.

Like other physicians and healers, homeopaths study cured cases that are published in peer-reviewed homeopathy journals to better understand the impact of the remedies on patients, as well as to keep abreast on new findings within the profession.

In some instances, patients are eager to self-prescribe homeopathic remedies, and there are many resources available to the layperson (books, magazines, Web sites, and computer programs). It is hoped that most self-prescribers or those who dabble with their family's first aid and acute health care problems understand the need for professional assistance when a problem is severe, long-lasting, or complicated.

Like other medications, homeopathic remedies also have recommended dosages. The strength, quantity, and frequency of the prescription are individualized to the patient as much as the remedy itself. Things that are taken into consideration when the dosage is made include the patient's age and size, type and severity of pathology, and other medications currently being taken.

Most homeopathic remedies are applied to small lactose pellets and taste sweet. The pellets are taken and allowed to dissolve under the tongue, away from food and drink. It is safe to give these small pellets to infants and those with difficulty swallowing.

What follows is a note about using homeopathic remedies after cardiac surgery and cardiac procedures. There is an increasing number of surgeons who recommend the administration of *Arnica montana* postsurgically or after other invasive procedures. Surgeons who use *Arnica* have reportedly noted a reduction in wound swelling and inflammation, as well as faster healing times in the involved areas. The general protocol is to administer *Arnica montana* 1 h after the patient is awake and again once a day for 3 d.

Other homeopathic remedies are sometimes indicated after surgery, depending on symptoms that arise (i.e., difficulty with urination or with normal bowel function, confusion or irritability after anesthesia, or extreme pain at the incision site). A homeopath would look at the patient and his or her individualized symptoms after surgery and prescribe accordingly. Some patients may present having self-prescribed combination remedies, which are available over the counter at health food stores and some pharmacies. These products have not undergone the accepted drug research protocols (provings) that single homeopathic remedies have and are not applied in a manner consistent with homeopathic theory. It is possible that the patient needs one of the remedies included in the combination remedy and will therefore have some effect, but it is generally not profound or long-lasting. Likewise, recently there have appeared "homeopathic combination patch" remedies that would raise the same concerns.

The use of homeopathy for cardiology patients can be considered regardless of whether tissue change is present. Most patients would benefit from constitutional care, and drug interactions or side effects are not seen. Patients generally enjoy the homeopathic interview and the decrease in symptoms and increased feeling of well-being offered by homeopathic care.

EDITORS' CONCLUSION

For the Western physician or other health care provider, knowledge of the clinical approach that patients will experience and the nature of the pharmaceuticals prescribed in a homeopathic practice are critical to providing advice to patients. Integrating homeopathic care within the context of the patient's selection of complementary homeopathic medicine will represent a challenge. However, because the major adverse event related to homeopathic medication is potential for the patient to fail to receive necessary traditional medical care, it is a challenge that must be met effectively. The cause of "head scratching" by medical scientists is the small number of clinical trials whose outcome supports the clinical efficacy of selected homeopathic treatments. As Dr. Merrell points out, larger well-designed and carefully controlled clinical trials are important to address meaningfully the issue of the clinical efficacy of homeopathic medicine.

RESOURCES

General

New England School of Homeopathy
356 Middle Street Amherst, Boston, MA 01002
413-256-5949
Fax: 413-256-6226
Website: www.nesh.com
E-mail: nesh@nesh.com

National Center of Homeopathy
801 North Fairfax, Suite 306
Alexandria, VA 22314-1757
703-548-7790
Fax: 703-548-7792
E-mail: info@homeopathic.org
Website: www.homeopathic.org

Certification and Regulation

American Board of Homeotherapeutics
(MD & DO licensees only)
2776 Hydraulic Road, Suite 5
Charlottesville, VA 22901
804-295-0362
Fax: 804-295-0798
Established 1960

American Institute of Homeopathy
801 North Fairfax, Suite 306
Alexandria, VA 22314-1757
888-445-9988
Fax: 888-445-9988
Organization of medical professionals who practice homeopathy; established 1844

Homeopathic Nurses Association
HC 81 Box 6023
Questa, NM 87556
505-586-1166
Fax: 508-223-1801
E-mail: wellnessnurse@5pillars.com
Website: www.homeopathicnurses.org

Homeopathic Pharmacopoeia Convention of the United States (HPCUS)
Box 2221
Southeastern, PA 19399-2221
601-783-0987
Fax: 601-783-5180
Website: www.HPUS.com
Established 1980; publishes the *Homeopathic Pharmacopoeia of the United States*

Books and Journals

Minimum Price Books
250 H Street
Box 2187
Blaine, WA 98231
800-663-8272
Website: www.minimumprice.com

Homeopathic Educational Services
2124B Kittredge Street
Berkeley, CA 94704
510-649-0294
Fax: 510-649-1955
Website: www.homeopathic.com
E-mail: Mail@homeopathic.com

REFERENCES

1. Snyderman R, Weil A. Integrative medicine: bringing medicine back to its roots. Arch of Intern Med 2002;162:4–7.
2. Eisenberg DM, Davis RB, Ettner SL, et al. Trends in alternative medicine use in the United States: 1990–1997: results of a national follow-up survey. JAMA 1998;280:1569–1575.
3. Jonas WB, Kinde K, Ramirez G. Homeopathy in rheumatic disease. Rheum Dis Clin North Am 2000;26:117–123
4. Merrell W, Shalts E. Homeopathy. Med Clin North Am 2002;86:47–61.
5. Hahnemann S. Essay on a new principle for ascertaining the curative powers of drugs, and some examinations of the previous principles. Hufeland's J 1796;2:391–439.
6. Ullman D. Discovering Homeopathy. North Atlantic Books, Berkeley, CA, 1991.
7. Eskinazi D. Homeopathy re-visited. Arch Intern Med 1999;159:1981–1987.
8. Boissel JP, Ernst E, Fisher P, et al. Overview of data from the homeopathic intervention over no treatment or placebo. In: Report of Homeopathic Medicine Research Group. European Commission, Brussels, 1996.
9. Integrated Health Care: A Way Forward for the Next Five Years, Foundation for Integrated Medicine, on behalf of the steering committee for the Prince of Wales' Initiative on Integrative Medicine, London, England. Cooper Publishing, Blaine, WA, 1997.
10. Nau JY. Le conseil de l'ordre des medicines reclame une reconnaissance officielle de l'homeopathi. Le Monde, February 13, 1998, p. 10.
11. Kent RT. Repertory of the Homeopathic Materia Medica, 6th American ed. B. Jain Publishers, New Delhi.
12. Jacobs J, Chapman EH, Crothers D. Patient characteristics and practice patterns of physicians using homeopathy. Arch Fam Med 1998;7:537–540.
13. Hahnemann S. Organon of Medicine, 6th ed. Cooper Publishing, Blaine, WA, 1982.
14. Siskind GW. Immunologic tolerance. In: Paul W, ed. Fundamental Immunology. Raven Press, New York, 1984, pp. 537–558.
15. Goodman LS, Goodman A. The Pharmacologic Basis of Therapeutics, 9th ed. McGraw-Hill, New York, 1996.
16. Kleijnen J, Knipschild P, ter Riet G. Clinical trials of homeopathy. Br Med J 1991;302:316–323.
17. Linde K, et al. Are the clinical effects of homeopathy placebo effects? A meta-analysis of placebo-controlled trials. Lancet 1997;350:834–843.
18. Linde K, Melchart D. Randomized controlled trials of individualized homeopathy: a state-of-the-art review. J Altern Complement Med 1998;4:371–388.
19. Ernst E. Classical homeopathy versus conventional treatments: a systematic review. Perfusion 1999;12:19–25.
20. Cuchorat M, et al. Evidence of clinical efficacy of homeopathy. A meta-analysis of controlled trials. Homeopathic Medicine Advisory Research Group. Eur J Clin Pharmacol 2000;56:27–33.
21. Walach H. Unspecifische Therapie-Effekte. Das Biespiel Homeopathie, PhD thesis, Psychologische Institut, Albert-Ludwigs Universitat, Freiberg, 1997. From Jonas WB, Kaptchuk TJ, Linde K. A critical overview of homeopathy. Ann Intern Med 2003;138:393–399.
22. Reilly D, Taylor MA, Beattie NG, et al. Is evidence for homeopathy reproducible? Lancet 1994;344:1601–1606.
23. Reilly D, Taylor MA, McSharry C, Aitchison T. Is homeopathy a placebo response? Controlled trial of homeopathic potency, with pollen in hayfever as a model. Lancet 1986;ii:881–886

24. Taylor MA, Reilly D, Lewellyn-Jones RH, et al. Randomized controlled of home-opathy versus placebo in perennial allergic rhinitis with overview of four trial series. Br Med J 2000;321:471–476.

25. Jacobs J, Jimenes LM, Gloyd SS, et al. Treatment of acute childhood diarrhea with homeopathic medicine: a randomized clinical trial in Nicaragua. Pediatrics 1994;93:719–725.

26. Jacobs J, Jimenes LM, Malthouse S, et al. Homeopathic treatment of acute child-hood diarrhea: results from a clinical trial in Nepal. J Altern Complement Med 2000;6:131–139.

27. Jacobs J, Springer DA, Crothers D. Homeopathic treatment of acute otitis media in children: a preliminary randomized placebo-controlled trial. Pediatr Inf Dis J 2001;20:177–183.

28. Chapman EH, Weintraub RJ, Milburn MA, et al. Homeopathic treatment of mild traumatic brain injury: a randomized, placebo-controlled clinical trial. J Head Trauma Rehab 1999;14:521–542.

29. Weiser M, Strosser W, Klein P. Homeopathic versus conventional treatment of vertigo: a randomized double-blind controlled clinical study. Arch Otolaryngol Head Neck Surg 1998;124:879–885.

30. Vickers AJ, Smith C. Homeopathic Oscillococcinum for preventing and treating influenza and influenza-like syndromes. Cochrane Database Systematic Rev, CD001957, 2000.

31. Jonas WB, Anderson RL, Crawford CC. A systematic review of the quality of homeopathic clinical trials. BMC Complement Alt Med 2001;1:12.

32. Linde K, Jobst KA. Homeopathy of chronic asthma. Cochrane Database Systematic Rev, pCD000353, 2000.

33. Jonas WB. The homeopathic debate. J Altern Complement Med 2000;6:213–215.

34. Ernst E, Pittler MH. Efficacy of homeopathic Arnica: a systematic review of pla-cebo-controlled trials. Arch Surg 1998;133:1187–1190.

35. Ramelet AA, Buchheim G, Lorenz P, et al. Homeopathic Arnica in post-operative haematomas: a double-blind study. Dermatology 2000;201:347–348.

36. Strausheim P, Borchgrevink C, et al. Homeopatisk behandling av migrene: en dobbeltblind, placebokontrollert sudie av 68 pasienter. Dynarmis 1997;2:18–22.

37. Walach H, Wausler W, Lowes T, et al. Classical homeopathic treatment of chronic headaches. Cephalgia 1997;17:121–126.

38. Whitmarsh TE, Coleston-Shields DM, et al. Double-blind randomized placebo-con-trolled study of homeopathic prophylaxis of migraine. Cephalgia 1997;17:600–604.

39. Homeopathy, National Center for Homeopathy, Washington, DC.

40. Clark JH. The Prescriber, Essex, Great Britain, Health Science Press, 1987.

41. Herscu P. Stramonium, with an introduction to analysis using cycles and segments. New England School of Homeopathy Press, Amherst, MA, 1996.

42. Herscu P. Provings, with a proving of alcoholus. New England School of Homeopa-thy Press, Amherst, MA, 1996.

43. Hahnemann S. The Organon of the Medical Art. In: Brewster O'Reilly W, ed. Birdcage Books, Redmond, WA, 1996.

44. Winston J. The Heritage of Homeopathic Literature: An Abbreviated Bibliography and Commentary. Tawa, Wellington, New Zealand, 2001.

15 Aromatherapy and Cardiovascular Disease

Jane Buckle, *PhD, RN*

CONTENTS

BACKGROUND
DEFINITIONS
SCIENTIFIC BASIS
CONTEMPORARY USE
CAUTIONS
CLINICAL AND SCIENTIFIC STUDIES AND EVIDENCE
CONCLUSION
REFERENCES

"Whatever the physiological problem with the heart, its function is affected by what each individual asks of their heart in terms of effort. This is determined by the person we are, by the way we live within our own body and by the relationship we do or do not make with it" (1).

BACKGROUND

The definition of aromatherapy is the controlled use of essential oils *(2)*. Essential oils are steam distillates obtained from aromatic plants. Aromatherapy is a fairly new complementary therapy, although its roots are in herbal medicine, one of the oldest known forms of medicine. Aromatherapy is an accepted part of nursing care in the United Kingdom, Switzerland, Germany, Australia, and Canada, and many nurses in the United States are beginning to use aromatherapy. Aromatherapy is particularly useful in cardiology (*see* Table 1), because the use of famil-

From: *Contemporary Cardiology*
Complementary and Alternative Cardiovascular Medicine
Edited by: R. A. Stein and M. C. Oz © Humana Press Inc., Totowa, NJ

Table 1
Essential Oils for Specific Diagnosis

Diagnosis	Essential oil	Research	Reference
Borderline hypertension	Ylang ylang	Freund, 2000	28
	Lavender	Saeki and Shiohara, 2001	30
	Rose	Nathan, 2000	31
	Neroli	Tiran, 1996	34
	Lemon	Tiran, 1996	34
	Clary sage	Tiran, 1996	34
Reducing fear and anxiety	Lavender	Hadfield, 2001	41
	Roman chamomile	Yamada et al., 1996	46
	Rose	Manly, 1993	51
Methicillin-resistant *Staphylococcus aureaus*	Tea tree	Nelson, 1997	22
	Lavender	Nelson, 1997	22
	Juniper	Nelson, 1997	22
	Peppermint	Nelson, 1997	22
	Lemongrass	Sherry et al., 2001	26
	Eucalyptus	Sherry et al., 2001	26
	Clove	Sherry et al., 2001	26
	Thyme	Sherry et al., 2001	26

iar smells and gentle touch can be deeply reassuring. Essential oils have many other properties that can be useful in cardiology—hypotensor, sedative, antiinflammatory, antispasmodic, analgesic, antibiotic, antifungal, and antiviral. This chapter covers the use of aromatherapy for borderline hypertension and for fear and anxiety associated with myocardial infarction (MI) or cardiac surgery and outlines interesting case and small clinical studies addressing the effect of essential oils on methicillin-resistant Staphylococcus aureus (MRSA).

Herbal medicine, which includes the uses of aromatics, dates back 6,000 yr and was, and is still, used in India, China, South America, Greece, the Middle East, and Europe. The renaissance of modern clinical aromatherapy occurred in France just before World War II. A physician (Jean Valnet), a chemist (Maurice Gattefosse), and a nurse (Marguerite Maury) were key figures. Each person used essential oils clinically—to help wounds heal and to fight infection rather than for the relaxing effect of a nice-smelling aromatic. Indeed, the first antiseptic, thymol, which was discovered by Lister, was obtained from thyme essential oil. In France, physicians use essential oils as an alternative to or enhancement of antibiotics. The use of synthetic scents, which has only appeared in the last few decades, is not part of clinical aromatherapy.

Aromatherapy was not mentioned in Eisenberg's 1993 landmark study *(3)*. This study showed nonconventional medicine to be a serious consumer-led commodity, with one in three Americans using complementary therapies. However, 5 yr later in Eisenberg's second study *(4)*, aromatherapy was used by 5.6% of the adult patient population ($n = 2055$ adults).

DEFINITIONS

Aromatherapy is the use of essential oils for therapeutic purposes that encompass mind, body, and spirit *(5)*. The name *aromatherapy* leads people to believe that the therapy is purely about smelling scents, but this belief is incorrect *(6)*. There are many different kinds of aromatherapy, ranging from a nice-smelling candle to the clinical application of essential oils for medicinal reasons *(7)*. Only the role of clinical aromatherapy has a place in a cardiology text.

The definition of essential oils is specific—they are "the steam distillates of aromatic plants" *(8)*. Therefore, any extract not obtained by steam distillation is not an essential oil and is relevant for use in aromatherapy. Essential oils are found in the flowers, leaves, bark, wood, roots, seed, and peels of aromatic plants and are stored in microscopic cellular containers of the plant, i.e., cells, glands, ducts, and hairs. Essential oils are highly volatile, complex mixtures of chemical constituents divided into functional groups, such as ketones, alcohols, terpenes, and esters. The proportions of these individual constituents vary according to the species of plant, climate where grown, and distillation process used. It is the chemistry of an essential oil that determines its therapeutic properties.

SCIENTIFIC BASIS

The pharmacologically active components in essential oils work at psychological and physical levels. Aroma effects can be rapid, and, occasionally, just thinking about a smell can have a powerful effect. This effect can be relaxing or stimulating, depending on the individual's experiences, as well as the chemistry of the essential oil used. Essential oils can be absorbed into and through the skin in minutes. They are lipophyllic (fat soluble) and nonpolar (do not mix with water) and are excreted through respiration, the kidneys, and insensate loss.

Each essential oil is composed of between 1 and 300 different chemical components. These separate olfactory stimulants travel via the nose to the olfactory bulb. From there, nerve impulses continue to the limbic system of the brain, an inner complex ring of brain structures below the cerebral cortex, arranged into 53 regions and 35 associated tracts. The limbic system also receives most sensory input and passes it on to the voluntary and involuntary motor centers. Gatti and Cayola *(9)* noted that odors produced an immediate effect on respiration, pulse, and blood pressure and, therefore, concluded that odors had, by a reflex action, produced a dramatic effect on the functioning of the central nervous system (CNS). Nearly 80 yr later, Singewald et al. *(10)* found that the locus coeruleus (situated in the limbic system) played a vital role in conditioned fear and inescapable shock.

The amygdala and the hippocampus, parts of the limbic system, are particularly important in aroma processing. The amygdala is believed to play a pivotal role in processing emotion, particularly the control of aggression, and in the formation of emotional memory. The amygdala also governs emotional response and affects survival behavior, because it is intimately responsible with a sensation of fear. Diazepam (valium) is believed to reduce the effect of external emotional stimuli by increasing gamma aminobutyric acid (GABA)-containing inhibitory neurons in the amygdala. Lavandula angustifolia (true lavender) has a similar effect on the amygdala, producing a sedative effect that is similar to diazepam *(11)*.

The hippocampus is where molecules in an aroma trigger learned memory and is involved in the formation and retrieval of explicit memories *(12)*. The hippocampus is believed to be the storage area for new experiences before they become permanent memories that are then thought to be stored in the cerebral cortex.

Smell is important to quality of life, beginning with a newborn baby's identification of its mother and continuing into old age, where studies have shown that the depression of residential elderly was reduced with fruit and flower aromas.

The effect of odors on the brain has been mapped using computer-generated topographics. Brain electrical activity maps (BEAM) indicate how subjects, who are linked to an electroencephalogram (EEG), psychometrically rated the odors presented to them. Smells can have a psychological effect even when the aroma is below the level of human awareness. Provided the olfactory nerve is intact, aromas will affect the brain even if the subject is anosmic.

CONTEMPORARY USE

Essential oils can be absorbed into the bodies through olfaction, applied topically or taken internally *(13)*. The components within an essential oil find their way into the bloodstream regardless of application method *(13)*. Inhaled aromas have the fastest effect, although components such as linalol (found in lavender) have been absorbed through massage and detected in the blood within 20 min *(14)*. The method of application depends on the time allowed, the desired outcome, the chemical components within the essential oil, and the patient's psychological needs. The effects of inhaled aromas do not last as long as the effect of topically applied aromas. However, it is difficult to analyze exactly what impact touch has in aromatherapy.

Inhalation

One of the simplest methods of application is direct inhalation. This means an essential oil is directly targeted to the patient. From one to five drops of essential oil are placed on a face tissue and inhaled for 5–10 min. This method is particularly useful for nausea.

Indirect inhalation includes the use of burners, nebulizers, and vaporizers that are heat, battery, or electrically operated and may include the use of water. Larger, portable aroma systems are available to control the release of essential oils on a commercial scale into rooms up to 1500 square feet. This is similar to environmental fragrancing, using synthetics, which is a common practice in hotels and department stores. Indirect inhalation can be useful for mood enhancement, stress reduction, and infection control.

Topical Applications

Essential oils can be used effectively in a compress. Add 4–13 drops of essential oil to a small basin (6 fl oz) of warm water. Soak a gauze swab in the mixture, wring out the swab, and apply it to the affected area (contusion or abrasion). Then cover the compress with plastic wrap to retain moisture. If a compress is being applied to a slow-healing wound, dilute the essential oils in a cold-pressed vegetable oil to prevent the wound from debraiding each time the compress is replaced.

Essential oils are absorbed into and through the skin through diffusion, in which the fat layer acts as a reservoir before the components in the essential oils reach the bloodstream. There is some evidence that massage or hot water enhances the absorption of the essential oils' components. The soothing effects of aromatherapy can be enhanced with the "m" technique®, a recognized, registered method of touch being used by nurses in the United States that is developed and published by the author *(15)*. This method of touch is quite different from massage, and it has proved useful in critical care settings, especially immediately before extubation, or before invasive procedures, such as cardiac catheterization. The technique, which is simple to learn and quick to do, uses structured stroking sequences in a set pattern at a set pressure. Please see resource guide for more information.

Aromatherapy using touch enhances nonverbal communication with patients. From one to five drops of essential oil are diluted in a teaspoonful (5 mL) of a cold-pressed vegetable oil, cream, or gel. The amount of essential oil absorbed from an aromatherapy massage using this dilution will normally be 0.025–0.1 mL (approx 0.5–2 drops) (15).

CAUTIONS

Aromatherapy is a safe complementary therapy if it is used within set guidelines. However, blanket use of essential oils is not recommended, because constant use of the same essential oil may produce sensitivity. This was reported in a woman who already had sensitivity to synthetic aromas and who put several drops of essential oil of lavender directly onto her pillow continuously for several weeks. She slept with the left side of her face on the area of the pillow on the lavender. After several weeks, she presented with acute eczema of her left cheek and forehead (16). She changed the pillow, ceased using lavender, and applied topical corticosteroids, and the eczema subsided.

Oral administration of essential oils should be avoided, unless the person is adequately trained, because there have been a few instances of poisoning from oral use. These fatalities have usually occurred when a large amount of a specific essential oil, such as eucalyptus, has been ingested by children (17).

Essential oils should be kept well away from the eyes. If essential oils get into the eyes, the eyes should be flushed with milk or carrier oil and then water. Essential oils that are high in phenols are aggressive and should not be used undiluted on the skin or for long time periods. Use care with patients who are receiving chemotherapy, because some essential oils may affect the absorption rate of certain chemotherapeutic drugs. Some essential oils, such as bergamot and angelica root, are photosensitive and should not be used topically if the recipient will be subjected to ultraviolet (UV) light.

Most essential oils have been tested by the food and beverage industry, because many essential oils are used as flavorings (18). Other research has been conducted by the perfume industry. Most of the commonly used essential oils in clinical aromatherapy have been given generally regarded as safe (GRAS) status. However, essential oils are concentrated and are generally diluted for topical use. Some essential oils, such as clove and red thyme, are high in phenols and should never be used undiluted on the skin. Some essential oils may cause dermal irritation and are better used by inhalation.

Essential oils should not be confused with herbal extracts, and the two substances cannot be used interchangeably. Herbal extracts are diluted and are often taken internally. Essential oils are concentrated and are not usually taken internally.

A good knowledge of plant taxonomy is important if the correct oil is to be used. Many essential oils have the same common names. Lavender is a common name that covers three different species of lavender and countless man-made hybrids that cannot be used interchangably. The botanical name indicates exactly which lavender by using the genus (rather like a surname) and the species (rather like a first name). The genus of lavender is *Lavandula*, and all lavenders begin with this word.

L. angustifolia is possibly the most used and researched essential oil and is recognized as a relaxant. However, the other two species of lavender have different properties. *L. latifolia* (Spike lavender) is a stimulant, expectorant, and mucolytic. *L. stoechas* is antimicrobial but should not be used for long periods of time, because it contains a large percentage of ketones, which can build up liver toxicity *(18)*. For aromatherapy to be used clinically, it is important to know the full botanical name of an essential oil. Please *see* Table 2 for a list of the botanical names of essential oils referred to in this chapter and Table 3 for examples of plant identification.

CLINICAL AND SCIENTIFIC STUDIES AND EVIDENCE

MRSA

Essential oils were used before synthetic antibiotics and antiseptics. Most essential oils and components of essential oils have some antibacterial, antifungal, or antiviral properties, and a large number of studies have indicated their effectiveness in vitro *(19–21)*. Peppermint, thyme, lavender, tea tree, and juniper essential oils are effective against MRSA in vitro *(22)*. A further article *(23)* also showed that *Melaleuca alternifolia* (tea tree) was effective against MRSA in vitro. It was tested against 64 methicillin-resistant and 33 mupirocin-resistant isolates of *S. aureus* and was effective in all cases, using dilutions of 0.25% and 0.50%. These results were duplicated in a UK study using similar methods. Chan and Loudon *(24)* conducted a further in vitro study on 28 isolates of MRSA and eight clinical isolates of coagulase-negative staphylococci at Manchester Royal Infirmary, England. The minimum inhibitory concentrations (MICs) were repeated three times and ranged from 0.25–0.5% tea tree. No resistant isolates were found. Many cos-

Table 2
Essential Oils in This Chapter

Common name	Botanical name
Angelica	*Angelica archangelica*
Bergamot	*Citrus bergamia*
Chamomile German	*Matricaria recutita*
Chamomile Roman	*Chamomelum nobile*
Clary sage	*Salvia sclarea*
Cimmamon	*Cinnamomum zeylanicum*
Clove	*Syzygium aromaticum*
Eucalyptus	*Eucalyptus globulus*
Lavender true	*Lavandula angustifolia*
Lavender spike	*Lavandula latifolia*
Lavender stoechas	*Lavender stoechas*
Lemon	*Citrus limon*
Lemongrass	*Cymbopogon citruatus*
Mandarin	*Citrus reticulata*
Neroli	*C. aurantium var amara flos*
Peppermint	*Mentha piperita*
Rose	*Rosa damascena*
Tea tree	*Melaleuca alternifolia*
Thyme	*Thymus vulgaris*
Ylang ylang	*Cananga odorata*

Table 3
Examples of Plant Taxonomy

Example 1:	Common name	Neroli
	Botanical name	*Citrus aurantium var amara flos*
	Genus	Citrus
	Species	Aurantium
	Variety	Amara
	Part	Flower (flos)
Example 2:	Common name	Lavender
	Botanical name	*Lavandula angustifolia*
	Genus	Lavandula
	Species	Angustifolia
	Part	Flowering plant

metic products contain 2–5% tea tree. Carson also found that although tea tree inhibited MRSA, it did not inhibit coagulase negative staphylococci and, therefore, preserved the skin flora.

The effective antimicrobial activity of an essential oil in vitro does not necessarily predict a similar action in human subjects. However, Caelli et al. *(25)* conducted a study with human subjects using 4% tea tree nasal ointment and 5% tea tree body wash against a control of 2% mupirocin nasal ointment and triclosan body wash on MRSA. The tea tree combination was better than the conventional one. Because of the small number of patients ($n = 30$), no statistical significance could be drawn.

A recently published case report in *BioMed Central Surgery* suggests a role for essential oils in MRSA osteomyelitis. Sherry et al. *(26)* reported on a chronic case of MRSA osteomyelitis. A 49-yr-old man had sustained an open fracture to his left tibia. He underwent debridement and insertion of an intramedullary nail and later a free-flap to the lower tibia, repositioning of the nail, and a femoral-popliteal bypass graft. Eight mo later, he underwent debridement of the flap, and 15 mo later he underwent a debridement of an infective focus of the left tibia. He subsequently developed chronic osteomyelitis (MRSA). Long-term antibiotic therapy with flucloxacillin and dicloxacillin had been unsuccessful.

Before a planned amputation a percutaneous incision was drilled in the lower tibia and washed and packed with calcium sulfate pellets impregnated with lemongrass, eucalyptus, tea tree, clove, and thyme in an ethanol base. A catheter was left to allow delivery of further delivery of essential oils. Three months later, the wound had healed, the culture was clear, and a plain X-ray showed resolution of the infective process with incorporation of the bone graft.

Chao et al. *(27)* demonstrated that airborne colonies of *S. aureus* and *Pseudomonas aeruginosa* were reduced by 44% and 96%, respectively, when a diffusion of essential oils (cinnamon, clove, rosemary, eucalyptus, and lemon) was diffused for 2 min before and during culture in a microbiology laboratory. After only 12 min of exposure, the bacteria was reduced 10-fold.

Borderline Hypertension

Many of the main classes of antihypertensive drugs are associated with adverse events, such as dizziness, headache, or rash. If essential oils were effective, a lower dose of conventional medication could be used. Freund *(28)* conducted a small pilot study on 13 patients with borderline hypertension (21–71 yr, five men and eight women). Baseline blood pressure was obtained, and patients rated their stress level based on a visual analog scale. Subjects were asked in inhale five drops of ylang

ylang essential oil for 15 min. Blood pressure was remeasured, and the
stress level recording was reassessed. The same group received a control
(plain vegetable oil with no pharmacological effect) at a different time.
The ylang ylang (*C. odorata*) group experienced a 50% greater drop in
systolic and diastolic pressures than did the control group. The stress
visual analog also indicated that the ylang ylang group felt 50% greater
reduction in stress. Freund went on to complete a further 100 patients and
found the results were similar to the first 13 patients. Ylang ylang has a
long anecdotal history of reducing blood pressure and is popular among
British midwifes to help reduce anxiety-induced hypertension in pregnancy *(29)*.

Inhaled *L. angustifolia* reduced systolic blood pressure significantly
in a small controlled Japanese study of normotensive women *(30)*. The
subjects inhaled essential oil of lavender, rosemary, or citronella in an
air-conditioned, temperature-controlled environment. Six drops of one
essential oil (0.3 mL) were added to 10 mL of hot water. The pot was kept
hot so the essential oil would evaporate. The three essential oils were
presented in a random order. Baseline measurements included blood
pressure, blood flow, and galvanic skin conduction (GSC), using a laser
Doppler-flow meter and a skin conductance meter and heart rate variability from a 3-min electrocardiogram (EKG) acquisition. The subjects
then entered the inhalation room for 10 min, where aroma pot was 30 cm
away from their noses. Between subjects, the room was left empty for 90
min to ensure no essential oil from the previous essential oil would
remain to confound the next essential oil. A control time of 10 min in the
room without any aroma was also recorded.

With *L. angustifolia* (lavender) the systolic blood pressure decreased
from a mean baseline level of 106 to 100 mmHg 10 min after inhalation.
GSC was significantly decreased 2 min after inhalation and remained
lower than the baseline level. Blood flow increased within 6 min of
inhalation and remained elevated until the end of the inhalation. The R-R
interval of the EKG did not change significantly. The high-frequency
component (HFC) value increased significantly at 5 min, and the low-
frequency component (LFC)/HFC ratio decreased.

With *Rosmarinus officinalis* (rosemary), neither heart rate variability
components nor GSC changed significantly. However, the systolic blood
pressure changed significantly from 102 +/– 2.2 – 112 +/– 2.00 mmHg.
Blood flow decreased from 38.0 +/– 4.4 to 31.2 +/– 3.2 mL/min/100 g
immediately after inhalation. However, both responses returned to
baseline immediately. The HFC did not indicate any change, but the
LFC/HFC ratio increased significantly from 0.34 +/– 0.03 to 0.95 +/–
0.13 s immediately after inhaling the rosemary.

With *Citronella nardus* (citronella), the blood pressure and blood flow did not change significantly; however, the R-R internal increased during inhalation and increased significantly at 10 min. GSC significantly decreased immediately after inhalation; however, citronella produced complicated effects on the autonomic nervous system that varied greatly. This divergence was directly related to whether the subject liked or disliked the smell of citronella. Citronella is a common aroma used in candles to deter mosquitoes.

Nathan *(31)*, an American midwife, found that both lavender and rose helped to reduce pregnancy-induced hypertension. Either essential oil was chosen and offered to the women an inhalation, or diluted, or topical application in the "m" technique®.

Rose may also be effective in hyperlipidemia. Kirov et al. *(32)* conducted a noncontrolled study on 32 patients with atherosclerosis with hyperlipoproteinemia and arterial hypertension, who were not on antihypertensive therapy. A total of 12 men and 20 women were given a twice-daily dose of rose orally in the form of a gelatin capsule containing 68 mg of Bulgarian rose oil, 30,000 IU of vitamin A, and up to 250 mg of sunflower seed oil. The mixture was called "girosital." Standard urinary and blood analysis were taken on days 1, 10, 20, 50, 80, and 110. Patients took rose essential oil twice daily for 110 d. The rose essential oil had a marked effect on total serum lipids that began on day 20. Patients were divided into three groups, depending on their initial total cholesterol. Basic hematological and biochemical parameters in the blood, serum, and urine remained normal.

The investigator commented that the results were similar to the effects of the drug Bezafibrate. Twenty years before Kirov's study, Shipotshliev *(33)* found that rose had a sedative effect on mice in various methods of application.

Other essential oils believed to help in reducing hypertension are lemon, mandarin, neroli, and clary sage *(34)*. A British midwife, Tiran, suggests that the following essential oils should be avoided in hypertension: rosemary, sage, hyssop, and thyme. Although there is no concrete evidence that rosemary, sage, hyssop, and thyme adversely affect hypertension, anecdotal evidence, clinical experience, and Saeki and Shiohara's study indicate caution.

Fear

Many cardiac patients are anxious or fearful, and these feelings can affect MI management and may be associated with sympathetic arousal and cardiac arrhythmia. Vlay and Fricchione *(35)* reported on the emotional disturbances of patients after infarction. Such emotional disturbance can manifest as depression, anger, frustration, or fear. Mood has a powerful influence on prognosis after acute MI (36). Despite all the reassurance that surgeons and nurses can give, most patients who are awaiting cardiac surgery experience anxiety, and some experience fear. The fear is mainly about uncontrolled pain. McCaffrey (37) found that a combination of pharmacological and nonpharmacological methods of pain control produced the best results. As mentioned in an earlier part of this chapter, fear and anxiety are governed by the amygdala (38), and the amygdala is influenced by aroma.

Gentle touch can do much to allay fear and anxiety (39). The effect of touch is greatly enhanced when the patient learns to associate relaxation with touch and specific aromas preoperatively (40). Smell and touch are two powerful nonverbal communicators and may help those patients who are unable to communicate verbally through lack of language or other skills.

Roman chamomile and lavender reduced anxiety in a small noncontrolled pilot British study by Hadfield (41). Eight patients with primary malignant tumors were given aromatherapy in a hand, foot, or neck massage during their first follow-up appointment after commencing radiotherapy. Patients completed Hospital Anxiety and Depression Scales (HADA) immediately before the aromatherapy and 24 h after the therapy. The results indicated a statistically significant reduction in all physical parameters.

Gould et al. (42) reported on the relaxing cardiac effects of chamomile tea with a group of 12 hospitalized patients who had undergone cardiac catheterization. They found that there was a small but significant rise in the mean blood pressure. However, they were more struck that 10 of the 12 patients fell into a deep sleep within 10 min of drinking the tea. Sleeping was a rarity during this procedure. Patients had not been premedicated and received no other sedation during the procedure. The chamomile tea had essentially no cardiac effect. This is not aromatherapy but a commonly accepted form of aromatic medicine (like coffee and tea). Essential oils are up to 100 times stronger than an herbal tea. Yamada et al. (43) found that chamomile essential oil reduced stress-induced increases in plasma ACTH levels in rats and suggested that essential oil of Roman chamomile might be useful against stress in humans. Avollone et al. (44) studied an aqueous extract of German chamomile flowers, and it behaved as both central and peripheral benzodiazepine receptor ligands, with anxiolytic effects. However, the compounds responsible for this action were unknown. Viola et al. (45) attempted to identify the compound in a further paper. German and Roman chamomile are different essential oils. Roman chamomile may be more useful in a cardiac unit, because it has a more pleasant aroma, as well as a long history of being used for its sedative and calming effects. The author has clinical experience using Roman chamomile essential oil for more than 25 yr to reduce anxiety and fear in human subjects and recommends its use in cardiology for anxious and fearful patients. A 5% dilution of Roman chamomile in sweet almond oil, used in the "m" technique® on the hand or foot is useful with anxious intubabated patients before extubation.

Lavender increased beta power in an EEG in a study by Diego et al. *(46)*. Beta power is related to the ability to relax. Forty subjects were randomly assigned to one of two groups that received rosemary or lavender. Subjects completed a State Anxiety Inventory, a visual analog mood scale, and a math computation test. A continuous EEG was recorded for 3 min before, during, and after the experiment. Results concluded that lavender was relaxing and rosemary was stimulating.

Dunn et al. *(47)* found that massage with lavender reduced the anxiety of 122 patients in an intensive care unit. Patients were randomly allocated to one of three groups: massage with lavender, massage without lavender, or rest. The group that received massage with lavender reported feeling a greater reduction in anxiety. Hewitt and Woolfson *(48)* conducted a similar controlled study on 100 patients in a coronary care unit. They found that a 20-min foot massage with lavender reduced heart rate, respiration, blood pressure, and anxiety. Patients were also randomly allocated to three groups. One group received massage plus lavender, one received massage alone, and the third "rested," without any massage or lavender. Data were obtained using questionnaires to document pain and wakefulness and by measuring heart rate, blood pressure, and respiratory rate. The results of this study showed a 50% reduction in anxiety, as well as a reduction in blood pressure, heart rate, and respiration in the group receiving massage with essential oils above the group just receiving massage.

A third study by Waldman et al. *(49)* also used the same format (three groups with either massage and lavender, massage without lavender, or rest) and agreed with the findings that lavender massage was more effective than massage and a useful anxiolytic.

A vanilla-like synthetic aroma was effective in reducing the anxiety and claustrophobia of magnetic resonance imaging (MRI). Redd et al. *(50)* conducted a controlled study on 57 patients with no psychiatric history or allergies who had not received any anxiety or pain medication in the preceding 48 h. Either 5% heliotropin (diluted in 25% dipropylene glycol and diethylpthalate) or plain air was delivered by nasal cannula. Patients completed a visual analog before, during, and after the imaging. Patients also completed a State-Trait Anxiety questionnaire before and

Table 4
Useful Addresses

National Association of Holistic Aromatherapy (NAHA) www.naha.org

Nationwide Training

American Holistic Nurses Association	Aromatherapy and
Flagstaff, AZ 86004	the "m" technique®
www.ahna.org	R J Buckle Associates LLC
	Hunter, NY 12442
	www.rjbuckle.com

Recommended Essential Oils Distributors

Elizabeth van Burens Inc.	Nature's Gift Ltd.
PO Box 7542	1040 Vheyenn Blvd.
Santa Cruz, CA 95061	Madison, TN 37115
Phone: 1-800-710-7759	Phone: 615-612-4270
www.evb.aromatherapy.com	www.naturesgift.com
Florihana France Ltd	Northwest Essence
Grasse, France	Gig Harbor, WA 98335
www.florial.com	www.northwestessence.com
Primavera	Nature's Gift
Novato, CA 94934	Madison, TN 37115
www.primaveralife.com	www.naturesgift.com

after the MRI. Results indicated that patients who liked the fragrance and inhaled heliotropin during the MRI felt a significant decrease in anxiety (63%). Those not receiving the heliotropin did not have a decrease in anxiety. The fragrance had no effect on pulse or blood pressure. This is not strictly aromatherapy, because the vanilla-like odor was synthetic and not derived from an aromatic plant. However, it is interesting to include.

CONCLUSION

Although there is some confusion concerning what aromatherapy really is, essential oils, when used clinically, have much to offer cardiology, whether as psychological support for fear and anxiety or to help reduce hypertension . For more information on clinical aromatherapy, please refer to Table 4.

REFERENCES

1. McCormick E. Psychological interventions for patients with heart disease. Br J Cardiol 1997;4:268–271
2. Buckle J. Clinical aromatherapy. Adv Nurse Practit 2002;10:67–69.
3. Eisenberg D, Kessler R, Foster C, et al. Unconventional medicine in the United States. N Engl J Med 1993;328:246–252.
4. Eisenberg D, Davis R, Ettner S, et al. Trend in alternative medicine in the USA 1990–1997. JAMA 1998;280:784–787.
5. Styles J. The use of aromatherapy in hospitalized children with HIV. Compl Ther Nurs 1997;3:16–20.
6. Schnaubelt K. Medical aromatherapy. Frog Ltd, Berkeley, CA, 1999.
7. Buckle J. Aromatherapy. In: Novey D, ed. Clinician's Complete Reference to Complementary & Alternative Medicine. Mosby, New York, 2000, pp. 651–667.
8. Tisserand R, Balacs T. Essential Oil Safety. Churchill Livingstone, London, UK, 1995.
9. Gatti, G, Cayola R. L'Azione delle essenze sul sistema nervosa. Rivista Italiana delle Essenze e Profumi 1923;5:133–135.
10. Singewald N, Kaehler S, Sinner C, Thurnher C, Kouvelas D, Philippu A. Seratonin and amino acid release in the Locus Coeruleus by conditioned fear and inescapable shock. 6th Internet World Congress for Biomedical Sciences. Presentation #27, 2000.
11. Tisserand R. Lavender beats benzodiazapines. Int J Aromatherapy 1988;1:1–2.
12. LeDeux J. The Emotional Brain. Simon & Schuster, New York, pp. 296–299.
13. Buckle J. Aromatherapy & chronic pain. Alt Ther Health Med 1999;5:42–52.
14. Jager W, Bauchbauer G, Jirovetz L, et al. Percutaneous absorption of lavender oil from a massage oil. J Soc Cosmet Chem 1979;43:49–54.
15. Buckle J. The 'm' Technique. Massage Bodywork 2000;52–64.
16. Coulson I, Khan S. Facial pillow dermatitis due to lavender oil allergy. Contact Dermatitis 1999;41:111.
17. Wilkinson H. Childhood ingestion of volatile oils. Med J Austr 1991;154:430–431.
18. Opdyke D L J. Safety testing of fragrances: problems and implications. Clin Toxicol 1977;19:61–67.
19. Deininger R. The spectrum of activity of plant drugs containing essential oils—their antibacterial, antifungal and antiviral activity. Proceedings from Wholistic Aromatherapy: a scientific conference on the therapeutic use of essential oils. San Franscico, CA, November 4–6, 1995, pp. 15–54.
20. Benouda A, Hassar M, Benjilali B. The antiseptic properties of essential oils in vitro, tested against pathogenic germs found in hospitals. Fitoterapia 1988;59:115–119.
21. Larrondo J, Agut M, Calco-Torras M. Antimicrobial actvity of essences of Labiates. Microbiology 1995;82:171–172.
22. Nelson R. In vitro activities of five plant essential oils against MRSA and vancomycin-resistant Enterococcus faecium. J Antimicrob Chemother 1997;40:305–306.
23. Carson C, Cookson B, Farrelly H, et al. Susceptibility of methicillin-resistant staphylococcus aureus to the essential oil of Melaleuca alternifolia. J Antimicro Chemother 1995;35:421–424.
24. Chan C, Loudon K. Activity of teatree oil on methicillin-resistant Staphylococus aureus (MRSA). J Hosp Infect 1998;39:244–245.
25. Caeli M, Porteous J, Carson C, Heller R, Riley T. Teatree oil as an alternative agent decolonization for methcillin-resistant Staphylococcus aureus. J Hosp Infect 2000;46:236–237.

26. Sherry E, Boeck H, Warnke P. Percutaneous treatment of chronic MRSA osteomyelitis with a novel plant-derived antiseptic. Available at: http:// www.biomedcentral.com/ 1471/2482/1/1. Accessed August 10, 1992.

27. Chao S, Young D, Oberg C. Effect of a diffused essential oil blend on bacterial bioareosols. J Essent Oil Res 1998;10:517–523.

28. Freund. The hypotensive effects of ylang ylang—a patient study. Unpublished dissertation, R J Buckle Associates LLC, Hunter, NY.

29. Price S, Price L. Aromatherapy for health Professionals. Churchill Livingstone, London, 1999, p. 186.

30. Saeki Y, Shiodara M. Psychological effects of inhaling fragrances. Int J Aromatherapy 2001;11:118–133.

31. Nathan A. Pregnancy-induced-Hypertension and the Use of Essential Oils of Rose and Lavender. Unpublished dissertation, R J Buckle Associates LLC, Hunter, NY.

32. Kirov M, Koev P, Popiliev I, et al. Girosital: clinical trial in primary hyperlipoproteinemia. Medico Biologic Information 1988;3:30–34.

33. Shipotshliev T. Pharmacological research into a group of essential oils and their effect on the motor activity and general state of white mice in separate application. Vet Med Nauki 1968;5:87.

34. Tiran D. Aromatherapy in Midwifery Practice. Balliere Tindall, London, 1996, p. 91.

35. Vlay S, Frichionne G. Psychological aspects of surviving sudden cardiac death. Clin Cardiol 1985;8:237–242.

36. Petty J. Surgery and complementary therapies: a review. Alt Therapies 2000;6:64–74.

37. McCaffrey M. Nursing approaches to non-pharmacological pain control. Int J Nurs Stud 1990;27:1–5

38. LeDoux J. The Emotional Brain. Simon & Schuster, New York, 1996.

39. Ingham A. A review of the literature relating to touch and its use in intensive care. Intens Care Nurs 1989;5:65–75.

40. Buckle J. Clinical Aromatherapy in Nursing. Arnold, London, 1997.

41. Hadfield N. The role of aromatherapy massage in reducing anxiety in patients with malignant brain tumors. Int J Palliative Nurs 2001;7:279–285.

42. Gould L, Reddy R, Gomprecht R. Cardiac effects of chamomile tea. J Clin Pharmacol1973;13:475–479.

43. Yamada K, Miura T, Mimaki Y, Sashida Y. Effect of inhalation of chamomile oil vapor on plasma ACTJ level in ovariectomized rat under restriction stress. Biol Pharm Bull 1996;19:1244–1246.

44. Avollone R, Zanoli P, Corsi L, Cannazza G, Baraldi M. Benzodiazepine-like compounds and GABA in flower heads of matricaria chamomilla. Physiother Res 1996;10:S177–S179.

45. Viola H, Wasowski C, Levi de Stein M, et al. Apigenin, a component of Matricaria recutita flowers, is a central benzodiazepine receptors ligand with anxiolytic effects. Planta Med 1995;61:213–216.

46. Diego M, Jones N, Field T, et al. Aromatherapy positively affects mood, EEG patterns of alertness and math computation. Int J Neurosci 1998;96:217–224.

47. Dunn C, Sleep J, Collett D. Sensing an improvement: an experimental study to evaluate the use of aromatherapy, massage and periods of rest in an intensive-care unit. J Adv Nursing. 1995;21:31–34.

48. Woolfson A, Hewitt D. Intensive aromacare. Int J Aromather 1992;4:12–14.

49. Waldman C, Tseng P, Meulman P, Whittet H. Aromatherapy in the intensive care unit. Care Crit Ill 1993;9:170–174.

50. Redd W, Manne S, Peters B, Jacobsen P, Schmidt H. Fragrance administration to reduce anxiety during MRI imaging. J Magnet Res Imaging 1994;4:623–626.

51. Manley C H. Psychophysiological effects of odor. Crit Rev Food Sci Nutr 1993;33:57–62.

16 A Physician's Guide to CAM and Cardiovascular Disease on the World Wide Web

Jacqueline C. Wootton, MEd

CONTENTS

Most medical Web sites and dietary supplement packages, alongside their disclaimers, urge users to discuss alternative treatment options with their doctors. Surveys show it is primarily the more educated, often better informed, and higher income patients that are seeking alternatives. Discussions about complementary and alternative medicine (CAM) potentially enhance the physician–patient relationship. The situation may also pose problems for health care professionals who have been cast in the challenging role of arbiters of an integrative approach to medicine, because that integrative model has scarcely begun to be defined or understood, and the evidence base on which it will build has only just

From: *Contemporary Cardiology*
Complementary and Alternative Cardiovascular Medicine
Edited by: R. A. Stein and M. C. Oz © Humana Press Inc., Totowa, NJ

begun to be gathered. In reality, conventional medicine and alternative and complementary therapies run parallel rather than in concert.

The situation is compounded by the speed of new information transfer and the contradictions of breaking research. Physicians can no longer rely on a conventional wisdom, imparted from their medical training and specialty knowledge and updated through conferences and current literature. The issues concerning information dissemination, even within conventional medicine, are illustrated by the decision in July 2002 to halt the Women's Health Initiative prevention trial when the preliminary findings demonstrated that the risks of taking estrogen plus progestin hormone therapy may outweigh the benefits. Professionals and consumers were largely convinced that hormone replacement therapy (HRT) would help prevent serious health problems, including heart disease in postmenopausal women. This had become the accepted position, transmitted through apparently authoritative sources that had assessed the available data.

Previous chapters have been concerned with systematically reviewing the current research data available on various CAM therapies used as adjuncts or alternatives to conventional care for cardiovascular disease (CVD). Even during the publication of this volume, new research findings will become available. This chapter provides categorized reference resources on the World Wide Web to aid the busy physician and other members of the health care team in updating that knowledge. However, Web-based resources are notoriously volatile, so the main rationale in this chapter is to provide guidelines and principles that can be used to find, assess, and cross-check information on the World Wide Web, both for professionals' use and for their use with patients.

GUIDELINES FOR EVALUATING CAM INFORMATION RESOURCES ON THE WEB

Despite recognized problems of exploitation and commercialism and deliberate misinformation that are present anyway in all walks of life, the Web is still an excellent information resource for professionals and the public. Many assessment tools have been developed to quality-evaluate Web resources. Many of these have been of short duration, were sometimes provided by an organization with vested interests, could be faked, or relied on voluntary compliance, such as the HONcode, the most widely known and respected code, developed by the Geneva-based Health On the Net Foundation. You can verify the authenticity of any site displaying the code by going to the HON code website at http://www.hon.ch/HONcode/Conduct.html.

The following brief guidelines have been compiled from common features of several sets of guidelines *(1,2)* and apply equally to all information resources on the Web. Where all or most of these principles are adhered to, the site can be deemed reasonably authoritative. This does not mean that the information is not open to debate in the same way that much received wisdom can always be overturned by new findings. Recent examples of such controversies include healthy diet and nutrition guidelines, in addition to the HRT example. Asterisks indicate essential features; other features are desirable for an ergonomic site with a clear structure. The essential principles are similar to those that apply to the review of journal articles, as used in the other chapters.

Site Ownership and Affiliations

- There should be clear information on ownership, affiliations, alliances, investors, or sponsors. All this information should be accessible from the home page.
- Product information and advertising should be clearly separated from information content. Most high-quality information sites do not sell products and advertisements.
  Restrictions on access to parts of the site should be clearly stated and easy to find.
  Clear information should be given on registration and password protection.

Editorial Identity

- Editors and reviewers of content should be clearly identified with affiliations.
- The criteria for selection of related links should be stated clearly.
- Where related links are reviewed this should be according to a clearly stated set of guidelines.

Some sites, in particular the health science library sites, aim for comprehensiveness and choose not to review or evaluate. This should be stated. Such resources are invaluable for gaining an overview of what information is available.

Ideally, reviewers should declare their financial interests.

Maintenance and Navigation of Site

- Dates of posting and updating should be clear.
- Links should be regularly maintained and monitored.
- Viewers should not be prevented from returning to a previous site.
- Sites should not frame other sites without permission/license.
- Sites should not automatically redirect viewers to another site or advertising material.

CATEGORIZED INFORMATION RESOURCES
ON CAM FOR CVD ON THE WEB

Most organizations now have Web sites that can be accessed for updating and finding new data; this is an advantage over print information that may date quickly. For clarity, the following resources are presented and categorized separately, in Tables 1–9. The URL is provided, along with a brief description of how the resource can be used to find CAM information pertinent to heart disease. Almost all of these Web-based resources are free and available without paid subscription. News and journal sites usually require free registration, and the health-information portals usually require paid subscription. This information is provided with the description. Already familiar information on conventional cardiology professional journals and professional associations has not been included.

Finally, a quick guide, especially targeted for your patients, is provided.

Table 1
Major Databases

Major Databases for Published Research

PubMed
http://www.ncbi.nlm.nih.gov/entrez/query.fcgi
PubMed is a service of the National Library of Medicine, providing access to more than 12 million MEDLINE and additional life science journal articles. A new feature, CAM on PubMed, developed in partnership with the National Center for Complementary and Alternative Medicine at NIH, provides a subset of more than 220,000 articles relevant to CAM. Go to PubMed and click on the "Limits" function (underneath the search box). From the Subsets pull-down menu, select "Complementary Medicine," and then search from within this subset by typing in relevant keywords, such as "heart" or "cardiovascular." Limit your search further with additional keywords and limits.

IBIDS
http://ods.od.nih.gov/databases/ibids.html
International Bibliographic Information on Dietary Supplements (IBIDS) is a database of published, international, scientific literature on dietary supplements, including vitamins, minerals, and botanicals, produced by the Office of Dietary Supplements at the National Institutes of Health (NIH). You can select from peer-reviewed and non-peer-reviewed literature for searches.

HerbMed
http://www.herbmed.org
HerbMed is a project of the nonprofit Alternative Medicine Foundation and presents categorized information on more than 160 medicinal herbs, compiled by pharmacologists and pharmacognosists. There is a dynamic updating feature that automatically generates live PubMed updates for each category of information. Search on heart AND cardiovascular and any other choice of keyword.

Phytochemical and Ethnobotanical Databases
http://www.ars-grin.gov/duke/
This site links to Dr. James Duke's US Department of Agruculture (USDA) databases, as well as other related databases.

Ongoing Clinical Research and Trials

CRISP
http://www.crisp.cit.nih.gov/
Computer Retrieval of Information on Scientific Projects (CRISP) is a searchable database of NIH-funded research and intramural research projects. It covers mainly conventional biomedicine but contains a growing proportion of CAM projects and clinical trials. The best search strategy may be to initially confine your search to the National Heart, Lung, and Blood Institute.

Table 1 (Continued)

CenterWatch
http://www.centerwatch.com/
This for-profit site provides a listing of more than 41,000 industry- and government-sponsored clinical trials, as well as new drug therapies recently approved by the Food and Drug Administration (FDA). This site is a resource both for patients interested in participating in clinical trials and for research professionals. The search function employs a drill-down strategy. Click on Trials Listings, then on Cardiology/Vascular Diseases, and scan for appropriate categories, such as Diet and Nutrition. There is no fee for searching.

ClinicalTrials.gov
http://www.clinicaltrials.gov
The National Library of Medicine at NIH has developed this site to provide patients and public with current information on clinical research studies at NIH. You can search the site or browse by topic.

Systematic Reviews

Cochrane Collaboration Database of Systematic Reviews
http://www.cochrane.org/
The Cochrane Collaboration is a global network of researchers who conduct systematic reviews of randomized clinical trials, including unpublished and difficult-to-locate research. The collaboration is organized into major disease review groups and cross-cutting fields. To view abstracts of relevant reviews, click on Abstracts of Cochrane Reviews and then Cochrane Heart Group for the listing. Some of the reviews have been undertaken in collaboration with members of the Field of Complementary Medicine. A complete list of CAM-related reviews can be found at the field's Web site:
http://www.compmed.umm.edu/Compmed/Cochrane/
Click on Reviews and Protocols in the sidebar for the pdf file listing.

Other Resources

Directory of Databases
http://www.rosenthal.hs.columbia.edu/Databases.html
Other databases relevant to CAM are listed and linked to in the directory of databases, maintained at the Rosenthal Center for Complementary Medicine at Columbia University, College of Physicians and Surgeons. They are categorized by topic and whether they are publicly available, require free registration, or available by paid subscription only.

These are global databases that have significant resources on complementary and alternative medicine (CAM) relevant to cardiovascular disease. All are freely available public domain resources.

Table 2
Health Science Library Meta-Directories

Ask NOAH
http://www.noah-health.org/
NOAH is a consortium of several New York libraries and institutions and provides rapidly updated, neutral information on a range of health topics. It is available in English and Spanish. Click on the relevant topics, Complementary and Alternative Medicine or Heart Disease and Stroke. The latter includes some complementary approaches to care.

Health Sciences Library System
http://www.hsls.pitt.edu/guides/internet/
This collection of Internet guides is compiled and maintained by the Health Sciences Library of the University of Pittsburgh. Click on Alternative Medicine.

HealthWeb
http://healthweb.org
Another useful meta-directory from a consortium of health science libraries, contracted by the National Library of Medicine (NLM).

MedlinePlus
http://www.nlm.nih.gov/medlineplus
MEDLINEplus, a project of the NLM provides evaluated resources on more than 500 diseases and conditions. There are a medical encyclopedia and dictionaries, health information in Spanish, extensive information on prescription and nonprescription drugs, health information from the media, and links to thousands of clinical trials. Click on Health Topics then A and scroll down to Alternative Medicine.

MedWeb
http://www.MedWeb.Emory.Edu/MedWeb/
Select Subject Index in the sidebar and then Alternative and Complementary Medicine. By selecting Focus Further, you access a further categorized listing.

An effective way to gain an overview of health resources on the World Wide Web is to use one of the Internet meta-directories that provides categorized listings of relevant sites. Health science libraries or consortia usually compile these free public domain resources. Directories include academic sites, online journals and newsletters, professional organizations, information services, and self-help and discussion groups. There is considerable overlap between the lists. Few of them provide crosslinking between complementary and alternative resources and conventional specialties.

Table 3
Other NIH and FDA Web Sites

NIH Institutes, Centers, and Divisions

National Heart Lung and Blood Institute, (NHLBI) NIH
http://www.nhlbi.nih.gov
Regular scanning of the professional resources yields latest research
information, clinical trials, practice guidelines, and research funding, some
of which will increasingly be related to CAM.

**National Center for Complementary and Alternative Medicine,
(NCCAM) NIH**
http://nccam.nih.gov
In 2002, NCCAM and NHLBI launched a joint multicenter clinical trial to
assess chelation therapy. Information can be tracked on either NIH Web site.
For other CAM clinical trials related to heart disease, click on Clinical Trials,
then NCCAM Clinical Trials—by Disease or Condition, then select
appropriate categories under the alphabetical listing.

Office of Dietary Supplements (ODS) NIH
http://ods.od.nih.gov
One of the ODS-funded centers, Purdue University and the University of
Alabama Botanicals Research Center for Age Related Diseases are studying
the effects of polyphenols on age-related diseases, including heart disease.
Try the search function for other related resources.

NIH Consensus Development Program
http://consensus.nih.gov/
The site provides the latest statements and state of the science for a range of
medical practice. Use the search feature to find relevant guidelines.

Food and Drug Administration—Dietary Supplements
http://www.cfsan.fda.gov/~dms/supplmnt.html/
The current Adverse Event reporting system is a simple recording of
consumer and practitioner complaints and has been subject to strong
criticism. The FDA has recognized that reports may be incomplete and open
to misinterpretation and is devising a new system for tracking and analyzing
adverse events reports, called CAERS. Follow this development on the Web
site.

Most of these are concerned with disease categories, but increasingly they cover
CAM approaches.

Table 4
Health News Sites

Yahoo!
http://news.yahoo.com/
Rather than just click on Health in the sidebar, scroll down to Full Coverage and select All Full Coverage. Then click on Health for Top Stories, or choose a category from the All Health Coverage listing, e.g., Alternative Medicine or Heart Disease & Circulatory Disorders. This will provide more in-depth coverage of the latest news or findings whenever it occurred, not just the late-breaking news.

CNN
http://www.cnn.com/
Click on health for the latest headlines. You can also establish an E-mail account on CNN Breaking News for instant alerts.

Health Scout News
http://www.healthscoutnews.com
Health Scout News is health news with a slant toward alternative therapies.

Search Engine Watch—News Search Engines
http://searchenginewatch.com/links/news.html
This Web site will guide you through many more options for news on the Web.

Any of the major news sites has a health section for quick updates on latest health news. Bookmark your favorite.

Table 5
Online Newsletters and Journals

Cardiology Today
http://www.cardiologytoday.com/
This monthly electronic newspaper is aimed at the clinician. Published by Slack, Inc.

Journal of Nuclear Cardiology
http://www2.us.elsevierhealth.co
/script/om.dll/serve?action=searchDB&searchDBfor=home&id=nc
Provides an electronic version for regular subscribers to the Mosby print journal but additionally a service for Rapid Publication Articles of current news and research.

Medscape
http://www.medscape.com/homeindex
Medscape, in conjunction with WebMD, provides medical information, electronic publishing, and educational tools. There is an initial, free registration, and then you can customize your home page and E-mail alerts according to your specialty and interests.

Online Journal of Cardiology
http://sprojects.mmi.mcgill.ca/heart/index.html
A fully online journal sponsored by McGill University.

Complementary and Alternative Medicine Journals
http://www.medbioworld.com/med/journals/complementary.html
MedBioWorld provides a comprehensive listing of all CAM journals print and online. No distinction is made between small self-published newsletters and peer-reviewed Medline-indexed journals.

In addition to the familiar professional print journals that generally require a paid subscription to access their online versions, there are online publications that offer rapid review and response to breaking research. These increasingly include CAM information.

Table 6
Information Portals

Intramedicine
http://www.intramedicine.com/
Intramedicine is relatively new portal focused on integrative medicine. The company provides clinical data on integrative therapies that have been scientifically validated, supported by a database of resources, including Chinese medicine formulas. The resources are available through paid registration. The only products for sale on the site are publications, courses, and electronic resources.

WebMD
http://my.webmd.com
WebMD has proved one of the enduring dot.com sites and provides current health news on the home page. There is a strong emphasis on health and wellness, including a section by Dean Ornish, MD, who developed the program to reverse heart disease by diet and lifestyle changes. Sponsors include pharmaceutical companies, and all information is interspersed by advertisements.

This is a very unstable group of websites that is continually changing and varying in quality. Many of these dot.coms went out of business with the downturn of the economy at the beginning of the 21st century, including the Dr. Koop site. Most of the portals also sell products. They generally try to keep people on their site by use of frames (providing information from other sites within a window so that it appears to be coming from their own site, with the goal of preventing visitors moving on to another site). Much of the licensed information is only available through paid subscription. A small cross-section of sites that provide CAM information resources is listed below. All have well qualified professional advisory boards.

Table 7
Search Engines

As search engine technology has become sophisticated, the commercial sites have become increasingly savvy about ensuring that their site gets a high ranking. The latest strategy is for commercial sites to "trade links" so they all increase their number of hits. Latest generation search engines, such as **Google**, use a search algorithm that works like citation analysis to identify "authoritative" sites. Unfortunately, authoritative has come to mean "popular," as more commercial sites jointly generate hits. Most serious and truly authoritative educational, governmental, and nonprofit sites do not play the game of increasing their ranking, so they may come lower down the listing of hits.

Nevertheless, **Google (http://www.google.com)** is still the fastest and most powerful search engine currently available, and any of the search engines, using automated search strategies, including natural language queries (such as **Ask Jeeves, Alta Vista, HotBot**, and **All the Web**), are generally superior to subject directories, such as **Yahoo!, Lycos**, or **Magellan**.

A new search engine, **Scirus (http://www.scirus.com)**, developed for Elsevier Science, may be worth exploring. It is science specific, so it focuses only on Web sites containing scientific or biomedical data. It locates peer-reviewed articles and offers a document delivery service.

Metasearch engines, such as **Metacrawler, Search.Com, Northern Light**, and **Dogpile**, query several search engines simultaneously and generate an enormous number of hits. The problem is that they may have reduced relevance if one of the included search engines returns results with low relevance.

Table 8
Integrative and Holistic Medicine Organizations

American Holistic Medical Association
http://www.holisticmedicine.org
Association for licensed physicians who practice holistic medicine.

American Holistic Nurses Association
http://ahna.org
AHNA embraces nursing as a lifestyle and a profession and provides a means to create bonds within the nursing community.

Global Academy—Institute for Integrative Medicine
http://www.theglobalacademy.org/int_medicine.asp
The Institute is working with a few selected institutions on strategic initiatives that can provide working models of an integrative approach to medicine, with international relevance.

Integrative Medicine
http://www.onemedicine.com/index.html
This company provides information services for healthcare professionals, consumers, and executives to combine the best of conventional and alternative medicine for optimal healthcare.

University of Arizona Program in Integrative Medicine
http://integrativemedicine.arizona.edu/
Andrew Weil, MD, heads this program that offers fellowships, associate fellowships, and research programs in integrative approaches to medicine.

There are many programs that combine conventional and CAM practices, but few, if any, have successfully developed truly integrative models of practice. The holistic medicine movement has been around since the 1970s and seeks to transform health care to address physical, environmental, mental, emotional, spiritual, and social health, contributing to the healing of the planet.

Table 9
Specific Modalities

This table is divided into the major CAM categories that are relevant to CVD:

1. Herbs, antioxidants, vitamins, and other dietary supplements
2. Diet, nutrition, and lifestyle
3. Mind–body therapies
4. Specific therapies associated with CVD

In each category, information is provided on professional associations, foundations, and other nonprofit organizations. Centers are listed where appropriate. Specific treatment clinics are generally too numerous to list.

CAM Research Center for Cardiovascuxlar Diseases
http://www.med.umich.edu/camrc/index.html
One NIH-NCCAM funded center, CAM Research Center for Cardiovascular Diseases, based at the University of Michigan, is investigating a range of modalities to treat and prevent cardiovascular disease (CVD). These include reiki, Hawthorn extract, herbal weight loss, and meditation. It is also investigating a model of care using CAM modalities. To update information, visit the Web site.

1. Herbs, Antioxidants, Vitamins, and Other Dietary Supplements
In a surprising development, large pharmaceutical companies are opening divisions to manufacture and market dietary supplements based on the drug model of a single active ingredient. Traditionally, herbalists use whole herbs, singly and in mixtures. New standardized methods for sustainable production of traditional herbals are being developed by small herbal companies.

Professional Associations

American Association of Naturopathic Physicians
http://www.naturopathic.org
Naturopaths are primary care doctors, not licensed in all states, who are trained to practice with herbs, minerals, and other dietary supplements. Contact the AANP for information on licensing and referrals.

American Herbal Products Association
http://www.ahpa.org/
This trades association promotes the manufacture and responsible commercial development of high-quality herbal products. The Web site provides information and discussion on legislative issues.

Association of Natural Medicine pharmacists
http://www.anmp.org/
AANP provides certification and training in natural medicines for pharmacists.

Table 9 (Continued)

Council for Responsible Nutrition
http://www.crnusa.org/
CRN represents its herbal and dietary supplement companies' interests to the
media, healthcare professionals, government policy makers, and consumers.

Foundations and Nonprofit Organizations

American Botanical Council
http://www.herbalgram.org/
ABC is an educational organization for public and professionals on the use and
regulation of herbs. Publishes HerbalGram, quarterly publication of news on
herbs and the industry.

American Herbalists Guild
http://www.americanherbalistsguild.com/
Provides a professional member referral list (by state), books and monographs,
a listing of its books, and a Directory of Herbal Education.

Herb Research Foundation
http://www.herbs.org
The foundation offers science-based information on the health benefits and
safety of herbs.

2. Diet, Nutrition, and Lifestyle

Diet is a key aspect of CVD prevention and treatment programs. Until recently,
the recommendation has been to decrease saturated fat and cholesterol and to
consume more vegetables, fruit, and whole-grain products. Professionals and
public alike are understandably confused by the latest claims that low-fat diets
and refined carbohydrates are at the root of the obesity problem in the United
States. The consensus is that amount of calories, with lack of exercise, is the
main culprit, leading to CVD and other obesity-related health problems. The
Dean Ornish program recommends a low-fat diet with other lifestyle
interventions, including support groups, meditation, and exercise. Exercise, in
the conventional sense, has not been included in the following Web sites,
although some forms of martial arts are included under C.

The Mediterranean Diet
circ.ahajournals.org/cgi/content/full/103/13/1823
A series of articles comparing the American Heart Association
recommendations with the controversial Mediterranean diet, high in cereals,
grains, vegetables, pulses, olive oil, garlic, fresh herbs, seafood and fruit and
that includes wine, meat, and poultry can be accessed from this site. Most can
be downloaded full text.

Table 9 (Continued)

Dean Ornish MD's Lifestyle Program
http://my.webmd.com/medcast_channel_toc/3068
Dean Ornish provides an advice column on the WebMD Web site that also
includes marketing of products. Click on The Diet War for continuing discussion
of the low-fat diet controversy.

Professional Associations

American Dietetic Association
http://www.eatright.org
This site provides education and career information. It is not clear which
organizations sponsor the activities of the association. There is a marketplace
for products alongside the information.

Foundations and Nonprofit Organizations

American Heart Association
http://www.americanheart.org
In addition to its advocacy activities, the AHA provides educational and specific
lifestyle-oriented information on preventing heart disease. Read the Annual
Report for information on funding. Partners include large pharmaceutical
companies that market CVD drug treatments.

Clinics and Centers

Center for Nutrition Policy and Promotion
http://www.usda.gov/cnpp/
This USDA center provides nutritional guidance based on the latest research.
However, the guidelines have been heavily criticized at a time of conflicting
nutritional claims.

George Ohsawa Macrobiotic Foundation
http://www.gomf.macrobiotic.net/
Macrobiotics is a way of eating and living that claims to be in harmony with the
natural order of all aspects of life—physical, emotional, mental, ecological, and
spiritual.

Kushi Insititute
http://www.kushiinstitute.org
The Kushi Institute provides educational and training programs, counseling,
and conferences based on their view that we are the result of our total
environment, the foods we eat, daily social interactions, lifestyle, and
environment.

Table 9 (Continued)

3. Mind–Body Therapies

Mind–body therapies are based on recognition of a relationship between mind and body. They are premised on the belief that the body's innate healing potential can be harnessed by mindful and meditational practices. Many mind–body practices derive from traditional medical systems, such as Chinese traditional medicine, Ayurveda, and Tibetan medicine, that are founded on the interconnection of mind, body, and spirit.

Biofeedback is one specific aspect of mind–body training that is part of mainstream medicine. Patients are trained to control brainwave activity to modify their own autonomic body processes. The technique can be used to retrain cardiovascular and respiratory functions. Hypnotherapy is also primarily mainstream.

Professional Associations

Association for Applied Psychophysiology and Biofeedback
http://www.aapb.org
Objective is research and the integration of biofeedback with other self-regulatory methods. Promotes high standards of professional practice, ethics, and education.

Biofeedback Certification Institute of America
http://www.bcia.org
Formed to establish and maintain professional standards for the provision of biofeedback services and to certify qualifying practitioners.

Foundations and Nonprofit Organizations

Mind Body Medical Institute
http://www.mbmi.org/Default.asp
President Herbert Benson, MD, developed the relaxation response for people suffering from stress-related illnesses. His courses are taught at Harvard Medical School.

National Institute for the Clinical Application
of Behavioral Medicine
http://www.nicabm.com/aboutus.html
NICABM supports the thoughtful consideration of the research and efficacy of behavioral medicine and where appropriate the integration of CAM treatment modalities into conventional care.

Table 9 (Continued)

Clinics and Centers

Center for Mind Body Medicine
http://www.cmbm.org/index.html
The center is a nonprofit, educational organization dedicated to reviving the spirit and transforming the practice of medicine through a compassionate, open-minded model of healthcare.

Duke Health—Heart Center
http://dukehealth.org/heart_center/new_clinical_trials.asp
See, in particular, the Behavioral Medicine Program.

Below are subcategories of organizations concerned with one aspect of mind–body therapies.

Consciousness, Subtle Energies, and Human Potential

Academy for Guided Imagery
http://www.interactiveimagery.com
This technique uses the imagination and the power of the mind for healing, growth, and improved physiological functioning. A practitioners listing is available.

Association for Humanistic Psychology
http://www.ahpweb.org/
Committed to holistic and interdisciplinary research and practices that lead to understanding, developing, and nurturing human potential.

Institute of Noetic Sciences
http://www.noetic.org/index.asp
The institute was founded on the vision of Apollo14 astronaut, Edgar Mitchell, to investigate consciousness and human potential through rigorous science.

International Society for the Study of Subtle Energies and Energy Medicine
http://www.issseem.org
ISSSEEM studies subtle energies known in traditional systems of medicine as chi, ki, prana, etc. Many CAM therapies are based on the concept of the flow of subtle energies through the physical body leading to changes that cannot easily be measured by conventional methodology.

Hypnotherapy

Anxiety, pain, and stress may be relieved through hypnotic trance as part of a treatment for many conditions. Hypnotherapists may be MDs or specifically trained therapists.

Table 9 (Continued)

American Academy of Medical Hypnoanalysis
http://aamh.com/
Nonprofit organization concerned with research, clinical training and education, and responsible practice of hypnotherapy. Provides practitioner listing.

American Association of Professional Hypnotherapists
http://aaph.org
Promotes the development of ethical methods, techniques, and standards in hypnotherapy.

American Society of Clinical Hypnosis
http://www.asch.net
Encourages scientific research, education, and high standards of practice by qualified health and mental health care professionals.

Music, Art, Dance, and Humor Therapy

These therapies may be used to improve physical and mental health.

American Art Therapy Association
http://www.arttherapy.org
Art therapists are professionals trained in both art and therapy.

American Association for Therapeutic Humor
http://www.aath.org
Therapeutic humor may stimulate an appreciation of the absurdity or incongruity of life's situations, relieving stress and promoting healing.

American Dance Therapy Association
http://www.adta.org
Dance and movement therapists integrate body, movement, and expression with counseling, psychotherapy, and rehabilitation.

American Music Therapy Association
http://www.musictherapy.org
Promotes the therapeutic use of music in rehabilitation and community settings.

Meditation, Yoga, Qigong

There are different ways of stilling the mind to allow wider awareness and clarity. Meditation may be used to attain altered states of consciousness; Qigong is a Chinese practice used to promote self-healing through meditation and controlled breathing; Yoga is a primarily Indian system of physical, mental, and spiritual development; and T'ai chi may be used as a gentle form of exercise.

Table 9 (Continued)

Center for Mindfulness in Medicine Healthcare and Society
http://www.umassmed.edu/cfm/
The Center at the University of Massachusetts Medical School, founded by Jon
Kabat-Zinn, PhD, has developed a program for stress reduction through
mindfulness meditation.

Chopra Center for Well-being
http://www.chopra.com
This commercial site and center places emphasis on mind-body modalities from
traditional Ayurveda—yoga, breathing, and massage therapy—to regain
balance in life.

East-West Academy of Healing Arts
http://www.eastwestqi.com
This nonprofit organization represents one particular style of qigong practiced
by founder Dr. Effie Poy Yew Chow.

Himalayan International Institute of Yoga, Science and Philosphy
http://www.himalayaninstitute.org
Nonprofit organization for the exploration of spiritual traditions, particularly
the teaching of classical yoga for modern life.

International Association of Yoga Therapists
http://www.iayt.org
IAYT operates as part of the Yoga Research and Education Center to support
Yoga teachers and therapists with an interest in Yoga as a healing modality.

Qigong Institute
http://www.qigonginstitute.org
Promotes understanding of qigong through education, research, and clinical
studies. The founder of this nonprofit has developed a large database of
published research on qigong.

4. Specific Therapies Associated with CVD

Specific therapies that are advocated for control and reversal of heart disease are
still highly controversial. They include chelation therapy, removal of dental
amalgams, coenzyme Q10, oxygen therapy for stroke recovery, and Chinese
medicine for reversing high blood pressure.

Professional Associations

American Academy of Environmental Medicine
http://www.aaem.com
The academy offers training for physicians on the effect of toxic substances in
the diet and environment that are potential stressors causing disease in
individuals.

Table 9 (Continued)

American College for Advancement in Medicine
http://www.acam.org
This nonprofit medical society is dedicated to educating physicians and other health care professionals about novel diagnostic, treatment, and preventive procedures. They have been associated particularly with chelation courses for coronary artery disease (CAD).

American College of Hyperbaric Medicine
http://www.hyperbaricmedicine.org
Promotes the use and investigation of hyperbaric oxygen therapy particularly for stroke patients.

Foundations and Nonprofit Organizations

American Association for Health Freedom
http://www.apma.net/about.htm
Formerly the American Preventive Medical Association, AAHF is the political voice for health care practitioners who use nutritional and other complementary therapies in patient care.

Committee for Freedom of Choice in Medicine
http://www.americanbiologics.com
This educational organization, also known as American Biologics, prepares position papers for legislative purposes and maintains a doctor referral service for patients seeking medical choice.

There are many CAM modalities that are not covered in the previous listings because they are not immediately relevant to CVD. However, a range of therapies in the categories of energy work (shiatsu, therapeutic touch, polarity therapy, reiki, reflexology, or bioenergetics), manual therapies (massage, rolfing, chiropractic, craniosacral therapy, and osteopathy), and acupuncture may have generally beneficial effects for heart disease or stroke patients. Information on these modalities may be found through the Health Science Library Meta-Directories or in a series of resource guides from the nonprofit Alternative Medicine Foundation (http://www.amfoundation.org/info.htm).

RESOURCES FOR PATIENTS—CAM THERAPIES
FOR HEART DISEASE ON THE WORLD WIDE WEB

It is important to recognize the difference between different types of sites. All have their uses, provided we are cautious. We all seek advice and opinions from family and friends. **Chat groups** can be used to broaden our network, but be aware that participants are offering individual testimonials not authoritative information. **Advice sites** provided by physicians and other practitioners, such as *Ask Dr. Weil*, provide a second opinion but should also be used with caution. If you know what you want to purchase, **commercial sites** provide a convenient outlet, but be wary of commercial sites that claim to provide impartial information. That applies also to some **nonprofit organizations** that may be supported by large pharmaceutical companies. Always check the *About Us* section to see what groups and sponsors are behind any information Web site.

Health Science Library sites provide as comprehensive an overview of sites as possible. **Government** and **educational sites** generally evaluate and select the sites they include. This is useful for mainstream medicine, but for CAM therapies where practitioners and researchers are breaking new ground and challenging accepted views, such sites may be seen as conservative. If it all seems rather daunting, just remember that it is really not so different from sorting out the junk mail and deciding which television channel to watch. If you find your searches return mainly commercial sites, you can filter unwanted information by adding *NOT .com* to your list of search terms.

The following are a few key Web sites to get you started.

Ask NOAH About—Heart Disease and Stroke
http://www.noah-health.org/english/illness/heart_disease/heartdisease.html
This site is compiled and maintained by a consortium of health science libraries in the New York area. The large amount of information is clearly organized and provides a useful explanation of technical terms. The section on Care and Treatment includes complementary therapies and there are resources for specific interest groups, including children. For more information on CAM, click on Health Topics in the top bar and select Complementary and Alternative Medicine.

InteliHealth: Merriam-Webster Medical Dictionary
http://www.intelihealth.com/IH/ihtIH/WSIHW000/9276/9276.html
It is important to understand the technical terms your physician and some of the information Web sites are using. This Aetna-sponsored site provides a searchable dictionary.

The Heart: An Online Exploration
http://sln.fi.edu/biosci/biosci.html
You may enjoy this educational site from the Franklin Institute Science Museum.

MEDLINEplus
http://www.nlm.nih.gov/medlineplus/coronarydisease.html
This is an evaluated site with selected listings from the National Library of Medicine at NIH. It provides the latest breaking news on new treatments and clinical trials, as well as educational materials on conventional and alternative approaches to treating and preventing heart disease.

National, Heart, Lung and Blood Institute
http://www.nhlbi.nih.gov/health/index.htm
This NIH site provides patient support resources for coronary heart disease and the Healthy People 2010 Projects. You can access the physician resources and select from the listing, e.g., Clinical Guidelines for various aspects of CVD or relevant research projects.

CAM Research Center for Cardiovascular Diseases
http://www.med.umich.edu/camrc/index.html
The CAM Research Center for Cardiovascular Diseases, based at the University of Michigan and funded by the National Center for Complementary and Alternative Medicine, is investigating a range of modalities to treat and prevent heart disease. These include Reiki therapy, Hawthorn extract, herbal weight loss, and meditation. Visit the site for updated information.

National Center for Complementary and Alternative Medicine
http://nccam.nih.gov/health/
Click on Health Information for latest information about complementary and alternative medicine and research news.

CenterWatch
http://www.centerwatch.com/
CenterWatch provides a service for patients seeking to be included in clinical trials. Click on Trial Listings, then Cardiology/Vascular Diseases, then scroll down to any relevant topics. Trials that are actively recruiting are hyperlinked; the number in brackets indicates the number of trials on that topic. It is worth drilling down and exploring many categories if you are interested in CAM-related trials.

REFERENCES

1. Gagliardi A, Jadad AR. Examination of instruments used to rate quality of health information on the internet: chronicle of a voyage with an unclear destination. Br Med J 2002;324:569–573.
2. Pandolfini C, Bonati M. Follow up of quality of public oriented health information on the world wide web: systematic re-evaluation. Br Med J 2002;324:582–558.

INDEX